Diagnostic Cytopathology

Diagnostic Cytopathology
A TEXT AND COLOUR ATLAS

Chandra Grubb
MB BS PhD MRCPath

Emeritus Consultant Cytopathologist, Bloomsbury Health District, London; Emeritus Fellow, International Academy of Cytology; Formerly Director, Royal Free Hospital/University College Hospital Department of Cytology, London and the Regional Cytology Training Centre, North-East Thames Health Region, London

CHURCHILL LIVINGSTONE
EDINBURGH LONDON MELBOURNE AND NEW YORK 1988

CHURCHILL LIVINGSTONE
Medical Division of Longman Group UK Limited

Distributed in the United States of America by
Churchill Livingstone Inc., 1560 Broadway, New York,
N.Y. 10036, and by associated companies, branches and
representatives throughout the world.

© Longman Group UK Limited 1988

All rights reserved. No part of this publication may be
reproduced, stored in a retrieval system, or transmitted in any
form or by any means, electronic, mechanical, photocopying,
recording or otherwise, without the prior permission of the
publishers (Churchill Livingstone, Robert Stevenson House,
1–3 Baxter's Place, Leith Walk, Edinburgh EH1 3AF).

First published 1988

ISBN 0-443-03050-2

British Library Cataloguing in Publication Data
Grubb, Chandra
　Diagnostic cytopathology: a text and
　colour atlas.
　1. Pathology, Cellular
　I. Title
　611'.01815　　RB25

Library of Congress Cataloging in Publication Data
Grubb, Chandra.
　Diagnostic cytopathology: a text and colour atlas/Chandra
Grubb.
　　p.　cm.
　1. Diagnosis, Cytologic. 2. Diagnosis, Cytologic—Atlases.
I. Title.
　[DNLM: 1. Cytodiagnosis—atlases. 2. Cytodiagnosis—methods. QY
95 G885d]
　RB43.G78　1988
　616.07'582—dc19　　　　　　　　　　　　　　87-27634

Produced by Longman Group (FE) Ltd
Printed in Hong Kong

Preface

Recent years have seen a virtually explosive increase in the demand for cytopathology services. The reasons are simple. Cytopathology can be applied to spontaneously desquamated cells in a large proportion of cases. Its scope has been greatly extended by technical advances in fibre-optic endoscopy and interventional radiology. The morbidity associated with invasive methods required to obtain cytological specimens is significantly lower than with methods employed to obtain a formal biopsy. Furthermore, cytology is rapid and cost-effective.

The demand is expected to be met by increasing numbers of trainee histopathologists whose curriculum now includes cytopathology, medical laboratory scientists whose traditional role as cytoscreeners of cervical smears is widened to include newer techniques, and pathologists whose interests were formerly confined to histopathology.

The provision of an expert cytopathology service rests on correct interpretation of cytological artefacts; this in turn, rests on study and experience. This book is intended to help towards that study. It has been designed as a text atlas in which the relatively new brush and aspiration techniques are included with exfoliative cytology in the consideration of organ systems. The specially prepared illustrations are of specimens submitted to a diagnostic and teaching laboratory and represent its day to day work. The two staining procedures favoured by most cytology laboratories and routinely used in the author's department are the Papanicolaou and the Romanowsky methods; both are represented in the book. Special staining methods, including immunocytochemical procedures, have been included where appropriate. The text has been designed to provide background information and teaching discussion in addition to descriptive legends. In some instances, selected cases have been included to reinforce a clinical or diagnostic point.

Guidelines to the cytodiagnostic approach to malignancy, applicable to all types of tumours and all tissue systems, have been placed in a separate introductory chapter.

Moraira, Spain   C. G.
1988

Acknowledgements

This book was made possible by a steady supply of meticulously prepared diagnostic specimens. For this, I am deeply grateful to all the medical laboratory scientific officers who worked with me in the joint Royal Free Hospital / University College Hospital Department of Cytology. Thanks are also due to my medical colleagues who drew my attention to specimens likely to be of interest and help to students of cytopathology. I am grateful to Mrs Frances Anderson and Mrs Margaret Cowper for typing the manuscript. The staff of Churchill Livingstone gave valuable advice on the format of the book.

Moraira, Spain
1988

C. G.

Contents

Introduction: Cytodiagnostic approach to malignancy 1

1. Female reproductive system 3
2. Breast 43
3. Respiratory tract 65
4. Serous effusions 113
5. Cerebrospinal fluid 141
6. Oesophago-gastrointestinal tract 146
7. Fine needle aspiration cytology of sub-diaphragmatic lesions 156
8. Urinary system 165
9. Male genital system 176
10. Lymph nodes 180
11. Bone 185
12. Skin and sub-cutaneous lesions 191
13. Thyroid 196
14. Cellular changes due to treatment 201

Index 209

Cytodiagnostic approach to malignancy

Diagnosis of malignancy is the major objective of cytopathology. A malignant tumour is characterized by uncontrolled growth, alterations to varying extent in the structural and functional differentiation of its component cells, and the capacity to spread beyond the limits of the tissue of origin.

The aberrant behaviour of cancer cells is more often than not reflected in abnormality of appearance. There is no single morphological or functional characteristic that identifies the cancer cell. Since a cytological smear virtually never carries evidence of invasion of surrounding tissues, cytodiagnosis of malignancy is based on assessment of deviation from the normal in respect of several cellular characteristics. The relevant morphological features are, in essence, features of unregulated growth and are seen principally in the nucleus. Defects of cell maturation are manifested by changes in cytoplasmic features. Abnormality of cell function is often demonstrable by appropriate cytochemical techniques.

NUCLEUS

Size

Enlargement of the nucleus, which should always be assessed against the nucleus of the corresponding normal cell, occurs in many benign proliferative cells and most neoplasms. In malignant cells, the increase in nuclear size is, as a rule, disproportionately great. It is seldom of the same order in all the cells in any one tumour and anisonucleosis and variable nuclear to cytoplasmic ratios are usual.

Chromasia

Malignant cells often have hyperchromatic nuclei. The hyperchromasia is particularly evident in spontaneously desquamated cells and in cells recovered from the surface of a tumour by abrasive methods. It is considered to be due in part to increased amounts of heterochromatin which stains deeply with conventional nuclear stains such as haematoxylin and in part to degenerative changes.

Some malignant cells appear normochromic or hypochromic; such cells are often met with in needle aspirations. The nucleus of a cell which is in the DNA synthesis or S-phase of its cycle contains increased quantities of euchromatin and nuclear proteins; these stain not at all or hardly with routine stains. The preponderance in some aspiration specimens of hypochromic malignant nuclei may be explained by the fact that intact, freshly aspirated tumour cells are more likely to be viable and capable of replication than degenerating cells from the surface of a tumour.

In practice, polychromasia of nuclei is commonly seen and is of greater significance than uniformity of staining reaction.

Chromatin pattern

The reticular arrangement of the chromatin punctuated by the occasional clump that is seen in the benign nucleus is seldom seen in cancer cells. In the malignant nucleus the chromatin is condensed into aggregates; these may be fine or more often coarse and are irregular in shape, size and distribution. The chromatin clumps may be so dispersed that variable sized areas of clearing become apparent in the nucleus. Disorganisation of the chromatin pattern is probably the single most important cytological criterion of malignancy. The chromatin pattern of a malignant nucleus is seldom reflected by its neighbours, each nucleus being aberrant in an individual anarchic fashion.

Patchy condensation of the chromatin beneath the nuclear membrane which appears unevenly thickened is frequently observed in neoplastic cells. The same appearance is also seen in association with inflammation especially in virus infected nuclei; it is not a feature of malignancy per se, but of degenerative change to which malignant cells appear to be particularly prone.

Shape and outline

Changes may occur in the shape and border of the malignant nucleus which may become elongated, convoluted, lobulated or assume bizarre forms. Nuclear pleomorphism is a well recognized feature of malignant tissue. Some extremely well differentiated or poorly differentiated tumours may be monomorphic.

Number

Multinucleation occurs in both benign and malignant cells. Whereas the multiple nuclei of a benign cell are more or less alike, those in a malignant cell show several of the features considered above. The diagnosis of malignancy is based not on the number but the character of the nuclei.

Macronucleolus

The presence or absence of a nucleolus is neither significant nor essential for the recognition of malignancy. Benign reactive cells often contain moderately large, single or multiple nucleoli which sometimes vary in shape. A macronucleolus, single or multiple, is more likely to occur in a neoplastic cell and a carefully judged nucleolar-nuclear ratio can be an aid to diagnosis.

Mitosis

Normal mitotic figures may be met with in benign and malignant lesions. These may be fairly abundant in benign proliferation as for example in foci of immature squamous metaplasia. Abnormal mitoses, whether morphologically obvious or determined by karyotyping, are of significance.

CYTOPLASM

Size and shape

Variations in the size and shape of malignant cells are common. Anisocytosis is generally evident in a group of tumour cells and cell pleomorphism may be gross in some cancers.

Differentiation

Specialized cytoplasmic structures elaborated by the normal cell to carry out its physiological function may undergo qualitative and quantitative changes in neoplasia. For example, a malignant cell is incapable of developing true cilia, although a pseudociliated appearance may occur due to the presence of uneven microvilli. A squamous carcinoma of the uterine cervix may synthesize abundant keratin although the normal ectocervical squamous lining is non-keratinized. At the other end of the spectrum, the squamous origin of the tumour may not be recognizable due to failure of cell maturation. Depending on the degree of differentiation, an adenocarcinoma may secrete moderate to excessive amounts of mucin or it may be mucin depleted.

Some differentiated tumours produce substances normally synthesized in fetal life. Examples of these are production of alpha-fetoprotein by a hepatoma and carcinoembryonic antigen by lung, breast and gastrointestinal carcinomas. Such products may be demonstrated in the cytoplasm of tumour cells by appropriate immunocytochemical techniques. Other tumours may produce ectopic substances not normally secreted by the tissue of origin.

Cell adhesion

The cohesiveness of cells is decreased in malignant tumours. As a result cancer cells may be dissociated from each other or they may break off in clumps or streaks. In some poorly differentiated carcinomas, cell borders are not well defined and the tumour cells may form an apparent syncytium.

1. Female reproductive system

The female reproductive system consists of the ovaries, the genital tract and the breasts. The genital tract comprises the two oviducts or Fallopian tubes, the uterus, the vagina and the vulva. The fimbrial ends of the Fallopian tubes are open to the peritoneal cavity close to the ovaries. The uterus is divided into the body or corpus uteri and a neck—the cervix uteri—part of which protrudes into the vagina (pars vaginalis). The Fallopian tubes and the uterine corpus constitute the upper genital tract; the cervix, vagina and vulva form the lower genital tract.

The entire tract has an outer wall of smooth muscle, an internal mucosal lining and an intervening layer of loose connective tissue. The muscle coat is thickest in the uterine corpus. The connective tissue of the cervix is rich in collagen fibres which interlace with the fibres of its muscle coat. The mucosal lining varies greatly in morphology and function in the different parts of the tract.

The vagina and the vaginal aspect of the cervix are lined by an identical protective, non-keratinized, stratified, squamous epithelium. The endocervical canal is lined by a simple mucus-secreting columnar epithelium which invaginates the musculocollagenous substance of the cervix to form deep branching crypts. The junction between the ectocervical squamous epithelium and the endocervical columnar epithelium (squamocolumnar junction) is an abrupt one and usually coincides with the external os, the opening of the endocervical canal into the vagina. At the internal os at the upper end of the canal, the endocervical mucosa merges into the endometrium, the mucosal lining of the body of the uterus. The Fallopian tubes are lined by ciliated and non-ciliated columnar cells.

THE OVARIAN CYCLE

From puberty to menopause, the reproductive system is subject to repeated hormonal cycles programmed to produce mature ova and to prepare a suitable environment in the endometrium for the implantation of a fertilized ovum. If pregnancy occurs, the cycle is suspended at this stage.

The ovary, at birth, contains numerous primordial follicles, each composed of a germ cell surrounded by a single row of flattened granulosa or follicular cells. The ovarian cycle is initiated after sexual maturity is reached. Under the influence of the follicle-stimulating hormone (FSH) of the anterior pituitary, several primordial follicles begin to mature. The granulosa cells multiply and the surrounding stromal cells are organised into a theca interna and a theca externa. Rising levels of circulating oestrogen secreted by the cells of the theca interna induce proliferation of the endometrium, inhibit FSH and initiate release of the luteinizing hormone (LH) by the anterior pituitary. As a rule only one follicle matures into a Graafian follicle; the rest undergo atresia and plasma oestrogen levels drop. The mature Graafian follicle ruptures to release an ovum and under the influence of LH is converted into a corpus luteum. The luteinized theca interna cells continue to secrete oestrogen; the granulosa cells enlarge into granulosa lutein cells and begin secretion of progesterone which promotes secretory activity in the endometrium. A feed-back mechanism operates via the hypothalamus whereby rising levels of progesterone inhibit the continued secretion of LH. The corpus luteum regresses into an inactive corpus albicans, production of oestrogen and progesterone ceases, the endometrium is shed in the menstrual flow and a new cycle commences.

The menstrual cycle is of variable duration but usually takes 28 days and is divided into the menstrual phase (days 1–4), the pre-ovulatory proliferative phase (days 5–14) and the post-ovulatory secretory phase (days 15–28). Ovulation usually occurs at or immediately prior to day 15 of a 28 day cycle. Although the histological and functional cyclical changes are most marked in the endometrium, subtler changes occur in parallel in the vaginal and cervical epithelia.

The specimens illustrated in this section are cervical scrape smears except where otherwise stated.

Squamous epithelium

The vaginal and ectocervical squamous epithelium of a woman in the child-bearing years may be divided into four strata:

1. Stratum germinativum or the basal layer consists of a single row of vertically orientated cuboidal cells.
2. Stratum spinosum profundum or the parabasal zone has several layers of larger polygonal cells.
3. Stratum spinosum superficiale or the intermediate zone is sub-divided into an inner zone of ovoid cells and an outer zone of large polyhedral cells.
4. Stratum superficiale or the superficial layer is made up of large flat polyhedral cells with pyknotic nuclei.

Cell division occurs in the basal germinal layer. Thereafter, the post-mitotic cells do not divide further but mature and move towards the surface. In the course of maturation, they undergo morphological and functional differentiation through the parabasal and intermediate stages into superficial cells which are continuously exfoliated. In a vital process the changes are gradual and cells will be met which appear to be transitional between arbitrarily separated strata.

The extent of maturation, the thickness of the different strata and the cohesiveness of the cells vary with the stage of the menstrual cycle. The date of ovulation preferred in some countries as day one of the menstrual cycle is a convenient and customary starting point for the study of changing cell patterns in smears. The cells seen, whether desquamated or scraped, come from the upper few layers; deeper layer cells are not normally recovered from an intact mature squamous epithelium.

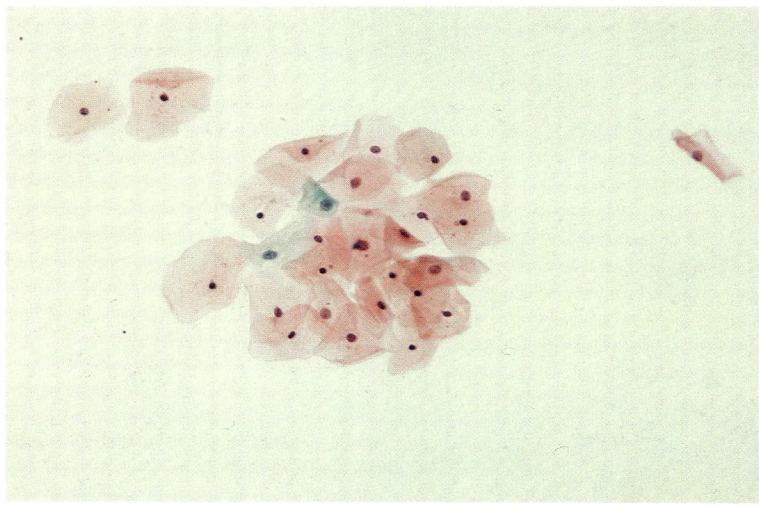

Fig. 1.1 Superficial and outer intermediate squamous cells

Papanicolaou ×183: mid-cycle vaginal smear

The superficial squamous cell is the end point in the differentiation of the oestrogen responsive squamous epithelium of the vagina and ectocervix. It is a large, flat, polyhydral cell, approximately 60 μm in diameter, generally eosinophilic and occasionally cyanophilic. Distanced from its sub-mucosal source of nourishment, it is characterized by a structureless pyknotic nucleus of 5 μm or less.

The outer intermediate squamous cell is the same size and shape, or it may be very slightly smaller. Its staining reaction is more frequently cyanophilic than eosinophilic. It is distinguished from the superficial cell by its nucleus which is larger, generally round, sometimes crenated, and in which a few granules of chromatin are discerned against a reticulated background.

The proportion of superficial cells, low at the commencement of a menstrual cycle, increase progressively during the proliferative phase and peaks at 60–80% of cell population at the time of ovulation. A sharp drop in number, reflecting the cessation of oestrogen production by the follicles that do not reach maturity, is followed by a smaller secondary peak which gradually tails off in the post-ovulatory phase.

The fully oestrogenized mid-cycle smear is typically sparse and the background is clear apart from normal bacterial flora. The cells are mainly dissociated and flat, eosinophilic, superficial cells dominate the picture.

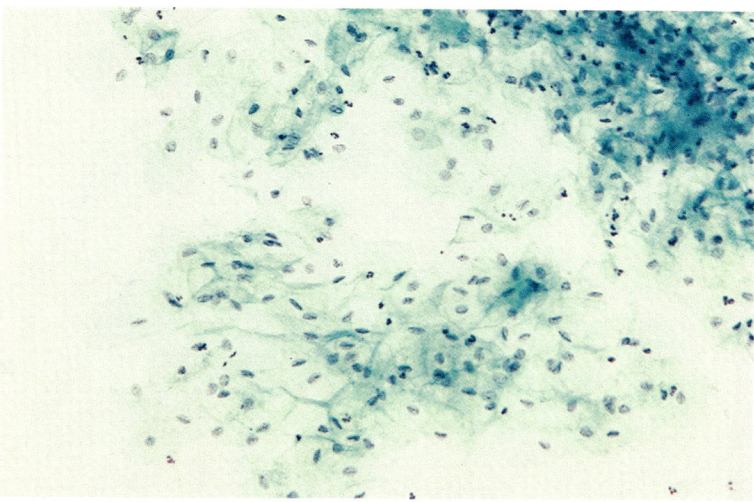

Fig. 1.2 Navicular cells
Papanicolaou ×183: mid-secretory vaginal smear

In the post-ovulatory luteal phase, the proportion of superficial and intermediate squamous cells is reversed. As progesterone levels rise and the secretory phase progresses, the smear becomes more cellular and consists mainly of sheets of closely adherent, inner intermediate cells, referred to as navicular cells on account of their boat-like shape. The individual navicular cell is smaller than the outer intermediate cell, has a thick rolled edge and a thinner centre. This appearance is due to an abundance of glycogen which is aggregated in the central part of the cell around or near the usually eccentric nucleus. The glycogen sometimes imparts a yellow-brown tinge to the Papanicolaou-stained cytoplasm (possibly due to the counterstain Bismarck brown). Navicular cells are most abundant in the midsecretory phase and in the early weeks of pregnancy.

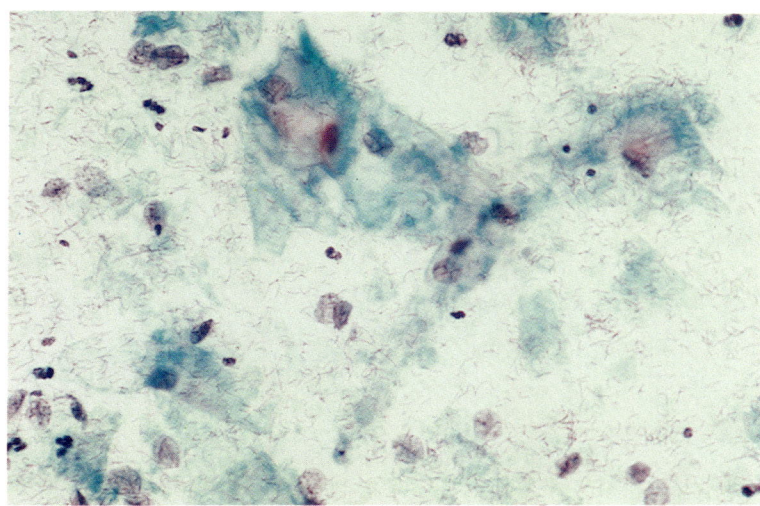

Fig. 1.3 Cytolytic pattern: Doderlein's bacilli
Papanicolaou ×458: pre-menstrual vaginal smear

In the last few days of the secretory phase which correspond with the formation of the inert corpus albicans, and the imminent dissolution of the endometrium, the intermediate squamous cells disintegrate and the smear is covered with fragments of cytoplasm and stripped nuclei. Slender commensal bacilli, present throughout the cycle, become more conspicuous amongst the cell debris. These bacilli, known as Doderlein's bacilli, form lactic acid by anaerobic metabolism of the epithelial glycogen and thereby produce and maintain the acid pH of a healthy vagina.

Endometrial cells

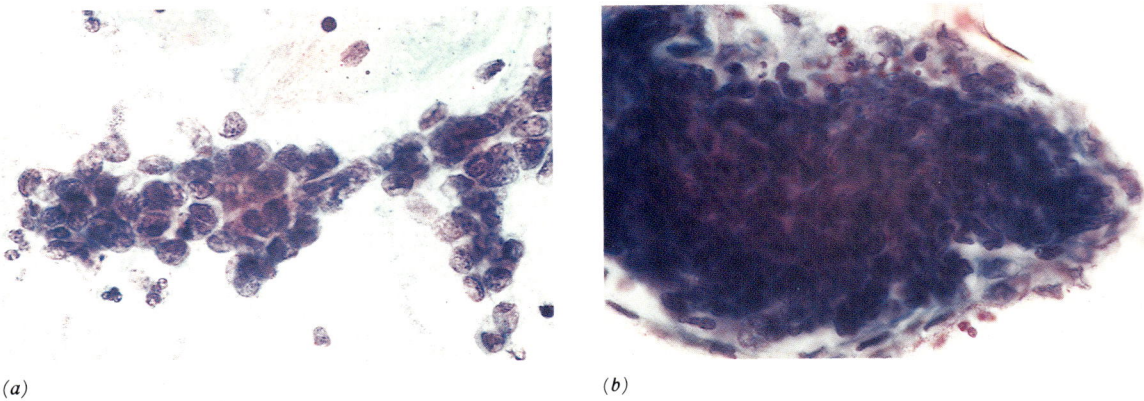

(a) (b)
Fig. 1.4 Menstrual smear
Papanicolaou × 525: vaginal smear (a) endometrial glandular cells (b) endometrial stromal cells

The menstrual smear contains blood, macrophages and two types of endometrial cells. The exfoliated glandular cell is two to three times the size of a neutrophil, and is usually round with a narrow rim of cytoplasm virtually filled with a hyperchromic granular nucleus (a). Degenerative changes are common and some nuclei may be pyknotic. The stromal cells are slender and elongated and have fusiform nuclei. Both types appear in a menstrual smear in substantial-sized clusters and the stromal cells are often seen on the periphery of a cone-shaped aggregate of cells, surrounding centrally positioned glandular cells (b).

Menstruation is preceded by ischaemic necrosis of the endometrium and endometrial cells are almost always present in a smear a day or two before the onset of overt bleeding. They are most abundant during the 3–5 days of the menstrual flow, but a few may persist to the 10th day of a normal cycle. They may be seen at mid-cycle on the rare occasion when rupture of the Graafian follicle is associated with a transient bleed. Desquamation of endometrial cells at times other than these is abnormal and may be caused by hormonal disturbances, underlying pathology or a local irritant such as an intra-uterine contraceptive device (IUCD). The end of menstruation is marked by an outpouring of histiocytes; this appearance is known as the exodus.

Endocervical columnar cells

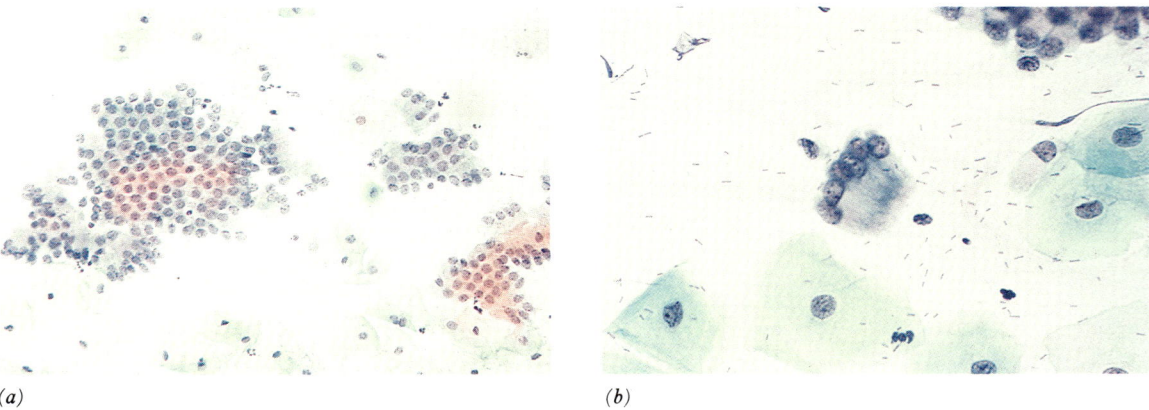

(a) (b)
Fig. 1.5 Mucus-secreting cells
Papanicolaou (a) ×133: squamocolumnar junction scrape (b) ×333: another field

A smear taken from the squamocolumnar junction contains endocervical, mucus-secreting columnar cells in addition to ectocervical squamous cells; in these micrographs the squamous cells are of the cyanophilic outer intermediate type. The columnar cells are tall, slender and cylindrical. They appear singly or, more commonly, in sheets. Viewed in profile, they appear in a palisade with basally-located nuclei (a), (b); in cross-section, they are arranged in a characteristic honeycomb pattern (a). Some alteration occurs in the height and distension of the columnar cells during the menstrual cycle, but is not of particular note; cyclical changes in the quality of their secretion is of greater significance. The mucus secreted is alkaline. During the proliferative phase, it is quite thin. At the time of ovulation, it becomes thinner still to facilitate the entry of the spermatozoa into the uterine cavity, and may flow into the vagina as a mid-cycle 'discharge'. In response to post-ovulatory progesterone, the mucus becomes viscid, plugs the external os and provides a protective barrier against invasion of the uterine cavity by infective organisms. In addition, the cervical mucus lubricates the vaginal epithelium and obviates the need for further squamous differentiation to the level of keratin formation.

NORMAL POST-MENOPAUSAL PATTERN

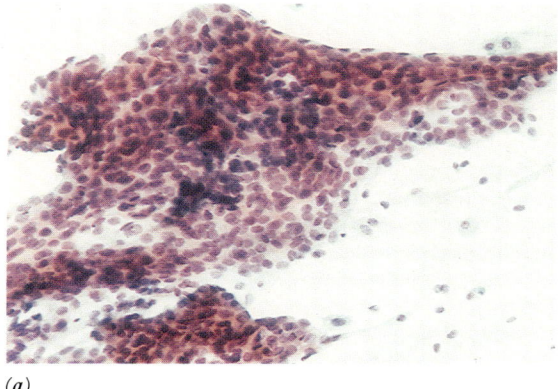
(a)

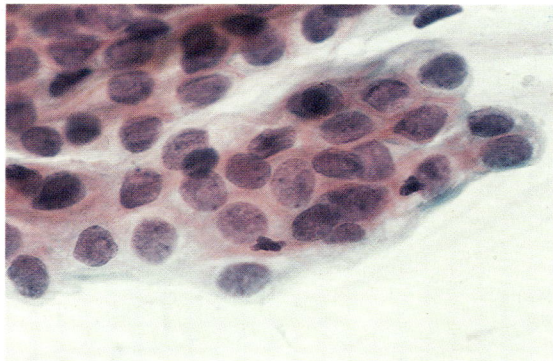
(b)

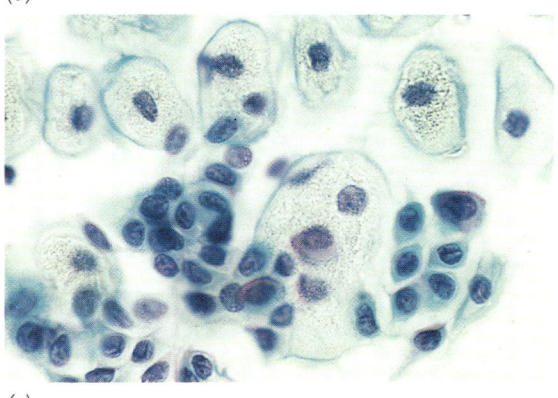
(c)

Fig. 1.6 Atrophic squamous cells
Papanicolaou (a) ×133 (b) ×525 (c) ×525: another case

Non-oestrogenized vaginal and ectocervical squamous epithelium is thin and less differentiated. In the post-menopausal years, the atrophic epithelium generally consists of a single row of basal cells and a few layers of parabasal cells. These are polygonal and appear in smears mainly in large sheets, single forms are few in number (a). The cytoplasm is fairly dense and often amphophilic (b); the relatively large nuclei have a reticulated chromatin. The cells disintegrate easily and a variable number of stripped nuclei are usually present (a).

Less commonly, the epithelium, although quite thin, shows a further stage of differentiation and the parabasal cells are accompanied by larger ovoid cells, similar to navicular cells (c).

The normal post-menopausal smear contains few or no superficial squamous cells. The atrophic epithelium may respond to external irritation and inflammation as in prolapse by reactive squamous differentiation. Superficial and intermediate squamous cells and/or anucleate squames may then be seen. The differentiation may progress to hyperkeratosis. In the absence of a local stimulus, superficial cells in excess of 10% of cell population are suggestive of an endogenous or exogenous source of oestrogen (see Fig. 14.16).

SQUAMOUS METAPLASIA

In addition to the effect on the mucosal lining of the genital tract, the female sex hormones, particularly oestrogen, induce expansion of the collagen-rich cervical stroma, thereby increasing its bulk. The cervix becomes everted at the external os and the lower end of the endocervical mucosa is exposed to the vagina. The sub-epithelial vasculature, visible through the simple columnar epithelium, imparts a red colour to the area around the os. This appearance, the result of anatomical cervical ectropion, is referred to in common clinical practice as cervical erosion, a misleading term as the cervical mucosa is in no way eroded.

The normal pH of the endocervical canal is alkaline. Exposure of the endocervical mucosa to the acid environment of the vagina stimulates the formation of a protective squamous epithelium. The process begins peripherally at the squamocolumnar junction and extends inwards until the exposed columnar epithelium is replaced by a newly formed metaplastic squamous epithelium. The cervix now has two epithelial junctions: a distal one between the native and metaplastic squamous epithelia and a proximal junction between the metaplastic squamous epithelium and columnar epithelium.

The formation of the metaplastic epithelium begins initially below an intact columnar cell layer. Opinions vary as to the origin of the progenitor cell. One theory is that of a bipotential, sub-cylindrical reserve cell which normally replenishes the columnar cell layer, but is capable of squamous differentiation if suitably stimulated. Another theory, advanced more recently, is that of a migrant stromal cell which crosses the basement membrane and comes to lie below the mucous layer.

Cervical ectopy occurs to some extent in each menstrual cycle, but is most marked at puberty, pregnancy, post-partum and with some steroid oral contraceptives. The maternal hormones may exert a similar effect on a female neonate (erosion of the new-born). Squamous metaplasia will be seen to be a normal physiological response to environmental changes. It is, however, less stable than native squamous epithelium, and may become the site of neoplasia. Cervical ectropion covered with columnar and metaplastic squamous epithelium is referred to as the transformation zone.

FEMALE REPRODUCTIVE SYSTEM 9

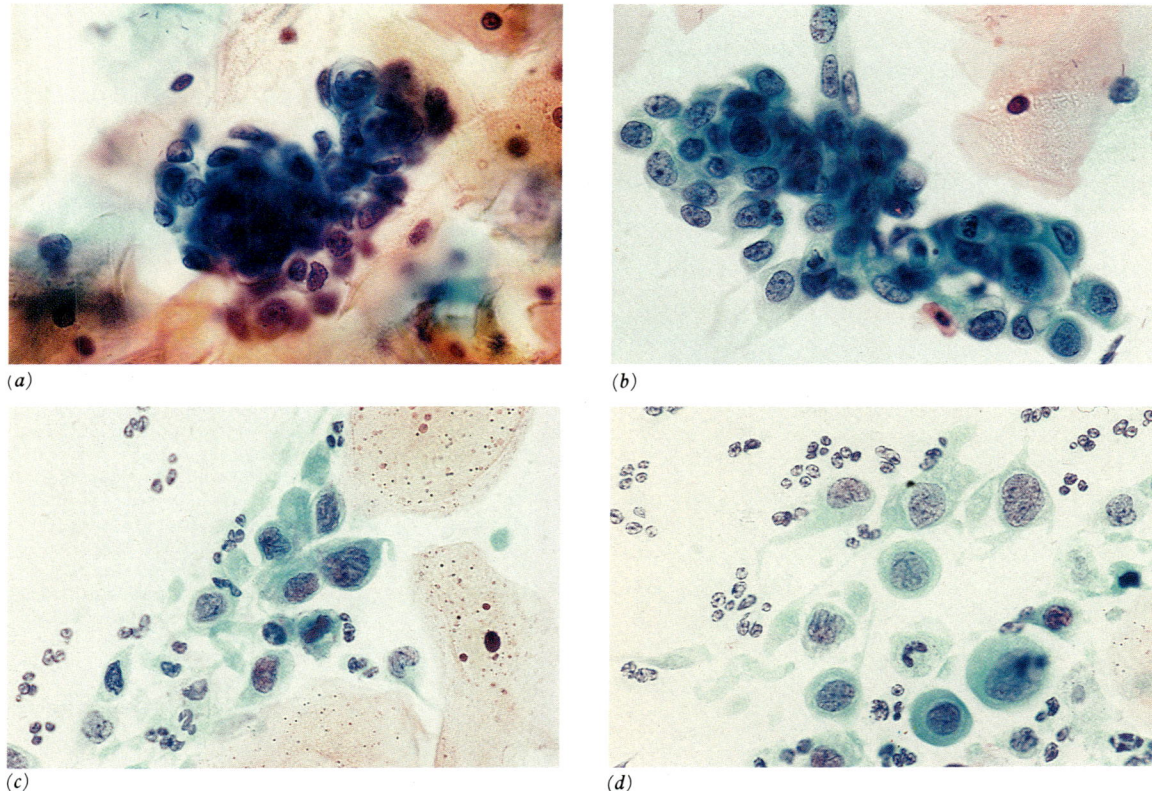

Fig. 1.7 Squamous metaplasia

Papanicolaou ×525 (a) reserve cell hyperplasia (b) immature squamous metaplasia (c) moderately mature squamous metaplasia (d) moderately mature squamous metaplasia

In the early stages of the histogenesis of squamous metaplasia, the sub-columnar progenitor cells multiply and become multi-layered (reserve cell hyperplasia). These cells are not often seen in smears. When present, they usually occur in tight clusters (a). The reserve cell is small with very scant delicate cytoplasm and resembles the exfoliated endometrial glandular cell. Its nucleus is about the size of the nucleus of an outer intermediate squamous cell and has abundant chromatin which is finely granular and evenly distributed. An occasional pinpoint nucleolus may be evident. Mitoses are often present.

As the reserve cell differentiates along squamous lines, it increases in size. The increase in the volume of the cytoplasm is proportionately greater and the nuclear cytoplasmic ratio is gradually reduced. In the early stages of squamous differentiation, the cells still tend to cohesion and the clumps may include a few glandular cells with circumscribed mucous vacuoles (b). With progressive differentiation cell dissociation becomes more frequent (c), (d). The cytoplasm loses some of its translucence and acquires a firmer texture (c), (d). Since alcohol fixation does not result in the same degree of cell retraction as routine histological techniques, inter-cellular bridges which identify early squamous differentiation in formalin fixed paraffin embedded sections, are not seen as such. In cytological smears, the spinal cells appear multiangular, and cell junctions follow the angular shapes of cohesive cells (b). The discrete cells may be irregular in shape; several have variable-sized cytoplasmic extensions or tails and have been fancifully described as spider cells (c), (d). Others are smooth and round or oval; these are parabasal squamous cells (d). As it seems highly unlikely that parabasal cells could be recovered from the lower levels of a thick, well-differentiated squamous epithelium, their presence in a smear is suggestive of an area of squamous metaplasia that has differentiated to the Malphigian zone.

The nucleus increases in size, but to a far lesser extent. Finely granular in reserve cells, it becomes vesicular (b); at this stage it resembles the nucleus of the endocervical columnar cell (compare with Fig. 1.5 b). With increasing squamous differentiation, the fine clumps of chromatin are replaced by bands, and the nucleus becomes coarser and is frequently irregular in shape (c), (d). A nucleolus barely visible in the reserve cell is constant and conspicuous though small in immature squamous metaplasia (b); thereafter it is inconstant and generally absent.

The final stages of squamous metaplasia, when the new epithelium closely approximates to native squamous epithelium, are not usually identifiable in smears.

POST-COITAL SMEAR

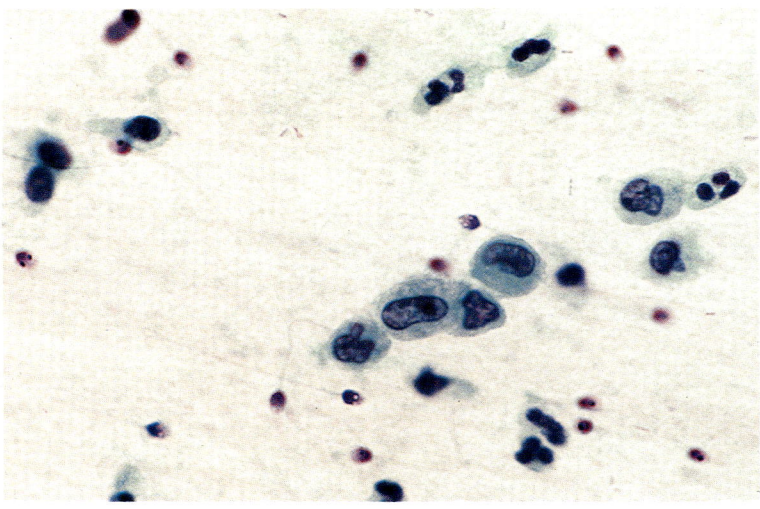

(a)

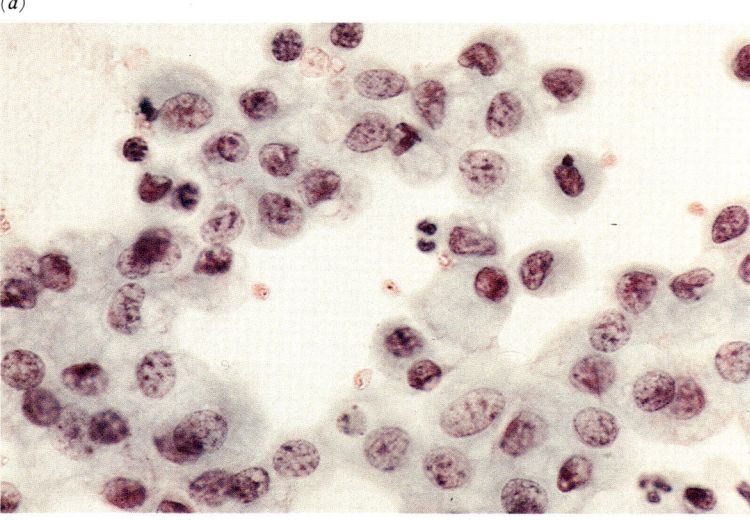

(b)

Fig. 1.8 Post-coital smear

Papanicolaou ×720 (a) spermatozoa: histiocytic cells: neutrophils (b) glandular cells

The post-coital smear often contains spermatozoa and a variety of glandular cells. The spermatozoon has a long tail and a pointed pear-shaped head (a). The distal half of the head is pale-staining, the portion adjacent to the tail is dark. It is likely that the variety of the cells seen closely associated with spermatozoa in a post-coital smear are derived from the various ducts in which semen is elaborated and through which it passes. The cells in (a) have indented nuclei and are histiocytic in appearance; however, they are cohesive and this suggests an epithelial lining origin. The cells in (b) form a large flat sheet, have finely vacuolated cytoplasm and vesicular nuclei and have the appearance of glandular cells. The smear contained many spermatozoa, not shown in this field.

INFLAMMATORY DISEASE

A certain number of neutrophils are always present in cervical mucus and their presence in a smear does not necessarily denote inflammation. Indeed, their absence from a cervical smear, except at mid-cycle, suggests inadequate sampling of the squamocolumnar junction. They are few in number at mid-cycle and abundant in a menstrual smear. In pregnancy, the cervical mucus is packed with polymorphs which may obscure epithelial cells in an ante-natal smear.

A mucopurulent discharge consists mainly of pus cells, and a smear obtained during an episode of acute inflammation may be unsuitable for screening for neoplasia. Inflammatory disease of some duration causes reactive changes in epithelial cells which are not themselves active participants in the inflammatory process. The reaction is manifested by degeneration and death of the cell when the damage is irreversible. Repair of the damaged tissue is effected by viable and healthy cells which show evidence of proliferative activity. Both nucleus and cytoplasm are affected.

Degenerative changes in the nucleus consist initially of condensation of the chromatin below the nuclear membrane which appears thick and dark. The chromatin aggregates may ring the entire nucleus or they may be punctate. Margination of the chromatin is extremely common in malignant cells, but is not a characteristic of malignancy per se. The nuclear outline becomes irregular and the chromatin on the membrane of a crenated nucleus may be seen as coarse bands across its surface. Nuclear death may be by total shrinkage of the chromatin (karyopyknosis), fragmentation (karyorrhexsis), or dissolution (karyolysis). Degeneration of the cytoplasm is indicated by hydropic vacuolisation of non-secretory cells, anomalous staining reactions and loss of integrity of the plasma membrane.

Proliferative activity is associated with some increase in the amount of chromatin and in the size of the nucleus. A mild degree of anisocytosis and anisonucleosis may be noted. One or more nucleoli, small but distinct, are present. The cytoplasm of an actively growing cell is generally deeply basophilic and dense in texture. A cell engaged in repair may succumb to injury and cells which show some morphological features of growth and some of degeneration are often seen in inflammatory disease.

Cellular changes associated with inflammation

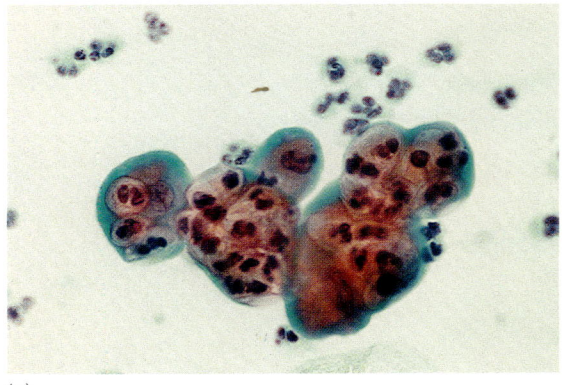 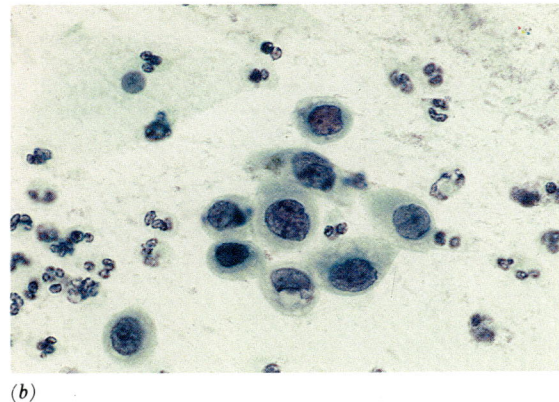

(a)   (b)

Fig. 1.9 Cervicitis

Papanicolaou ×525 (a) parabasal squamous cells (b) parabasal squamous cells: another case

The parabasal squamous cells in (a) are abnormally dense, display polychromasia and are infiltrated by neutrophils; an invading polymorph may be distinguished from a superimposed one by its surrounding phagosomal vacuole. The nuclei are hypochromic due to central depletion of chromatin which is deposited on the crenated nuclear membrane. The cells in (b) have normochromic, normal textured cytoplasm, but contain hydropic vacuoles. The nuclei are moderately hyperchromic and the chromatin is condensed into bands of variable length and thickness. Note that the bands of chromatin can be traced to the nuclear margin in at least one direction.

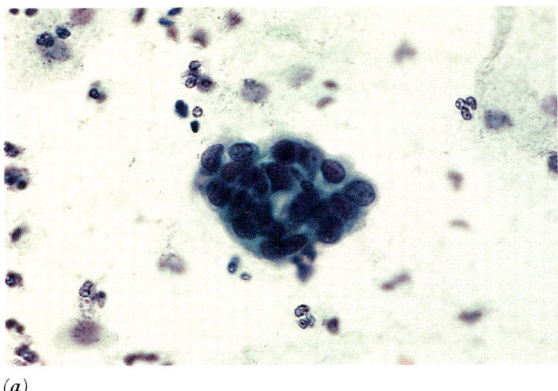 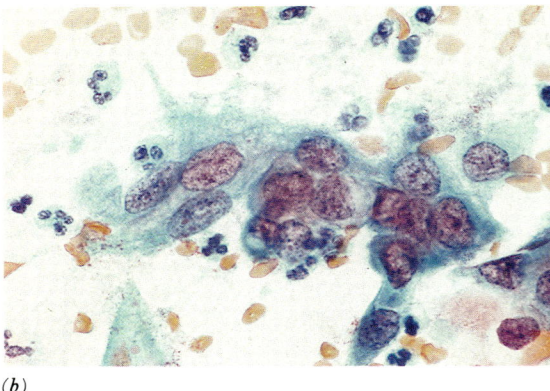

(a)   (b)

Fig. 1.10 Cervicitis

Papanicolaou ×525 (a) immature squamous metaplasia (b) moderately mature squamous metaplasia: another case

Squamous metaplasia may develop in response to inflammation, in the absence of hormone-induced cervical ectopy. Two cases of cervicitis with reactive metaplasia are illustrated in these micrographs. The cells in (a) are immature and approximate in size and arrangement to reserve cells (compare with Fig. 1.7a). The cytoplasm, however is more basophilic and firm, and the nuclei more hyperchromic. The background consists of polymorphs and amorphous debris, whereas in physiological reserve cell hyperplasia, the background is clear, normal commensals are present, and the accompanying cells are mature squamous cells.

The moderately mature metaplastic cells in (b) show advanced degeneration. The cytoplasm is flimsy and contains hydropic vacuoles. The cell periphery is ragged and intercellular borders are ill-defined. The sparse chromatin is seen as granules and uneven bands against a homogenous background of violet coloured nuclear sap.

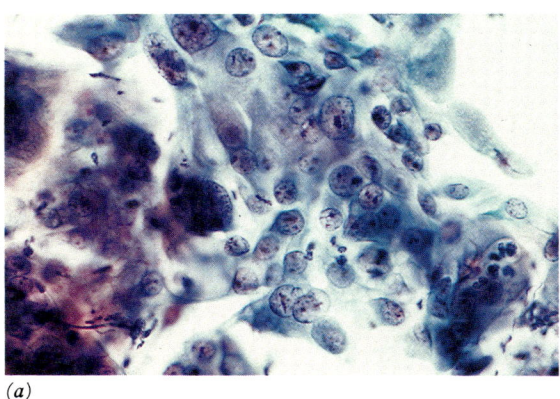 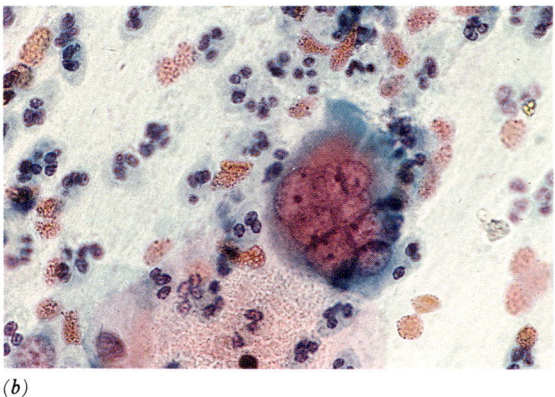

(a)   (b)

Fig. 1.11 Endocervicitis

Papanicolaou (a) ×333: hyperplastic columnar cells (b) ×525: degenerate multinucleate columnar cells

Compare the hyperplastic endocervical columnar cells in (a) with the normal columnar cells in Figure 1.5 (b) and note the disorderly arrangement of the reactive cells. A moderate degree of anisonucleosis is evident. The cytoplasm is relatively normal. The nuclei contain a variable number of small eosinophilic nucleoli. In contrast, the multinucleated endocervical cell in (b) is mucus depleted and polychromic. The nuclei contain little chromatin and appear pink due to virtual lack of haematoxylin uptake.

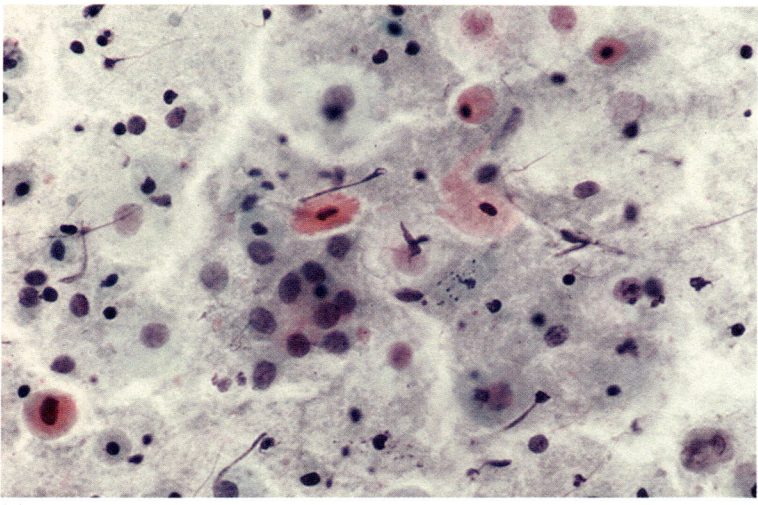

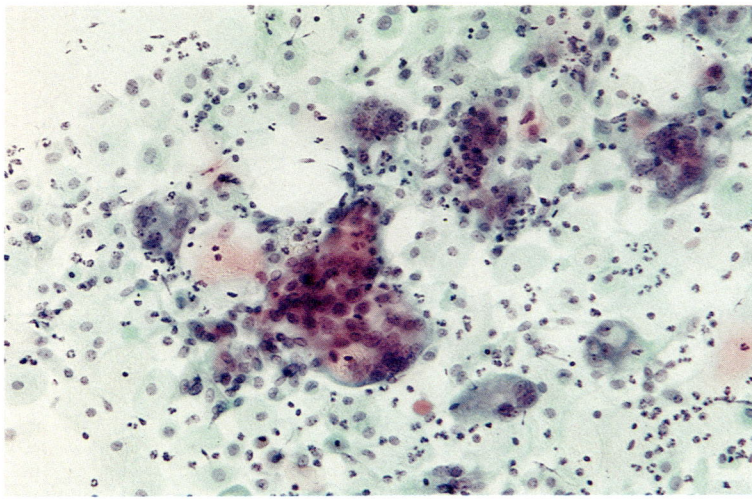

Fig. 1.12 Atrophic vaginitis
Papanicolaou (a) ×458: anomalous staining (b) ×183: multinucleate cells

Post-menopausal atrophy of the squamous epithelium may lead to atrophic vaginitis. The condition is caused by insufficiency of hormonal support to the epithelium and responds to oestrogen therapy; it is rarely due to a specific pathogen. The cells tend to dissociation, appear attenuated and the majority are somewhat amphophilic (a). A common feature of atrophic vaginitis is the presence of eosinophilic parabasal cells which vary from the occasional to half or more of the cell population. In a Papanicolaou-stained smear, degenerate cytoplasm often displays an anomalous staining reaction and eosinophilia of parabasal cells in atrophic vaginitis should not be misinterpreted as pathological dyskeratosis. The nuclei are generally degenerate. The condensed chromatin of a pyknotic or fragmented nucleus may be pulled out in long threads which mimic condensed mucus threads. When karyolysis occurs, the cell appears as a blue blob, the ghost nucleus being represented by a central circumscribed zone of pallor.

Another common finding in extreme senile atrophy and vaginitis is the presence of variable sized multinucleated cells which resemble giant histiocytes. Similarity between their nuclei and the nuclei of parabasal cells suggest an epithelial syncytium rather than a phagocytic macrophage.

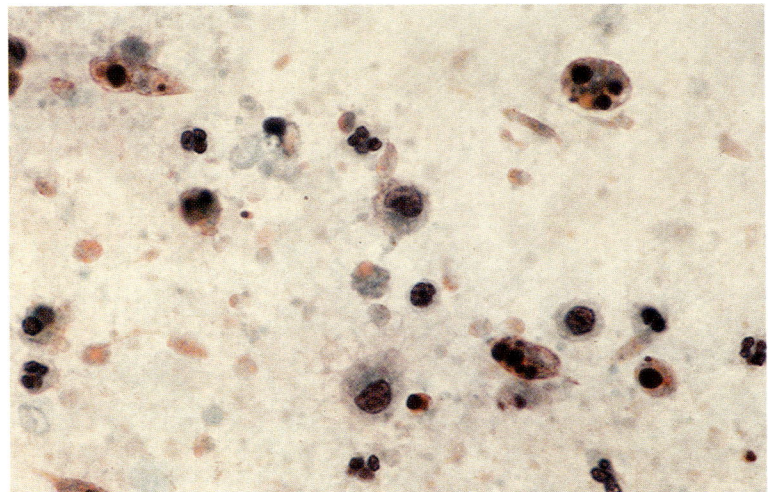

Fig. 1.13 Apoptosis
Papanicolaou ×720

A form of cell death, not related to injury and necrosis but considered to form part of a cell population regulatory process, has been termed apoptosis. Fragments of cytoplasm, which vary in size from the dot-like to small cuboidal cell size, are seen concentrated in one or two microscopic fields or even part of one field. The staining reaction is also variable. Several fragments are devoid of nuclear material, others contain highly condensed pin-point granules of chromatin, yet others resemble small cells undergoing karyorrhexis. The appearance has been noted by the author in post-coital smears, in cases of endometrial carcinoma and in atrophic vaginitis.

Fig. 1.14 Follicular cervicitis
Papanicolaou (a) ×183 (b) ×720

In chronic cervicitis, the cervix may contain lymph follicles with germinal centres. Chance scraping of a follicle produces a characteristic cytological picture. Numerous small discrete cells are seen streaked across two or three contiguous low power fields (a). High power examination shows an admixture of lymphoid cells (b): small mature lymphocytes with condensed hyperchromic nuclei, larger prolymphocytes with small nucleoli, large lymphoblasts with more open pale nuclei and one or several nucleoli, and an occasional histiocyte with a reniform nucleus and phagocytosed intra-cytoplasmic debris. Mitotic figures occur in reactive lymphoid hyperplasia; one is seen near the centre of the field (b).

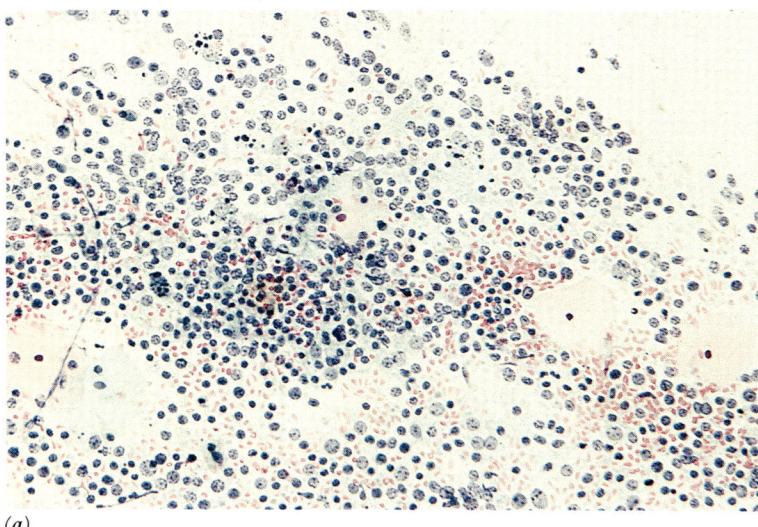

(a)

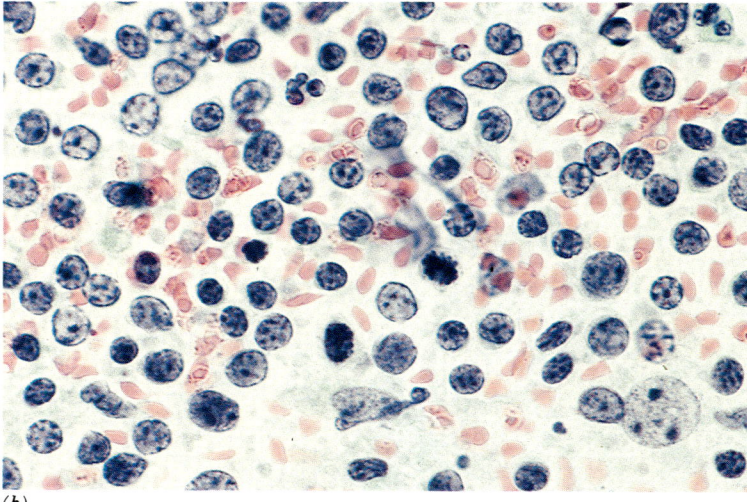

(b)

Flora and fauna

A number of pathogens that invade the genital tract may be recognized in smears. Several are sexually transmitted and some of these have a probable role as aetiological agents in the causation of cervical squamous neoplasia.

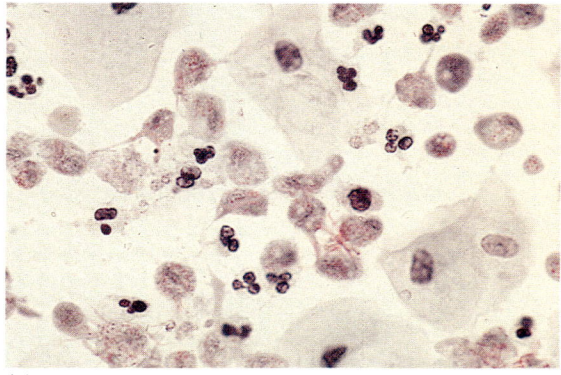
(a)

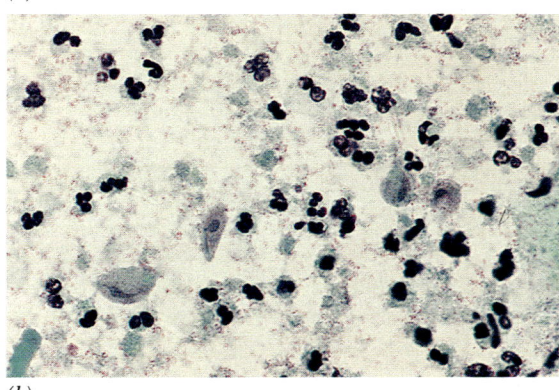
(b)

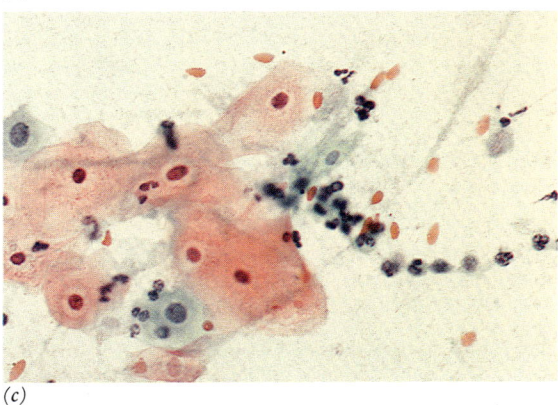
(c)

Fig. 1.15 Trichomonas vaginalis (TV)

(a) Papanicolaou ×525: flagellated forms (b) ×525: acute TV cervicitis (c) ×333: chronic TV cervicitis

One of the commonest pathogens met with is Trichomonas vaginalis, a flagellated unicellular protozoon with a size range of 10–30 µm. The flagellae illustrated in (a) are rarely evident in an alcohol-fixed smear and are not required for correct identification. The parasite usually appears as a greyish-blue, pear-shaped body with a single ovoid or crescentic nucleus (b). Some may contain a dusting of fine intracytoplasmic granules (a). Visualization of the nucleus is essential to discriminate between the parasite, fragments of cytoplasm and degenerate karyolytic parabasal squamous cells which are particularly common in atrophic smears.

Trichomonas vaginalis is usually, but not invariably sexually transmitted and causes an initial acute vaginitis and cervicitis associated with a frothy discharge. The smear at this stage shows many parasitic forms, large numbers of neutrophils and much proteinous debris (b). A chronic phase may follow and in persistent or recurrent infestation, the epithelium shows degenerative changes which consist of pseudo-eosinophilia of intermediate squamous cells which often contain small perinuclear haloes (c). Although this appearance is commonly associated with trichomonal infestation, it is not specific. The parasites may be few in number at this stage and a diligent search may be necessary for the identification of the organism and firm diagnosis. Trichomonads are more easily identified by their motility in a wet preparation of a fresh vaginal discharge.

16 DIAGNOSTIC CYTOPATHOLOGY

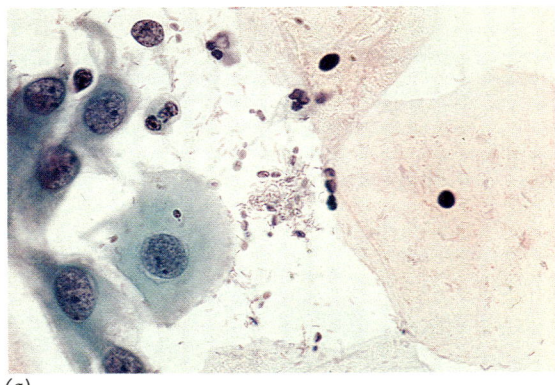
(a)

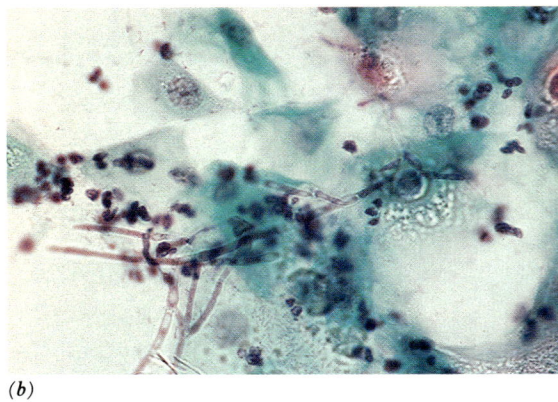
(b)

Fig. 1.16 Candida albicans

Papanicolaou ×525 (a) blastospores (b) hyphae

The widely prevalent yeast, *Candida albicans* is one of the normal flora of the body (see p. 76), and dormant spore forms may be present in a routine smear from an asymptomatic woman. The vegetative stage, developed when spores bud into blastospores (a) pseudo-hyphae and branching septate hyphae (b), is a common cause of vulvovaginitis, which presents with intense itching and a thick, curd-like discharge. Vegetative forms of *Candida albicans* are particularly common in smears of some women on steroid oral contraceptives and in pregnancy. Although, not one of the usual venereally transmitted pathogens, it may, on occasion, be conveyed to the male partner and cause penile irritation.

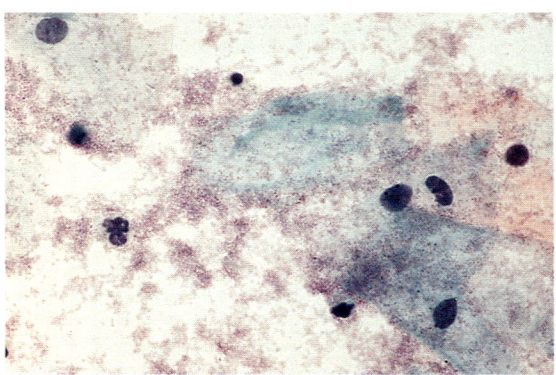

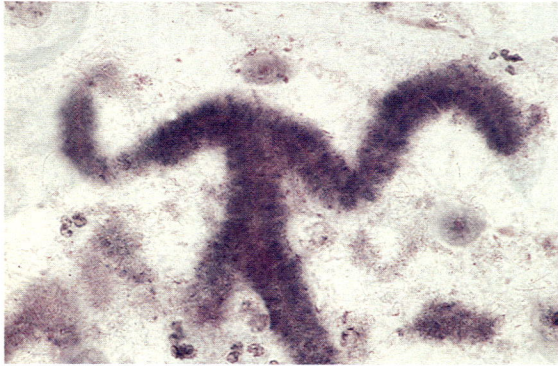

Fig. 1.17 Gardnerella vaginalis

Papanicolaou ×525

Gardnerella vaginalis, a sexually transmitted coccobacillus, is associated with a thin, foul-smelling discharge and a characteristic smear pattern. The smear contains myriads of coccobacilli and the cell population consists almost exclusively of intermediate squamous cells covered with the bacteria; leucocytes are conspicuous by their absence. Although the cells overlaid with the coccobacilli have been designated 'clue' cells, the appearance is suggestive, but not pathognomic of Gardnerella infection which should be proved by appropriate bacteriological studies.

Fig. 1.18 Actinomycetes spp.: Entamoeba gingivalis

Papanicolaou ×525

An opportunistic infection of the uterine cavity may be caused in a woman fitted with an inert intra-uterine contraceptive device by *Actinomyces israeli*, a filamentous bacterium which branches freely and resembles fungal hyphae. The bacterial filament is 1 μm in width and is studded with numerous punctate coccal forms. The characteristic morphology of Actinomycetes species seen in a smear is non-specific as to type. The only pathogenic member, *A. israeli*, is difficult to culture in the laboratory but may be correctly identified by immunofluorescent demonstration of specific antigen-antibody reaction. The bacterium may occur in smears of asymptomatic subjects; in others, it may cause pelvic inflammatory disease. Actinomycetes encrusted IUCD has been known to rupture through the uterine wall into the abdominal cavity, producing an actinomycetoma.

A non-pathogenic unicellular protozoon, Entamoeba gingivalis (seen opposite 12 o'clock and 3 o'clock) sometimes occurs in tandem with actinomycetes.

FEMALE REPRODUCTIVE SYSTEM 17

Fig. 1.19 Herpesvirus simplex (HVS)

Papanicolaou ×720 (a) early infection (b) recurrent infection

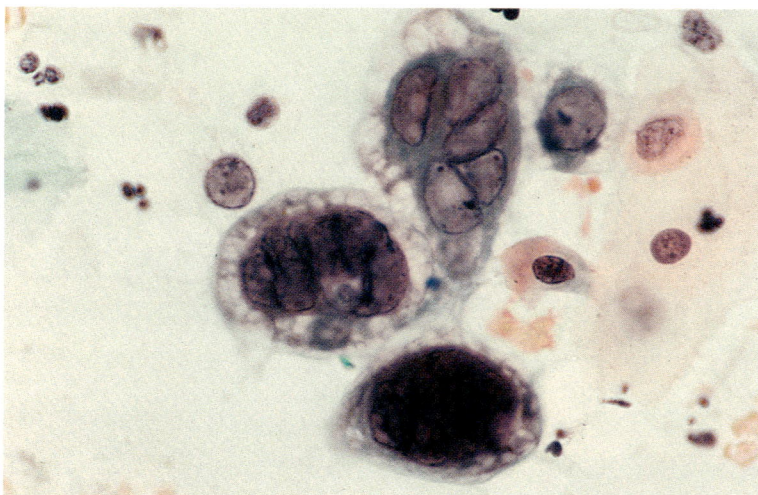

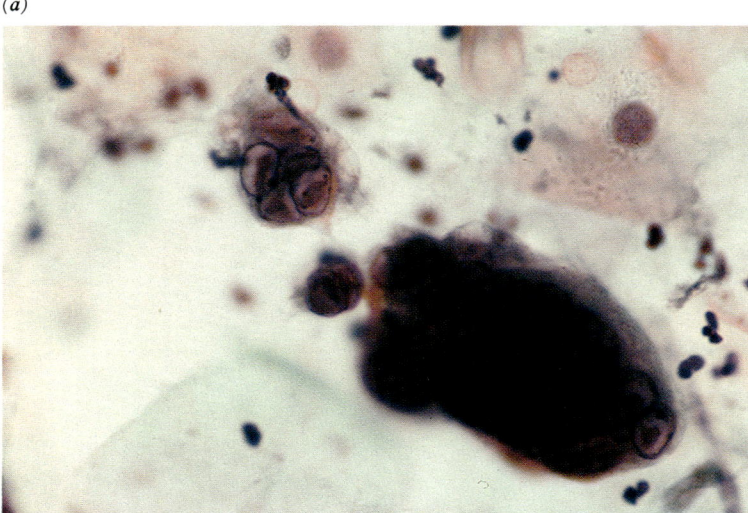

Infection of the lower genital tract by herpesvirus simplex may be due to HVS type 1, but is more often caused by the sexually transmitted type 2, referred to as Herpes genitalis. Characteristic cytopathic effects are seen in both squamous and endocervical columnar cells. The infected cell may be mononuclear, but more often contains several nuclei which mould one another (a). The nucleus has a ground-glass appearance due to accumulation of intranuclear viral particles; the chromatin, pushed to the periphery, sharply demarcates the nuclear margin. One or two clumps of chromatin may be seen attached to the inner surface of the nuclear membrane, in simulation of a Barr body (a). The large dense intranuclear inclusions illustrated in (b) are considered to appear in a recurrent infection or in a reactivated phase of a latent infection. The pathognomonic cytopathic appearance is obtained from the fluid and the base of an intact herpetic vesicle, and is quickly lost once the vesicle has ruptured and become secondarily infected.

HVS type 2 has been proposed as a major aetiological agent in the causation of squamous carcinoma of the cervix because of a statistically significant correlation between the disease and high titres of circulating antibodies to the virus. It is now thought that it may play a subsidiary or synergistic role, or is possibly an opportunist which favours malignant tissue.

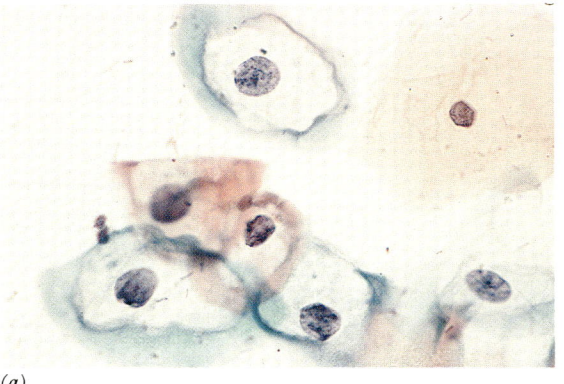
(a)

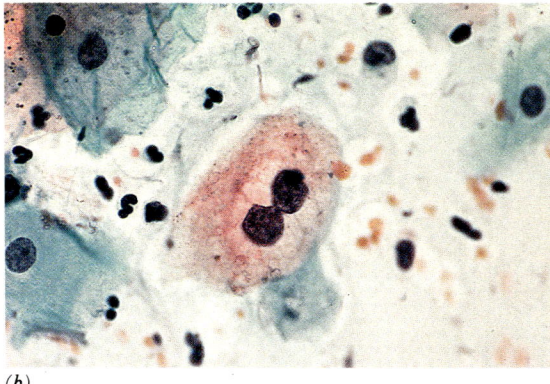
(b)

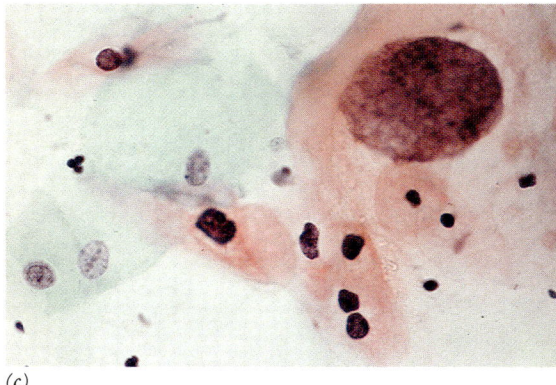
(c)

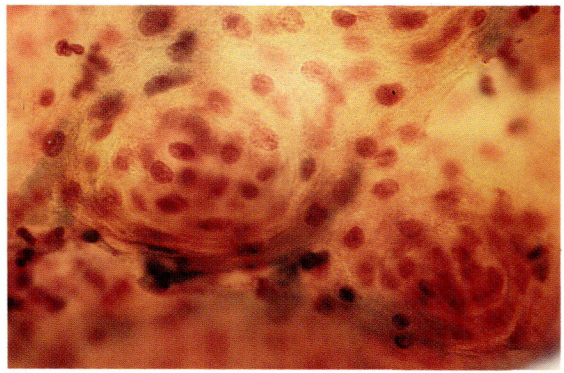
(d)

Fig. 1.20 Human papilloma virus (HPV)

Papanicolaou ×525 (a) koilocytes (b) binucleate koilocyte (c) dyskeratosis: giant nucleus (d) parakeratosis (e) hyperkeratosis

Interest has centred in recent years on a family of sexually transmitted viruses, known to cause papillomas and warts, and appearances previously attributed to mild epithelial dysplasia or non-specific inflammation are now recognized as the finger-print of the human papilloma virus (HPV). The pathognomonic change is seen in intermediate squamous cells and consists of a large perinuclear vacuole which imparts a concave appearance to the cytoplasm: hence the affected cell is referred to as a koilocyte (a). The vacuole is substantially larger than the perinuclear halo seen in trichomonal vaginitis (compare with Fig. 1.15c). The nucleus may be enlarged, irregular and hyperchromic, binucleation is a common feature (b). Additional but non-specific changes include individual cell keratinization, dyskeratosis and degenerate giant nuclei (c). The papilloma group of viruses may cause a flat condyloma, also referred to as a plane wart, or an exophytic papillomatous condyloma acuminatum, with a parakeratotic or a hyperkeratotic surface. Koilocytes are not usually recovered from keratinized lesions. The appearance illustrated in (d) is suggestive of a lesion with a parakeratotic surface, that in (e) of a hyperkeratotic lesion. Cells with small nuclei and keratinized cytoplasm (d) and anucleate squames (e), arranged in a concentric manner, similar to epithelial pearls, are seen within a three-dimensional sheet of surface cells.

The plane wart is not visible to the naked eye. It may be identified colposcopically, but distinction from a focus of

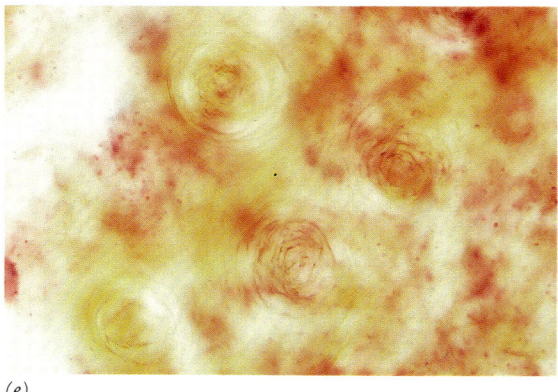
(e)

intra-epithelial neoplasia may not be possible. The two lesions may exist synchronously, or condylomatous and neoplastic changes may be present in the same lesion. DNA sequence of HPV types 6, 11, 16 and 18 have been demonstrated in the cells of intraepithelial and/or invasive squamous cell carcinoma of the cervix. From this evidence, it has been suggested that HPV, in association with synergistic factors, plays a major role in the causation of cervical cancer.

FEMALE REPRODUCTIVE SYSTEM 19

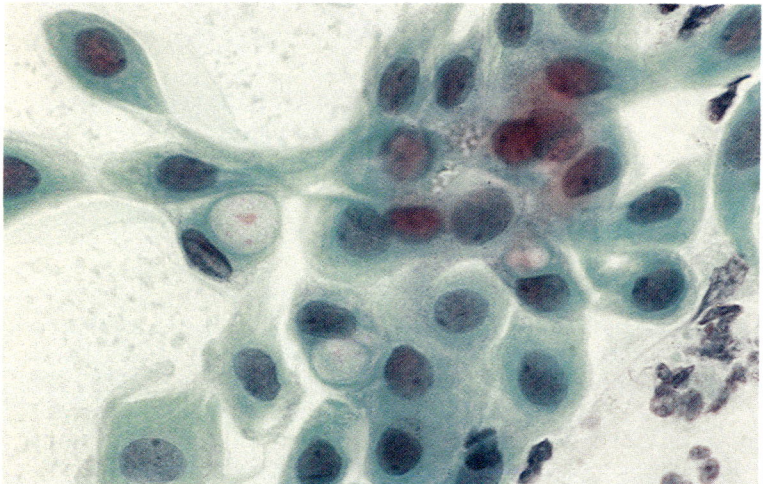

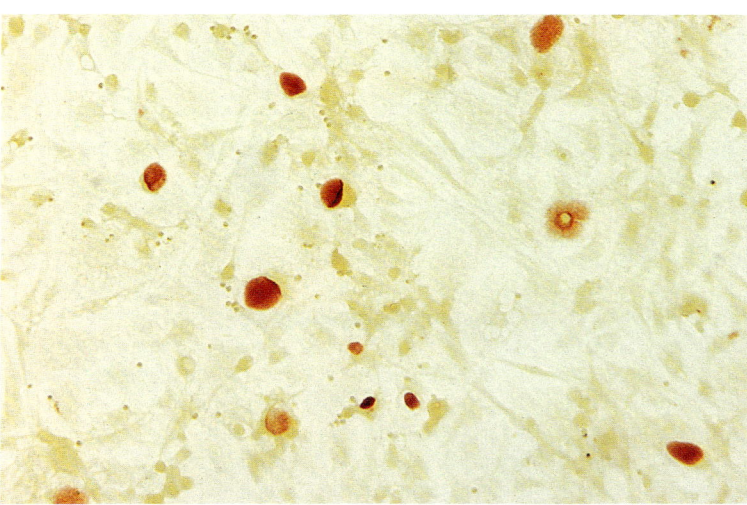

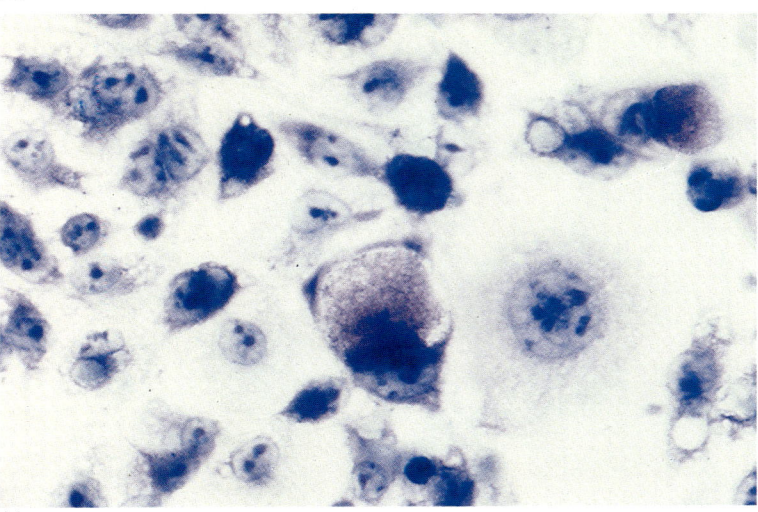

Fig. 1.21 Chlamydia trachomatis

Papanicolaou ×720 (a) cervical smear (b) mouse McCoy cells infected with C. trachomatis from endocervical discharge; Lugol's iodine (c) mouse McCoy cells infected with C. trachomatis; control culture; Giemsa

Another sexually transmitted pathogen which has been mooted as a possible aetiological agent in cervical carcinoma is *Chlamydia trachomatis*, an obligatory intra-cellular organism, previously regarded as a large virus and now considered to be a bacterium. *C. trachomatis* consists of two main groups and 15 immunotypes, three of which cause lymphogranuloma inguinale. Twelve immune sub-types are associated with infection of columnar cells; infection of the conjuctiva results in trachoma; of the male urethra in non-gonoccocal urethritis, epididymitis and Reiter's syndrome; of the female genital tract in mucopurulent endocervicitis, Bartholinitis, salpingitis and urethral syndrome. Passage of a fetus through an infected cervix may lead to neonatal inclusion conjunctivitis, and infant pneumonia.

The appearance illustrated in (a) has been claimed by some workers to be diagnostic of chlamydial infection. It consists of one or more clear cytoplasmic vacuoles within which one or several fine or large eosinophilic inclusions are seen. The claim has been rejected by other workers who consider the appearance to be non-specific. Culture for *C. trachomatis* was negative in the case illustrated. It is generally accepted that direct microscopic examination is inefficient and Chlamydial infection is best confirmed by tissue culture in mouse McCoy cells. The colonized cells are filled with numerous intracytoplasmic inclusions which stain brown with iodine (b) and violet with Giemsa (c).

PRE-INVASIVE AND INVASIVE CARCINOMA

Cervical intraepithelial neoplasia (CIN)

The CIN classification, currently preferred to the earlier terms, such as epithelial dysplasia and carcinoma in situ, refers to the spectrum of potentially invasive neoplastic changes in squamous epithelium where the basement membrane is unbreached. The malignant transformation is believed to occur in pre-existing metaplastic squamous epithelium, on the surface or in the endocervical crypts, which has become atypical. The junction between the native and neoplastic epithelium is often as abrupt as the squamocolumnar junction.

CIN is graded according to the degree of morphological and structural abnormality. Grade 1 corresponds to the former mild dysplasia, grade 2 to moderate dysplasia and grade 3 to severe dysplasia and carcinoma in situ.

Cytological evidence of malignancy is seen primarily in the nuclei and these are abnormal in all grades of CIN. The difference between the different grades lies mainly in the degree of squamous maturation. Just as the normal post-mitotic germinal cell undergoes maturation and becomes aligned and organized into recognizable strata, so may the cancerous germinal cell. The capacity for differentiation is, however, altered to a lesser or greater extent in neoplasia.

CIN 1 or mild dysplasia displays a considerable degree of squamous differentiation. The neoplastic cells retain their basaloid character for a third or so of the thickness of the epithelium and then mature and become stratified. The cells of the outermost zone attain the size and shape of intermediate squamous cells. In CIN 2, maturation does not progress beyond the inner intermediate or outer parabasal levels, the lower two-thirds of the epithelium remaining immature. CIN 3 is characterized by little or no maturation, and the full thickness of the epithelium is made up of poorly-differentiated or undifferentiated cells which form a single multi-layered stratum; in some cases a little enlargement or some flattening of the surface cells may be evident. CIN 1 and 2 are generally thicker than CIN 3 on account of their more abundant cytoplasm.

Cytological assessment of the grade of the lesion has its basis in the fact that a cervical scrape smear contains cells from the outer few layers of the epithelium. The degree of differentiation of the neoplastic focus may be deduced from the type of the predominant abnormal cell. The term dyskaryosis was coined by Papanicolaou to denote a cell with a malignant nucleus and a more or less normal cytoplasm (*dys*: bad, abnormal; *karyon*: kernel). In CIN, the differentiated cell closely resembles its benign counterpart. Intermediate type cells with nuclei which carry stigmata of neoplasia (intermediate cell dyskaryosis) indicate an epithelium which has differentiated to this level: the smear pattern would therefore be suggestive of CIN 1. Conversely, predominance of dyskaryotic parabasal or basal cells would indicate a minimally differentiated focus or CIN 3. Moderately mature dyskaryotic cells would be suggestive of CIN 2. An intraepithelial carcinoma may be uniformly of one grade along its full extent; focal variations are common and the entire spectrum of epithelial atypia may be present in a single case.

Histological examination of biopsy should be regarded as mandatory to define precisely the nature of a neoplastic lesion and for confirmation of the presumptive cytological diagnosis. Cytohistological discrepancy may be due to an incorrect diagnosis or an inappropriate sample. Colposcopic assessment and a colposcopically-directed biopsy obtained from the highest grade is a useful intermediary procedure.

FEMALE REPRODUCTIVE SYSTEM 21

Fig. 1.22 CIN 1: intermediate squamous cell dyskaryosis
Papanicolaou (a) ×183 (b) ×720

Dyskaryotic squamous cells often appear in streaks or groups and stand out against the benign cells on account of their large nuclei. One of several such streaks present in a cervical smear from a case of CIN 1 is illustrated in (a). At high magnification, the cells are seen to have the size, shape, texture and staining reaction of cyanophilic outer intermediate squamous cells (b). The nuclei are disproportionately large and variable; most show degenerative changes in the form of irregular outlines, compaction of chromatin and intense hyperchromasia. The better preserved cells to the left of the field have smooth normochromic nuclei.

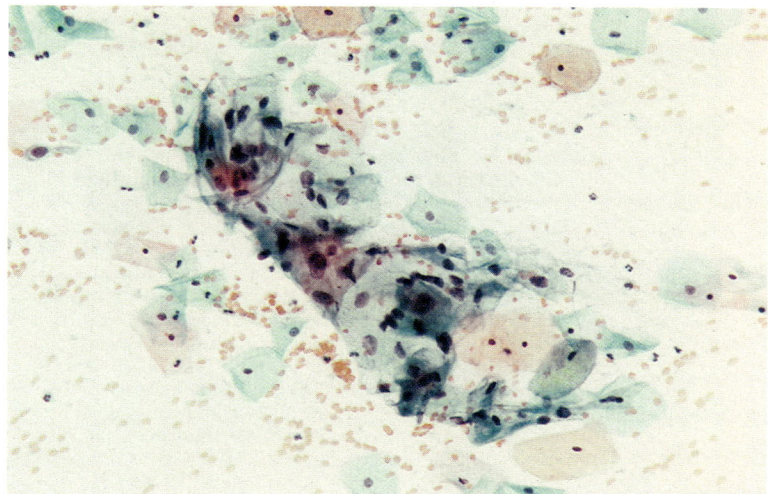
(a)

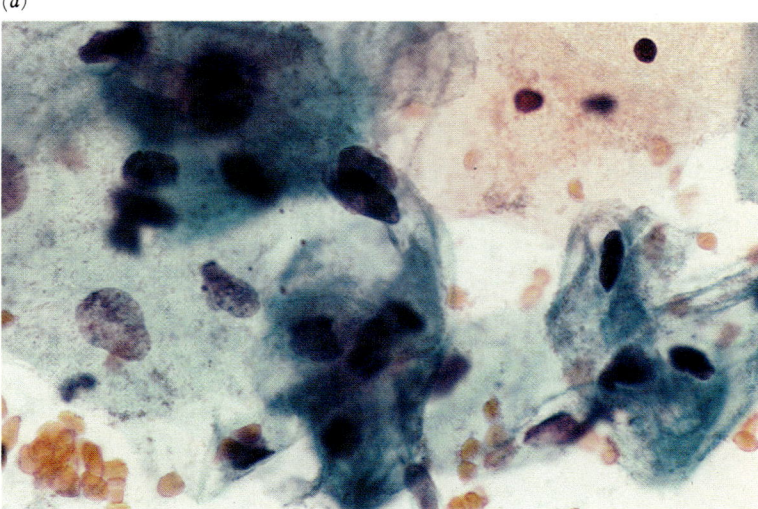
(b)

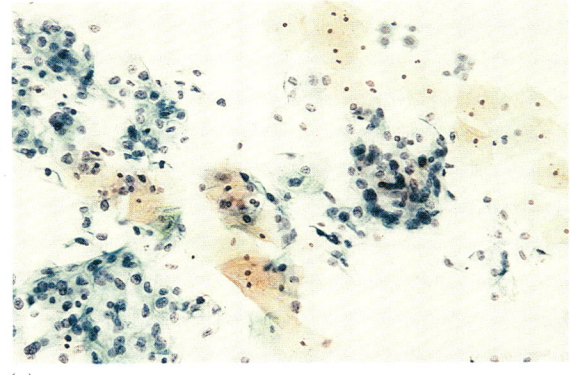

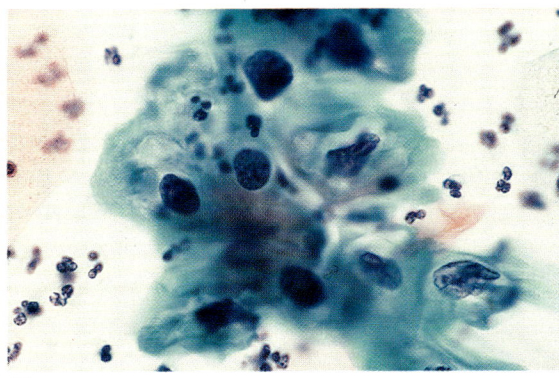

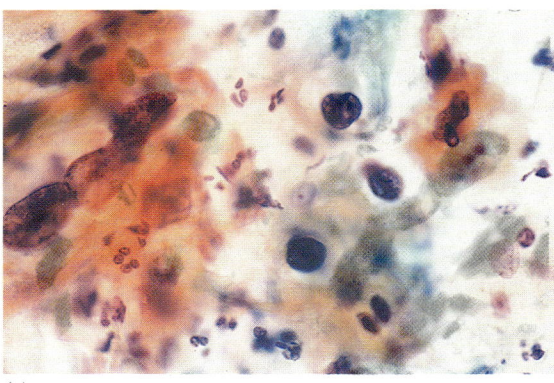

Fig. 1.23 CIN 2: flat condyloma acuminatum. Navicular cell dyskaryosis: koilocytosis.

Papanicolaou (a) ×133 (b) ×525 another case (c) ×525: same case as (b); another field

A case of CIN 2 and a plane wart is demonstrated in (a). The field shows a binucleate koilocyte in the centre, some benign superficial cells and a large number of dyskaryotic inner intermediate, and outer parabasal squamous cells. Compare the degree of maturation with that of the intermediate cells in Fig. 1.22a and the undifferentiated cells in Fig. 1.25a. The nuclei are variable in shape, size and staining reaction.

Cells from another case in which evidence of CIN 2 and wart virus atypia were present in the same focus are seen in (b) and (c). Cytoplasmic maturation is to the level of navicular cells which contain the large perinuclear vacuoles characteristic of koilocytes. The degree of nuclear enlargement and the increase of the chromatin content is, however, greater than occurs with HPV infection and is consistent with dyskaryosis. The intense hyperchromasia and extreme irregularity of the nuclei indicate advanced degeneration. The orangeophilia of the cells in (c) differs from degenerative anomalous eosinophilia and suggests abnormal keratinization. Dyskeratosis occurs in papillomas and in some cases of CIN.

FEMALE REPRODUCTIVE SYSTEM 23

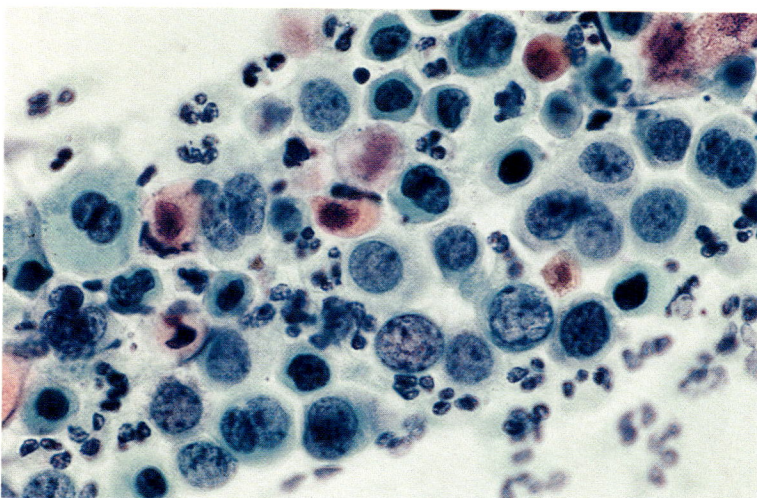

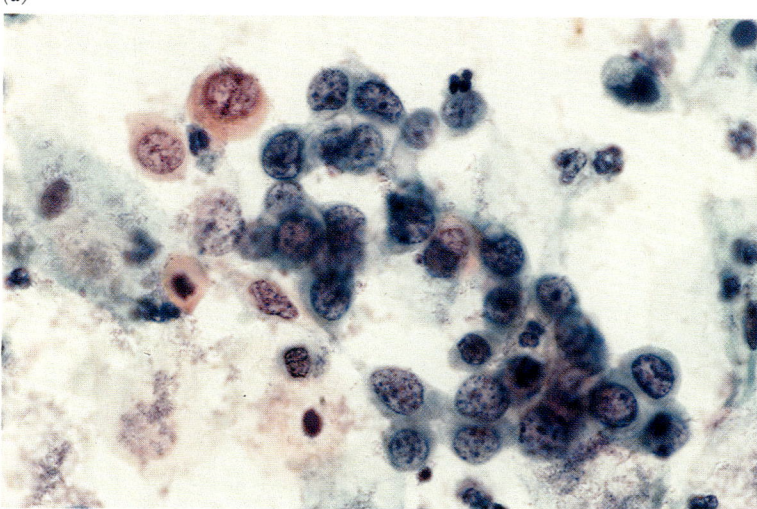

Fig. 1.24 CIN 3: Parabasal squamous cell dyskaryosis
Papanicolaou ×720 (a) discrete cells (b) cohesive cells: another case

Cells from a CIN 3 may be undifferentiated or they may show cytoplasmic features of markedly limited maturation. These micrographs illustrate two examples of the latter type. The dyskaryotic round or oval small cells have the appearance of parabasal squamous cells. This type of cell is often discrete (a) but may occur in aggregates (b). The abnormally large nucleus may be surrounded by a band of dense cytoplasm (a) or it may occupy almost the entire cell (b). Compare these cells with the benign parabasal squamous cells in Figure 1.7(d) and note the increased chromatin content of the neoplastic cells, the condensation of the chromatin into small granules and some coarse clumps, the random distribution of the chromatin and in (b), the clearing of the background nuclear sap.

Degenerative changes are present in both cases, but are more advanced in (a). Several nuclei have undergone pyknotic change and are irregular, structureless and dark (a). Several cells show anomalous eosinophilia (a), (b). In three eosinophilic cells in (b), the nuclei have a diminished chromatin content and appear pale due to a reduced uptake of haematoxylin. Note the occasional pin-point nucleolus in (b).

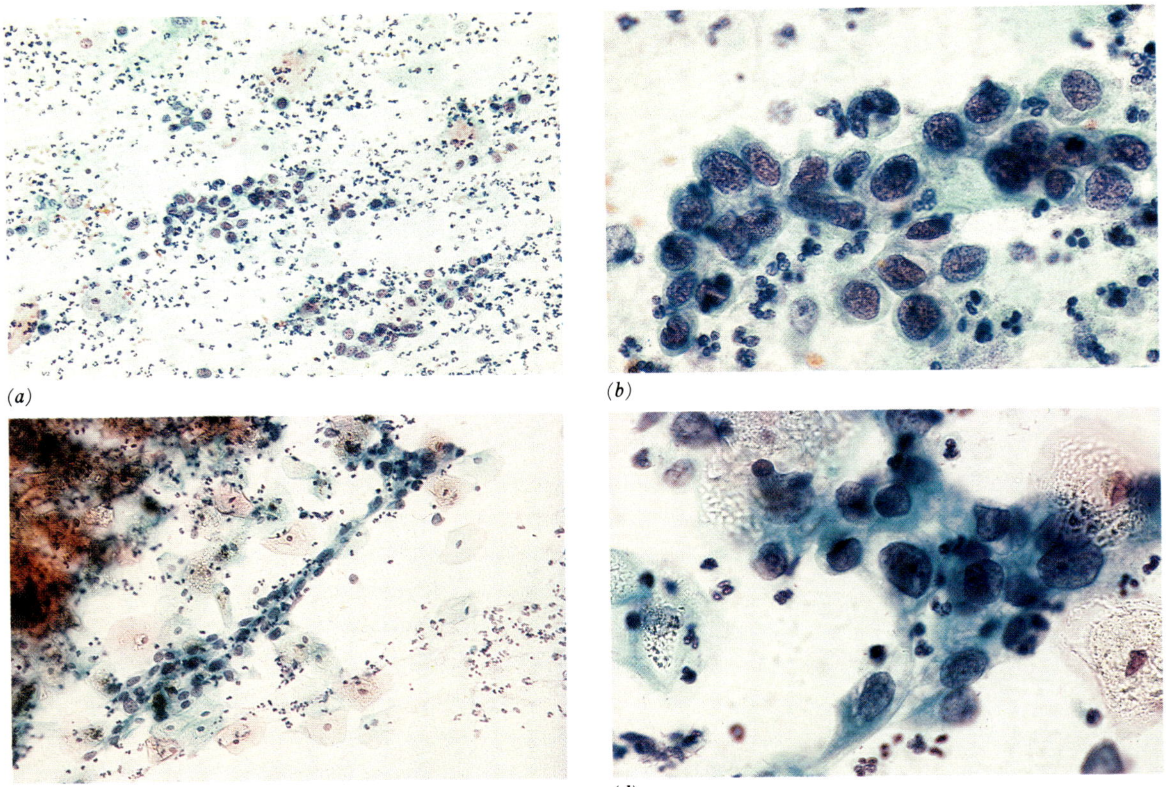

24 DIAGNOSTIC CYTOPATHOLOGY

Fig. 1.25 CIN 3: undifferentiated cell dyskaryosis
Papanicolaou (a) ×133 (b) ×525: same field as (a) (c) ×133: another case (d) ×525: same field as (c)

These micrographs illustrate two cases of CIN 3 composed of undifferentiated cells. At low magnification, the cells in (a) appear to consist of relatively uniform normochromic nuclei. At a higher magnification (b), a small amount of cytoplasm and a slight degree of anisocytosis becomes evident. The cells from the second case contain more cytoplasm (c), and the nuclei are larger, variable and hyperchromic (d). In both cases, the cytoplasm is flimsy and pale, intercellular borders are just discernible here and there, the free edges are ill-defined and the nuclei are haphazardly embedded in an apparent syncytium of cytoplasm. In the absence of a clear cell outline, the nuclear-cytoplasmic ratio cannot be judged; however, the total nuclear mass is excessive for the volume of cytoplasm. Micronucleoli are present in (b).

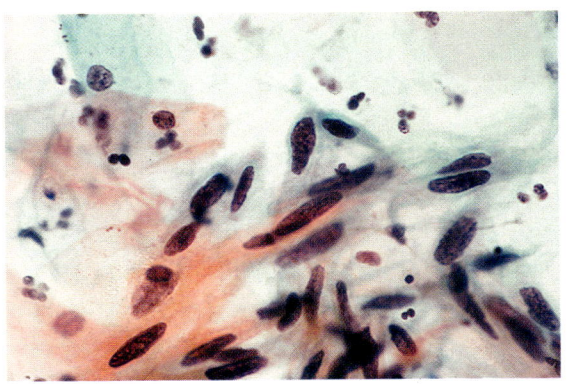

Fig. 1.26 CIN 3 Fibre-shaped and parakeratotic cells
Papanicolaou ×525

The flattening of surface cells that occurs in some cases of CIN 3 is reflected in a smear by the presence of elongated, fibre-shaped cells. The nucleus generally follows the shape of the cell, may be cigar or spindle-shaped and is usually hyperchromic. Occasionally the cytoplasm of the nucleated surface cell is prematurely keratinized (parakeratosis). Fibre cells and abnormally keratinized cells are more common in invasive lesions and the presumptive cytological diagnosis in a case of CIN 3 with parakeratosis is likely to be at variance with the definitive histological diagnosis.

Cervical invasive squamous cell carcinoma

The cellular presentation of an invasive carcinoma is different from that of an intraepithelial lesion in 75–85% of cases. Except for some early cases or cases in which the surface epithelium is intact, smears of an invasive carcinoma carry evidence of tissue necrosis, inflammatory exudate and altered blood (cancer diathesis). The differentiated squamous cells from an invasive lesion rarely resemble their benign counterparts. They are usually larger, abnormal in shape and display a moderate or marked degree of pleomorphism. Poorly-differentiated invasive carcinoma cells are often smaller than cells from a CIN 3 and within the limits of the small size, evince some variation from cluster to cluster. Some poorly-differentiated invasive carcinomas, however, are monomorphic and in the absence of a cancer diathesis, distinction between an invasive and an in situ lesion may not be feasible.

Approximately three out of five squamous cell carcinomas of the cervix are moderately differentiated and are referred to as the large cell non-keratinized type; one fifth are keratinized and one fifth are poorly differentiated. As in CIN, cytological assessment of the grade is based on the type of the predominant cell; it is of limited specificity as the area sampled is not necessarily representative of the entire tumour.

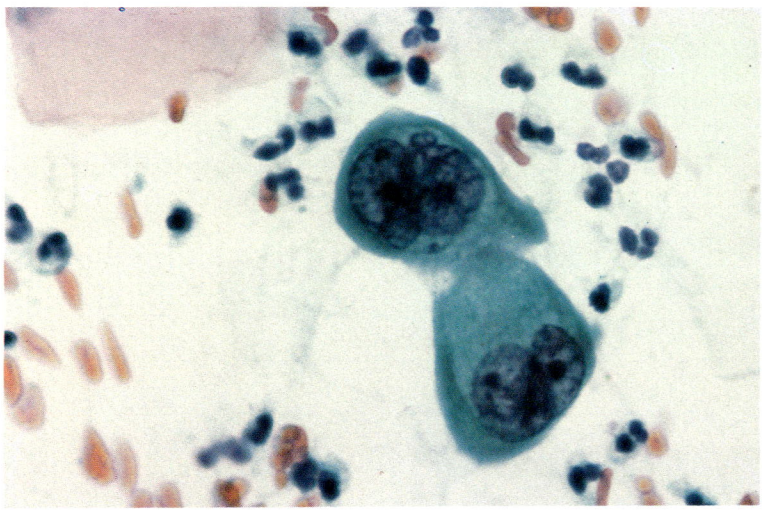

(a)

Fig. 1.27 Moderately differentiated squamous cell carcinoma

Papanicolaou ×720 (a) large non-keratinized cells (b) spindle shaped cells

This type of tumour is composed of large non-keratinized cells, usually with gross nuclei which may be round, crenated or convoluted (a). Moderate to large nucleoli are almost always present. The cytoplasm is cyanophilic and firm, the cell outline clearly defined. Keratinized cells are not seen, but a few poorly-differentiated carcinoma cells with thin cytoplasm and tenuous intercellular borders may be present (b). The elongated spindle-shaped nuclei bear some resemblance to the nuclei of flattened surface cells of CIN 3 (compare with Fig. 1.26).

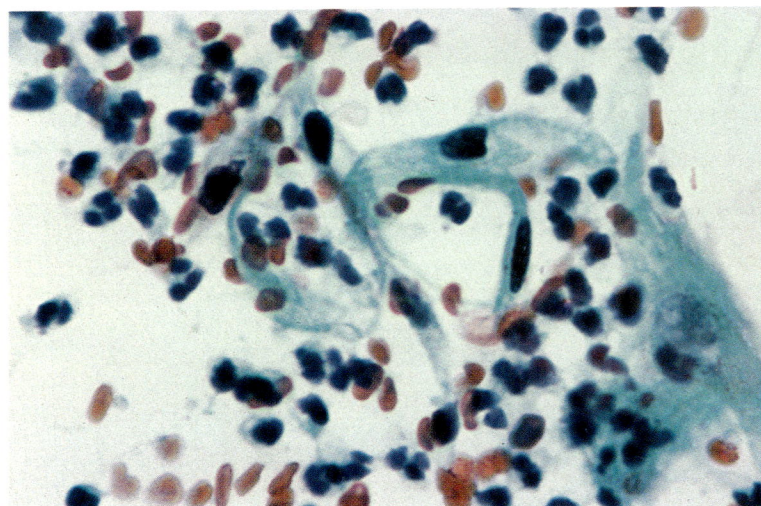

(b)

26 DIAGNOSTIC CYTOPATHOLOGY

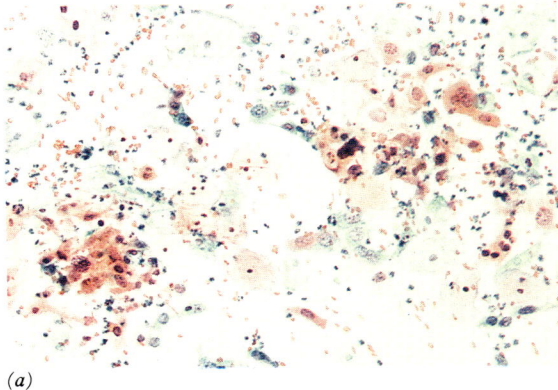

(a)

Fig. 1.28 Well differentiated squamous cell carcinoma

Papanicolaou (a) ×133 (b) ×525: same field as (a) (c) ×525: another field; same case as (a) and (b) (d) ×133: another case (e) ×525: another field; some cases as (d)

A well-differentiated squamous cell carcinoma contains many keratinized cells and has areas of epithelial pearl formation. The pearls form within islands of tumour tissue and are not often met with in a smear. Keratinized cells, on the other hand, are seen in abundance and are conspicuous on account of their orangeophilia (a), (d). The keratin imparts a hard texture to the cell which becomes optically dense and has a sharply demarcated border (b), (c). Round forms occur (b), but abnormality of shape is particularly common in a keratinized carcinoma (b), (c). Cells referred to as caudate or tadpole cells have an expanded or bulbous head and one or more tail like extensions of the cytoplasm (c). The cell may be mononuclear (b), binucleate or multinucleate (b), (c). The nuclei invariably show degenerative changes (b), (c), (d), occasionally, a fully keratinized cell becomes anucleate.

The keratinized cells are usually accompanied by some less-differentiated cells. Moderately mature cyanophilic carcinoma cells, recognizably squamous in type are seen in (b) and (c). The manner of cell attachment in (c) is suggestive of well-developed intercellular bridges and is reminiscent of moderately mature metaplastic squamous cells (see Fig. 1.7c). Note that cytoplasmic tails may be seen in non-keratinized cyanophilic cells.

Differentiated squamous cells are incapable of replication and every squamous cell carcinoma has malignant germinal basaloid cells from which the differentiated cancer cells are derived. Some poorly-differentiated or undifferentiated carcinoma cells may also be recovered in a scrape smear of a keratinizing carcinoma (e). A correct cytological diagnosis would take the abundance of keratinized cells (d) into account. Remnants of necrotic tumour cells and a heavy inflammatory exudate (cancer diathesis) are seen in (d).

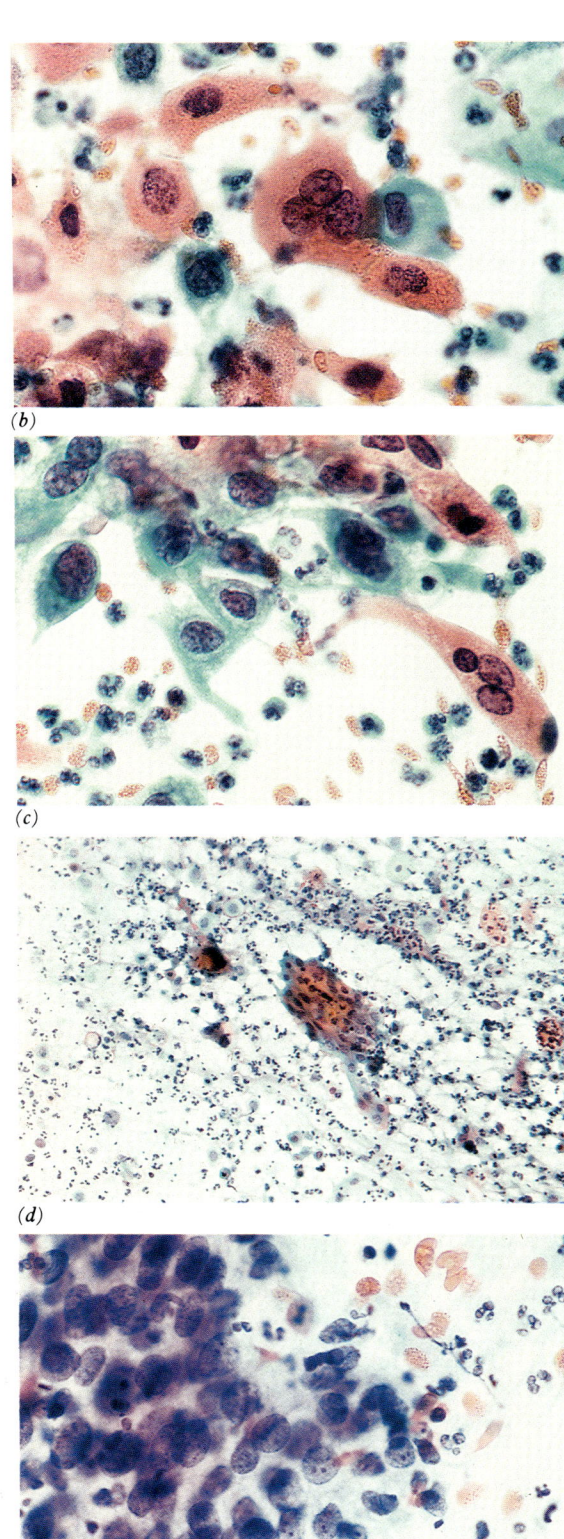

FEMALE REPRODUCTIVE SYSTEM

Fig. 1.29 Poorly-differentiated invasive squamous cell carcinoma

Papanicolaou ×720 (a) fibre-like cells (b) same smear as (a); another field (c) another case

The poorly-differentiated malignant squamous cells in (a) are also elongated and fibre-like and have hyperchromic ovoid nuclei. They are however, smaller and more slender than the cells in Figures 1.26 and 1.27 (b), their nuclei are markedly variable in size and the longest nucleus in the field is seen to fill the entire width of the cell and slightly expand it. This type of feathery cell does not occur in CIN and is diagnostic of an invasive carcinoma. The other cells from the same case are small, oval and cohesive (b). Note again the fineness of the cytoplasm and apparent absence of intercellular borders that characterizes immature squamous cells. A large number of moderately hyperchromic nuclei are crowded into a small amount of cytoplasm. The nuclear chromatin is granular. In another example of a poorly-differentiated squamous cell carcinoma, the nuclei are hypochromic and the chromatin is finely stippled (c). Nucleoli are present in both cases but unlike the nucleoli in moderately differentiated tumours (see Fig. 1.27), these are small and inconspicuous.

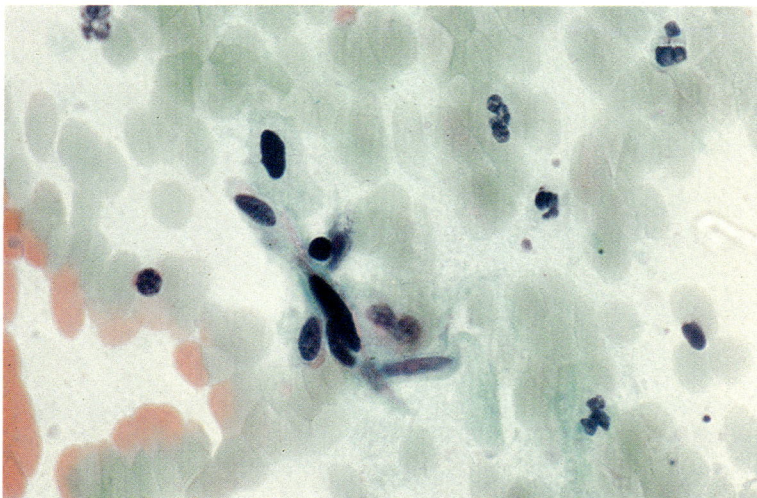
(a)

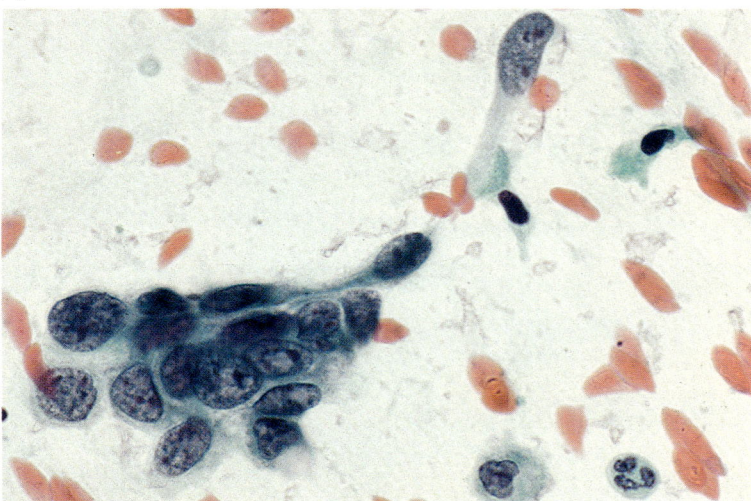
(b)

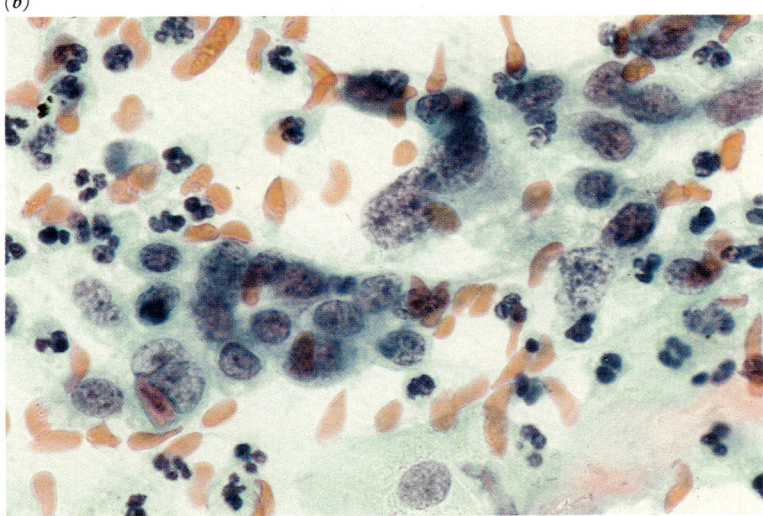
(c)

Problem cases and micro-invasive squamous cell carcinoma

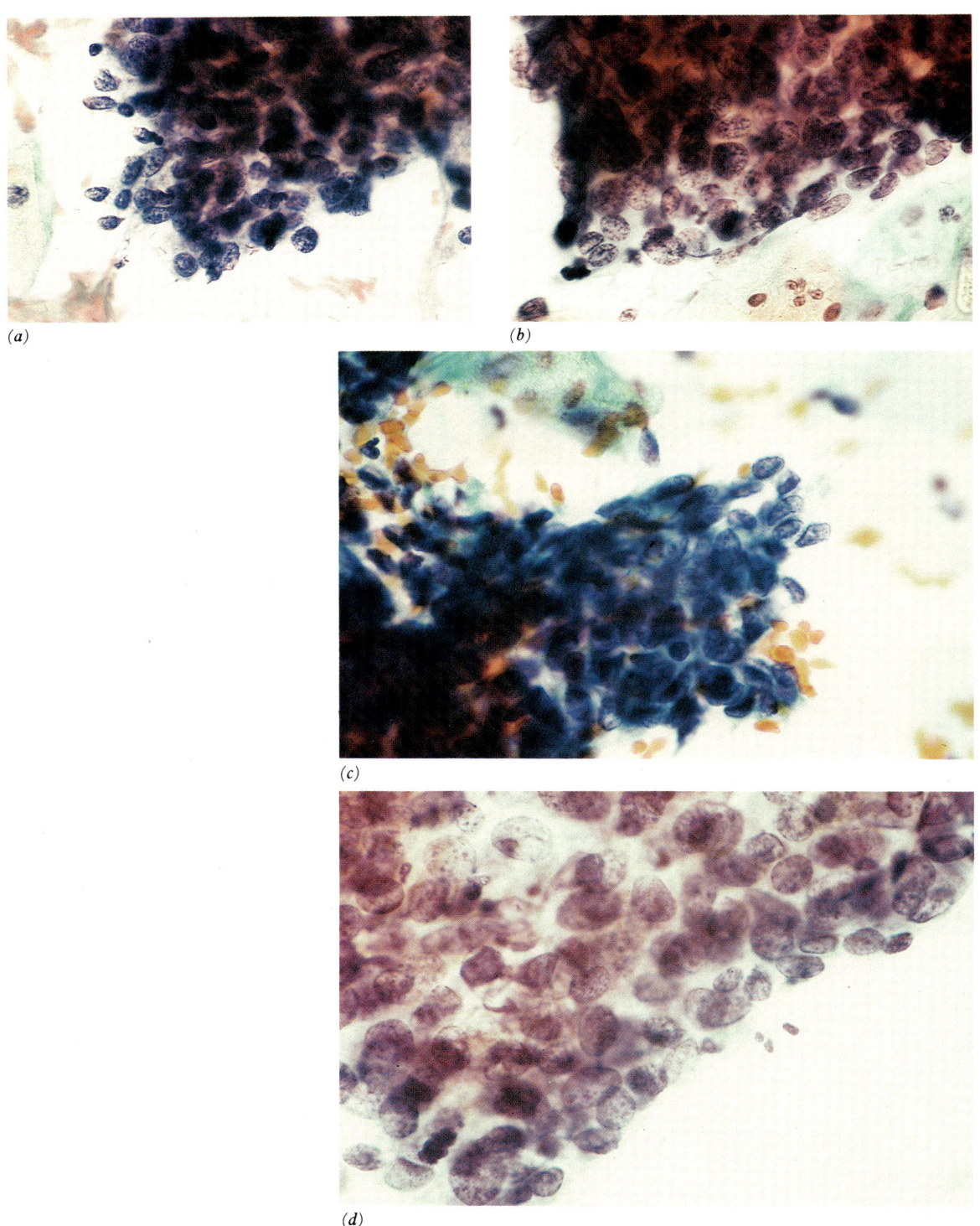

(a)

(b)

(c)

(d)

(e) (f)

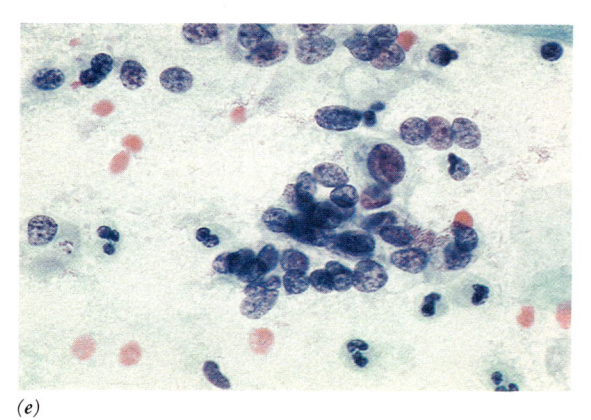

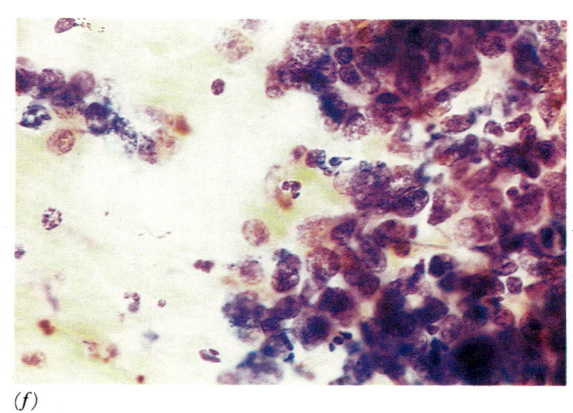

Fig. 1.30 Undifferentiated cells *(illustrations opposite and above)*

Papanicolaou (a) ×525: reserve cell hyperplasia (b) ×525: reserve cell hyperplasia: another case (c) ×720: CIN 3 (d) ×720: CIN 3: another case (e) ×525: poorly-differentiated invasive squamous cell carcinoma (f) ×525: poorly-differentiated invasive adenocarcinoma

Three areas of diagnostic difficulty may be encountered when the lesion sampled is made up of small undifferentiated cells.

In the first instance, discrimination between benign reserve cell hyperplasia and a CIN 3 may prove difficult. The colposcopic biopsy histology diagnoses in the cases illustrated were reserve cell hyperplasia in (a) and (b) and CIN 3 in (c) and (d). The cytological assessment in (a) (b) and (c) was undecided between CIN 3 and immature metaplasia, the CIN 3 in (d) was correctly identified. The cells in all four cases are small, tightly packed and show features of proliferation. The nuclei fill the cells and the chromatin is finely granular. Repeat colposcopy and a careful follow-up over a period of time is advisable in such a situation as the cytohistological discrepancy may be due either to incorrect cytological interpretation or due to the biopsy not being obtained from the correct area.

The second problem that may arise is distinction between CIN 3 (d) and an invasive monomorphic poorly differentiated squamous cell carcinoma (e). In the absence of a cancer diathesis, the cellular presentation may be similar.

The third source of diagnostic uncertainty is a poorly-differentiated adenocarcinoma (f), the cells of which may closely resemble poorly differentiated malignant squamous cells.

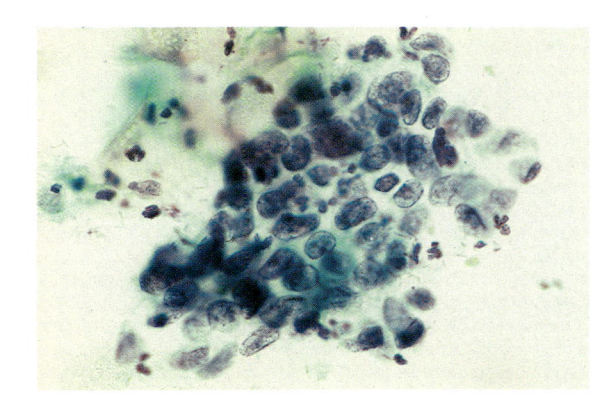

Fig. 1.31 A case of CIN 3 and endocervical carcinoma in situ

Papanicolaou ×525

A CIN 3 may occur in conjunction with an in situ or invasive endocervical carcinoma. In the example illustrated, a cytological diagnosis of CIN 3 was submitted. Colposcopy biopsy confirmed the CIN and revealed an endocervical carcinoma in situ. The neoplastic endocervical cells were tall and cylindrical. The poorly differentiated malignant cells in this micrograph do not contain secretory vacuoles and are arranged in an untidy sheet with ragged edges. The appearance is suggestive of a squamous cell origin.

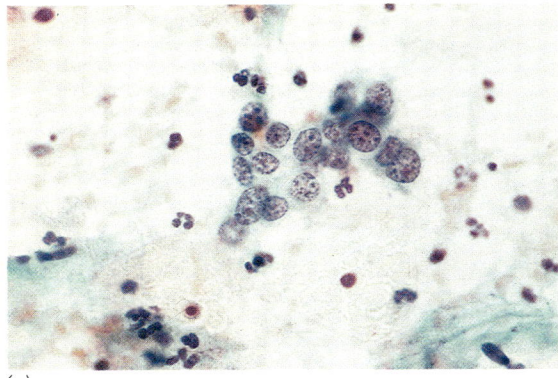

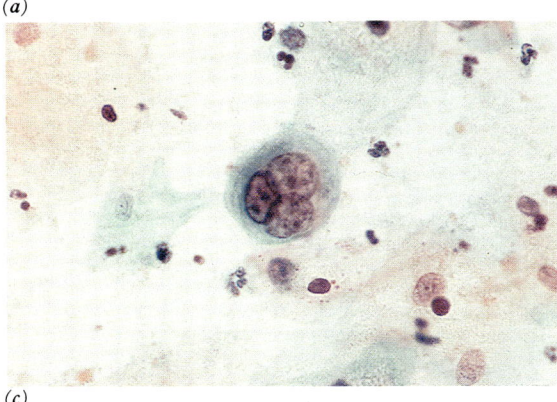

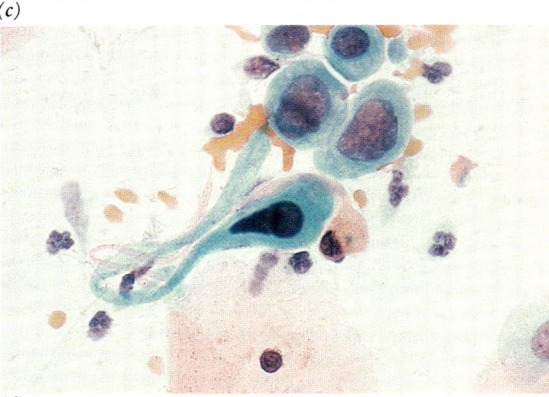

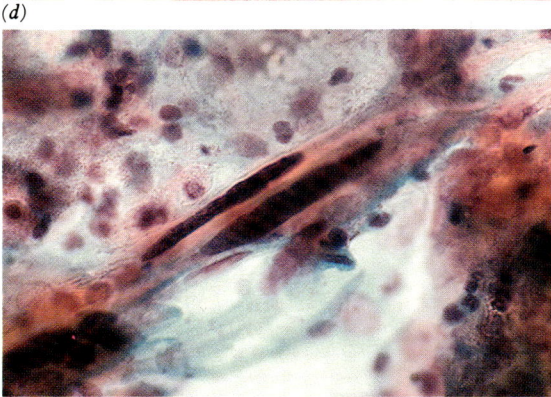

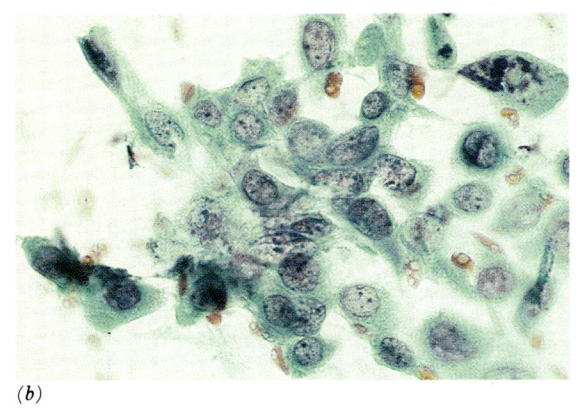

Fig. 1.32 Microinvasive squamous cell carcinoma of the cervix

Papanicolaou ×525 (a) poorly differentiated dyskaryotic squamous cells (b) same case as (a); another field (c) same case as (a), (b); another field (d) another case (e) another case

It is generally agreed that the treatment of microinvasive carcinoma need not be different from that of CIN 3. The precise definition of what constitutes a microinvasive carcinoma as distinct from an invasive carcinoma, continues to be the subject of debate and has been revised more than once. The term is provisionally accepted to describe lesions in which the penetration of the basement membrane by a single or multiple non-confluent tongues of neoplastic cells is no greater than 3 mm deep from the base of the epithelium. A definitive diagnosis of microinvasion requires histological examination of a biopsy of adequate size and depth, and is facilitated by the well established observation that the invading cells are usually better differentiated than the overlying CIN from which they are derived. The cytological presentation may be indistinguishable from CIN 3.

In some cases of microinvasive carcinoma, foci of better differentiated cells, similar to the invading cells, are present within the CIN, some of them close enough to the surface to be recoverable in a smear. The CIN may appear exceptionally pleomorphic or it may contain dyskeratotic cells which are arranged in whorls and form incipient or actual squamous pearls. The neoplastic epithelium acquires an appearance which has been described as restless. The smear pattern may be similar to that seen in an invasive carcinoma.

In about 50% of cases, a different picture is seen, and a cytodiagnosis of probable microinvasive carcinoma is feasible. The overall appearance of the smear is compatible with CIN 3, but a small number of malignant cells inconsistent with a typical intraepithelial lesion are present in addition. Variants of the suggestive picture are illustrated by three cases in which a cytological diagnosis of a probable microcarcinoma was confirmed by cone biopsy histology. None of the smears showed a cancer diathesis. All contained poorly-differentiated dyskaryotic squamous cells: these are shown from one case in (a). The other cells in this case are large pleomorphic cohesive cells (b) or of the large non-keratinized type (c) more commonly seen in a moderately differentiated invasive squamous carcinoma. In the second case shown, the CIN 3 cells were accompanied by a few better differentiated malignant squamous cells and an occasional bizarre caudate cell (d). In the third case, the cells that do not fit a CIN 3 are large and keratinized and contain grossly abnormal spindle shaped nuclei (e).

Squamous cell carcinoma of the vagina

Squamous cell carcinoma of the vagina is rare and extension from a cervical or a vulval carcinoma is more common than a primary tumour. The vaginal epithelium may be the site of intraepithelial neoplasia. Vaginal intraepithelial neoplasia (VAIN) usually occurs in association with CIN, but not necessarily at the same time. It is graded in the same manner as CIN and may, on occasion, progress to invasive disease. The incidence of VAIN is lower than that of CIN.

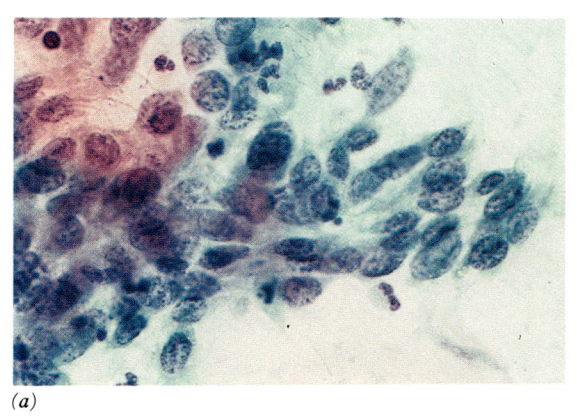

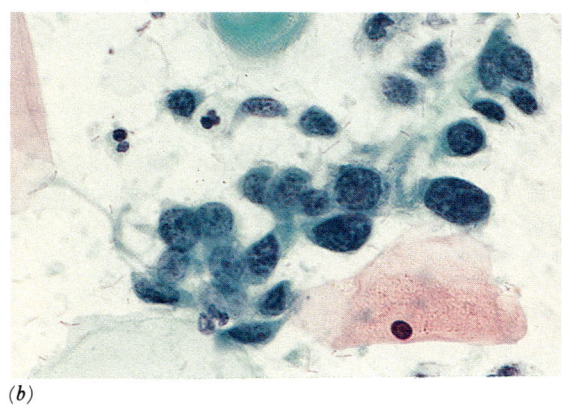

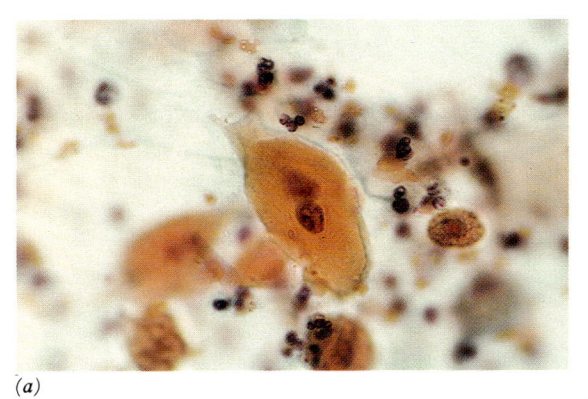

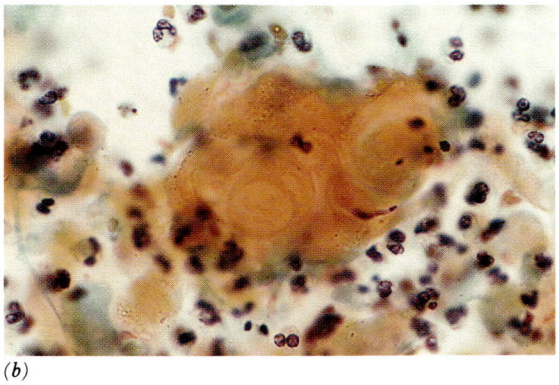

Fig. 1.33 Poorly differentiated squamous cell carcinoma
Papanicolaou ×525 (a) vaginal smear (b) same smear; another field

In the case illustrated in these micrographs, a smear of the vaginal vault showed dyskaryotic parabasal squamous cells 12 months after a simple hysterectomy with an adequate vaginal cuff had been carried out for CIN 3; intervening smears had been normal. A focus of VAIN was identified and extirpated. Multiple foci of intraepithelial neoplasia appeared subsequently and a partial vaginectomy was performed. Six years after the hysterectomy, a cytological diagnosis of poorly-differentiated invasive squamous cell carcinoma (a), (b) of the vagina was confirmed. The tumour had penetrated the bladder wall and identical cells were recovered from a specimen of urine (see Fig. 8.11a).

Fig. 1.34 Well differentiated squamous cell carcinoma
Papanicolaou × 525: (a) vaginal smear (b) same smear; another field

A case of primary squamous cell carcinoma of the vagina in which the smear pattern is typical of a highly-differentiated tumour is illustrated. The cells in (a) show features met with in some keratinized malignant cells. The cytoplasm has a bright glistening appearance and is refractile under the microscope; the refractility is enhanced by lowering the condenser. In (b) several adherent cells arranged in a circular manner are fully keratinized, have lost their nuclei and merged together to form a malignant epithelial pearl.

Adenocarcinoma

Adenocarcinoma of the endocervix accounts for 10% of cervical carcinomas and is not frequently encountered in routine gynaecological cytology. The endocervix may be the site of an in situ carcinoma, this is presumed to be a precursor of an invasive lesion. A significant increase in the incidence of a rare variant—clear cell carcinoma—was noted some years ago in young girls and was traced to the effect of diethylstilboestrol (DES) administered to the patient's mother in the early weeks of pregnancy. Pre-natal exposure to DES is also associated with a high incidence of adenosis and clear cell carcinoma of the vagina.

The greater majority, by far, of adenocarcinomas seen in routine exfoliative cytology are of endometrial origin. These tumours are most frequent in the post-menopausal years and abnormal bleeding is a common and relatively early symptom. Malignant endometrial cells are more likely to be recovered from a posterior vaginal fornix pool smear if the bleeding is heavy or recent; when this is not the case, the cells may be arrested in the cervical mucus and are equally likely to be present in a cervical smear in which they appear better preserved. Exfoliation of tumour cells may not occur, or it may be sparse. The cells may undergo necrotic change in vivo or after they have been shed and may not be easily identifiable. The sensitivity of diagnosis of endometrial carcinoma is consequently considerably lower than of cervical tumours which are generally scraped under vision. Direct sampling of the endometrial cavity by jet wash or aspiration has been advocated for cases of post-menopausal bleeding and for screening women receiving hormone replacement therapy. The techniques are not always acceptable to a woman with an atrophic genital tract and this has limited their application.

Adenocarcinoma of the Fallopian tube is extremely rare. Tumour cells may find their way into the vagina or cervical canal; whilst their malignant character is usually obvious, the site of origin cannot be determined from the cellular appearance.

Malignant cells from an ovarian carcinoma are occasionally seen in a vaginal or cervical smear. These are generally from a disseminated cancer, but on rare occasions, cells from a carcinoma limited to the ovary may pass down the oviducts and uterus and appear in an otherwise normal smear.

Except in the case of the Fallopian tube, it is often possible to suggest the likely source of the adenocarcinoma cells from the smear pattern and so direct attention to the site requiring further investigation. There is however, a considerable overlap of histological variants seen in the different parts of the genital tract. Endometrioid type cells are characteristic of a corpus carcinoma, but may form tumours in the endocervix and ovary. Mucous tumours, common in the endocervix and ovary, may develop in the endometrium. For this reason, clinical considerations are of particular importance in the diagnosis and localization of a genital tract adenocarcinoma.

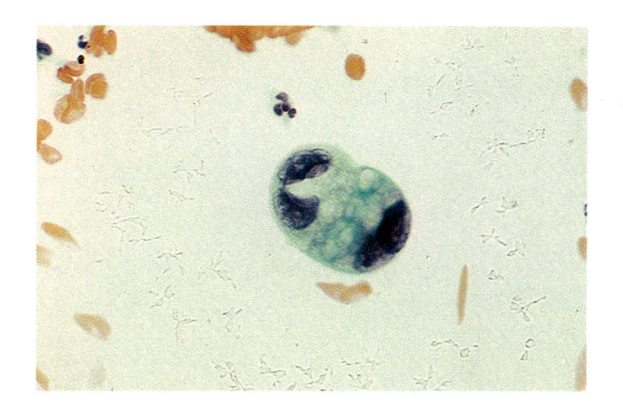

Fig. 1.35 Endocervical adenocarcinoma
Papanicolaou ×525

The salient diagnostic features of an adenocarcinoma are illustrated by a case of endocervical adenocarcinoma. The two large carcinoma cells are closely adherent. The periphery is notched on the upper surface at the point of junction of the two cells, the lower border is continuous, rounded and smooth. The cytoplasm contains abundant variable sized secretory vacuoles. The nuclei are pushed to the periphery and their outer borders coincide with the outer limit of the cells. The lower left nucleus has a cup-shaped depression characteristically seen in mucous-secreting cells. The nuclear-cytoplasmic ratio of a secretory cell, whether benign or malignant, varies inversely with the degree of distension of the cytoplasm and is fairly low in these cells. The degree of nuclear hyperchromasia is accentuated by the compression of the nuclei.

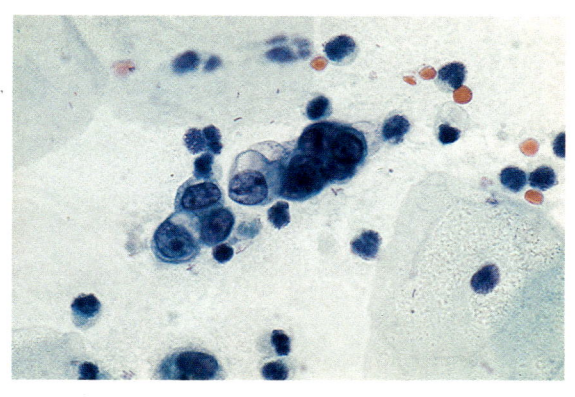

Fig. 1.36 Endometrial adenocarcinoma
Papanicolaou ×525

Compare the size of the tumour cells from this case of a well-differentiated endometrial carcinoma with neutrophils and with the malignant endocervical cells in the preceding micrograph, and note their smaller size. The arrangement is essentially similar to that in Figure 1.35. There are, however, many more cells in the endometrial cluster and the drawing in of the outer border at the several points of cell junction has produced a scalloped outline, often seen in a typical group of adenocarcinoma cells. The degree of cytoplasmic distension is variable and is reflected in the variation in the nuclear-cytoplasmic ratio. Small but distinct nucleoli are present.

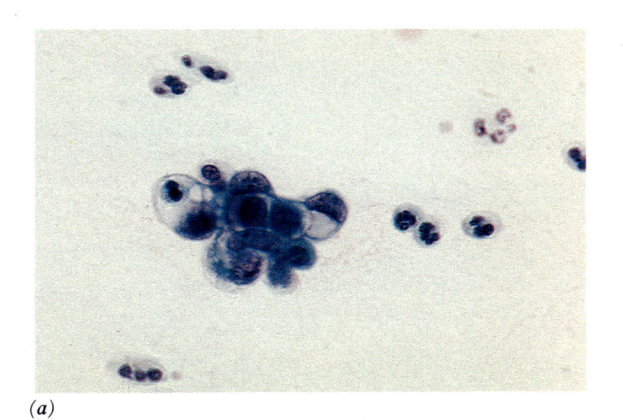

(a)

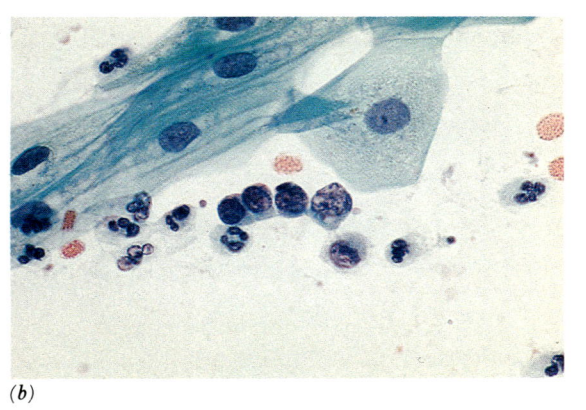

(b)

Fig. 1.37 Endometrial adenocarcinoma
Papanicolaou × 525: (a) secretory cells (b) same smear; another field

A closely similar malignant cluster with a scalloped border is seen in (a). Note again that several nuclei are displaced by secretory vacuoles to the edge of the cluster. Nucleoli are absent or insignificant. A neutrophil is seen within one cell. Foci of leucocytic infiltration are common in endometrial carcinomas. A tumour cell packed with and obscured by numerous neutrophils should not be included in a diagnostic assessment as benign inflammatory disease may show a similar appearance.

A different pattern of exfoliation is seen in (b). Five tumour cells with a high nuclear-cytoplasmic ratio and granular chromatin are streaked across the centre. In size, they appear slightly larger than neutrophils. The partially detached cell at lower right has an eccentric kidney-shaped nucleus and resembles a small histiocyte. Cells from a benign endometrial hyperplasia with cellular atypia have a similar appearance and pattern of exfoliation and in the absence of a typical adenocarcinoma cluster, distinction between malignancy and benign hyperplasia is often difficult.

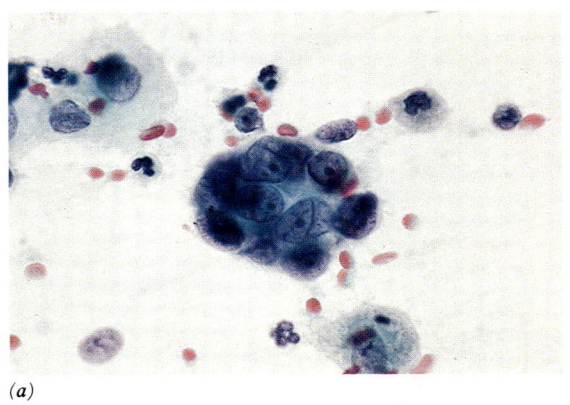

34 DIAGNOSTIC CYTOPATHOLOGY

(a) 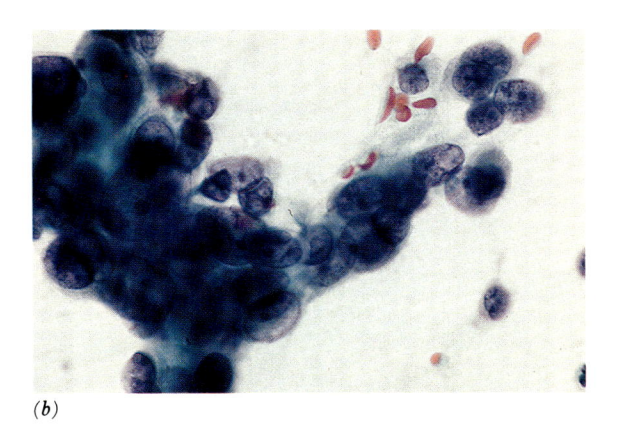 (b)

Fig. 1.38 Endometrial adenocarcinoma

Papanicolaou ×525 (a) secretory cells (b) same smear; another field

A less well differentiated endometrial carcinoma is illustrated in these micrographs. The rosette-shaped arrangement of the cells in (a) is indicative of a glandular tumour. The individual cells are larger than in the two preceding examples of endometrial carcinoma, the nuclei are more variable in size and display a moderate degree of polychromasia. The nuclear cytoplasmic ratio is very high and nucleoli, although not as large as in a non-keratinized invasive squamous cell carcinoma, are prominent.

In the other group (b), the cells are arranged in a sheet and the three dimensional appearance of a round cluster is absent. Cytoplasmic vacuolisation is not evident. The smooth outlines of several nuclei and their eccentric location on the edge of the sheet is suggestive of an adenocarcinoma.

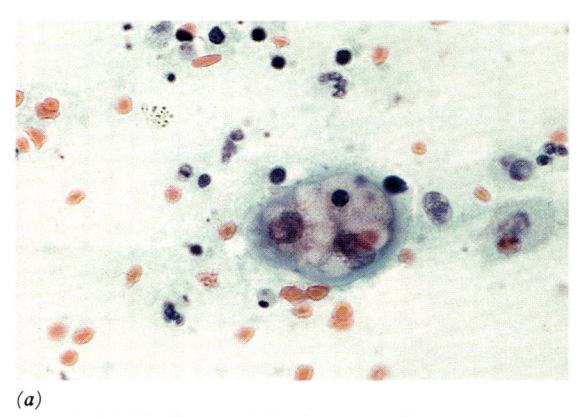

(a) 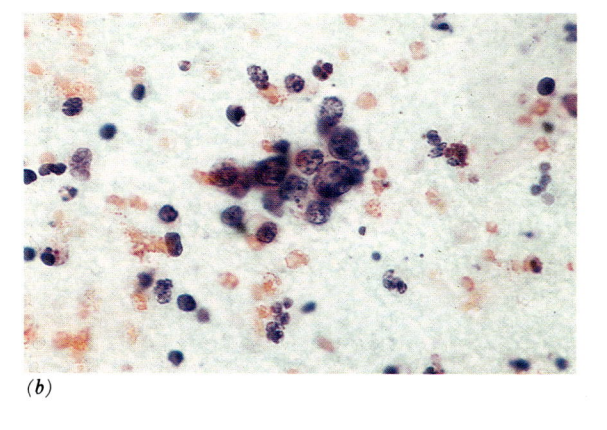 (b)

Fig. 1.39 Endometrial adenocarcinoma

Papanicolaou ×525 (a) large secretory cells (b) small cells: same smear; another field

The cells in (a) are typical of an adenocarcinoma. In size and in abundance of mucous vacuoles, they resemble the malignant endocervical cells in Figure 1.35.

The clump of tightly packed, degenerate endometrial cells with hyperchromic granular nuclei seen against a background of neutrophils, erythrocytes and breakdown products of blood (b) is not dissimilar to cells seen in a menstrual smear. Exfoliation of identifiable endometrial cells in association with adenocarcinoma cells is suggestive of involvement of the endometrium in the disease process. Assumption of a primary endometrial carcinoma would be reasonable, although secondary deposits which have destabilized the endometrium cannot be ruled out.

In the absence of typical tumour cells (a) a diagnosis of malignancy, based on the cells in (b) is less certain even in a case of post-menopausal bleeding. In a case of dysfunctional bleeding, it would be hazardous.

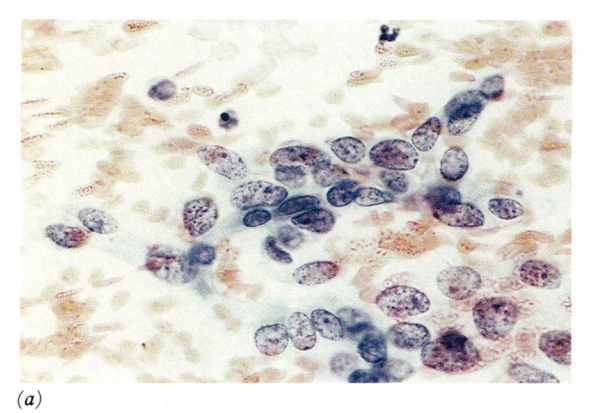

Fig. 1.40 Endocervical adenocarcinoma

Papanicolaou (a) ×525 (b) ×133: same smear; another field

Compare the cells in (a) with Figures 1.24(b) and 1.28(e) and note the similarity in disposition and arrangement of these cells with poorly differentiated squamous cells. The significantly helpful artefact of a smooth cluster with a round or scalloped border and depth of focus is most evident in spontaneously desquamated cells which travel through or lie in a fluid or semi-fluid medium. It is often absent from a scrape smear of an endocervical carcinoma and contributes in part to the difficulty encountered in distinguishing between flat malignant glandular cells and poorly-differentiated malignant squamous cells.

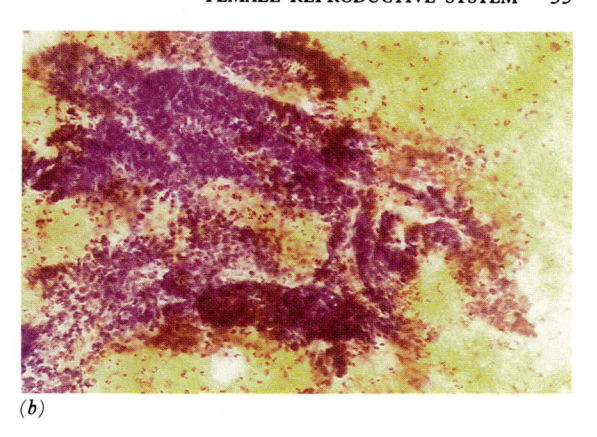

The correct diagnosis in this case is suggested by the architecture of the tumour tissue, better appreciated at a low magnification (b). In the upper left part of the field, the cells form a solid mass, towards the lower right, they open out to line branching cavities and the appearance is reminiscent of endocervical crypts. An endometrial carcinoma may yield a similar picture in a specimen obtained directly from the uterine cavity.

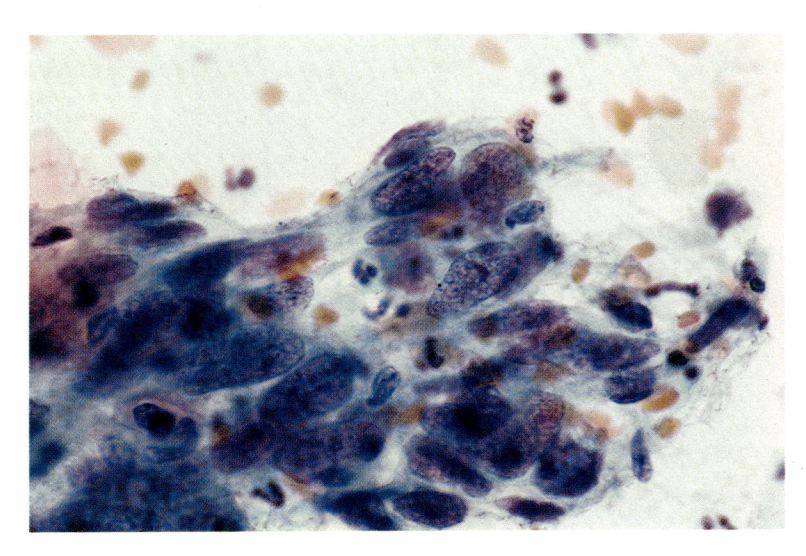

Fig. 1.41 Endocervical adenocarcinoma

Papanicolaou ×720

This micrograph illustrates malignant cells from an extremely poorly-differentiated adenocarcinoma of the cervix. The cells are anaplastic and any suggestion of acinar formation is absent. The ovoid nuclei bear some resemblance to the nuclei of some soft tissue tumours. Intercellular borders are absent and the nuclear chromatin pattern is disorganized. The very occasional mucous vacuole demonstrated in the biopsy specimen was not appreciated in the smaller amount of tissue in the smear.

36 DIAGNOSTIC CYTOPATHOLOGY

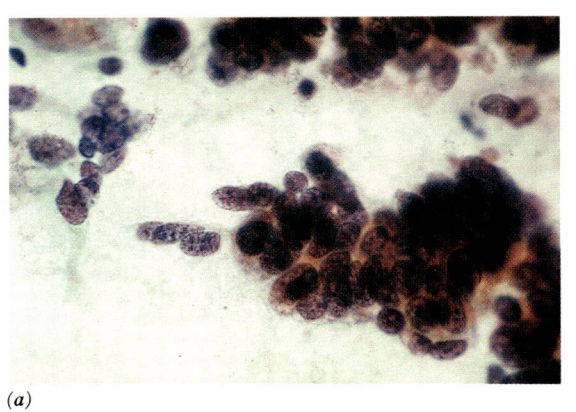

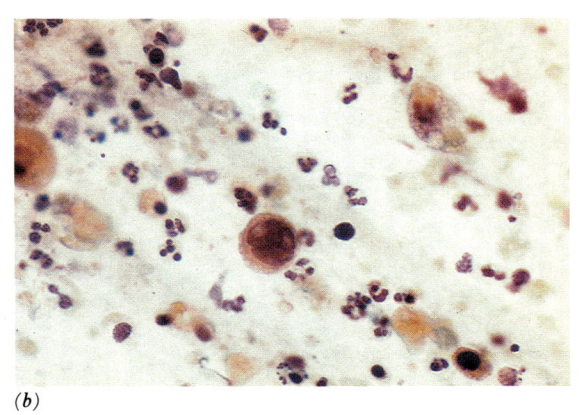

(a) (b)

Fig. 1.42 Endocervical adenocarcinoma: cancer diathesis

Papanicolaou ×525 (a) well preserved carcinoma cells (b) tumour necrosis: same smear; another field

Foci of necrosis, leucocytic infiltration and bleeding are common in cancers and provide the cytopathologist with important ancillary evidence of the invasive nature of the lesion. In addition to frank carcinoma cells (a), the smear contains proteinous debris, many leucocytes and degenerated or fragmented necrotic tumour cells (b). The appearance is referred to as a 'cancer diathesis'. Intact red blood cells indicative of fresh blood, possibly drawn by the instrument used to obtain the specimen, are of no significance; altered blood and fibrin from an episode of past bleeding, are useful adjuncts.

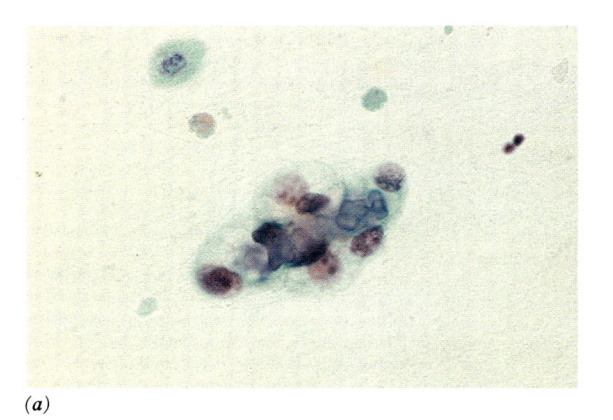

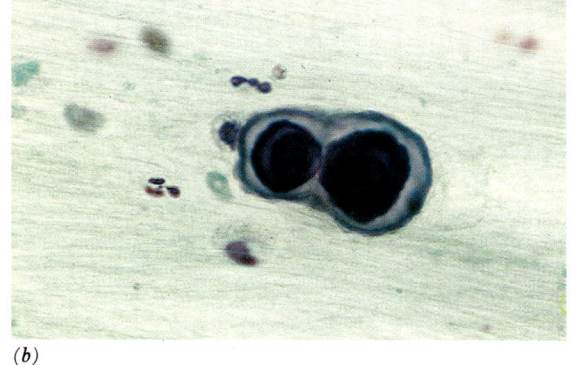

(a) (b)

Fig. 1.43 Ovarian carcinoma

Papanicolaou ×525 (a) adenocarcinoma cells (b) psammoma bodies

A cluster of adenocarcinoma cells is seen in (a) and psammoma bodies in (b). A psammoma body or a calcospherite is an organised structure, somewhat variable in appearance, but usually consists of a central area of density surrounded by dark, often wavy, concentric rings separated by pale zones. It is formed when minerals, chiefly calcium, are deposited in a focus of necrotic cells, and occurs commonly in papillary tumours. In the genital tract, they may occur in a papillary endometrial carcinoma, this type of tumour is, however, relatively uncommon. The ovary, on the other hand, is the most frequent site of a papillary carcinoma and the commonest source of psammoma bodies. A cytological diagnosis of a probable primary ovarian carcinoma was proved correct in this case.

FEMALE REPRODUCTIVE SYSTEM 37

Fig. 1.44 Ovarian carcinoma

Papanicolaou (a) ×720: vaginal smear; psammoma bodies (b) ×720: vaginal smear; papillary tumour cells

A vaginal vault smear, shown in these micrographs, carries evidence of a recurrence of a serous cystadenocarcinoma of the ovary, treated 10 years earlier. Psammoma bodies are seen in (a). The tumour cells in (b) are ringed round pale fibrous tissue. A papillary tumour forms fronds which consist of a central fibrovascular core with an external lining of neoplastic cells. In a smear, the tips of the fronds may be seen and are identified by the presence of the fibrous core. Psammoma bodies are often abundant in serous papillary tumours of the ovary; these may be benign or malignant.

(a)

(b)

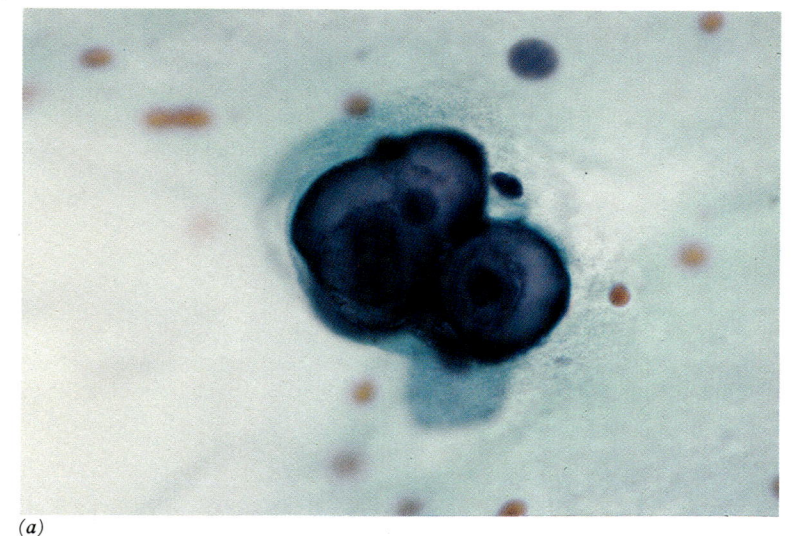

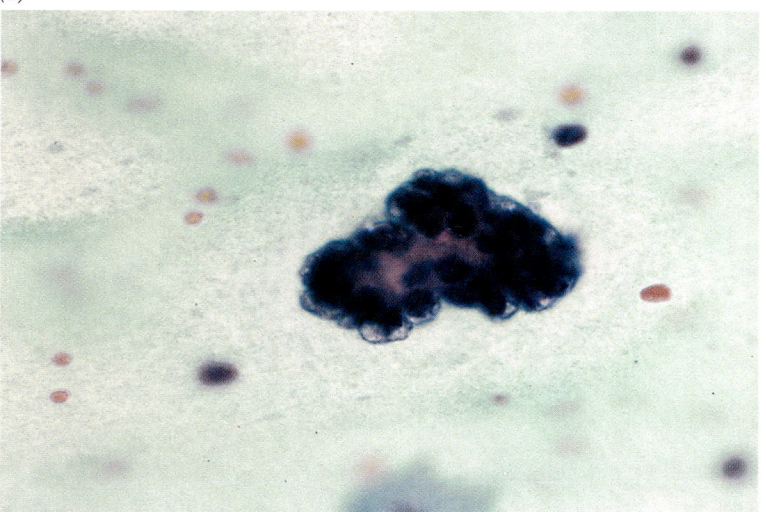

Fig. 1.45 Colon carcinoma metastatic to vagina

Papanicolaou ×720

This vaginal smear shows typical mucus-secreting adenocarcinoma cells and was obtained from a patient with a past history of a primary carcinoma of the colon, the genital tract being normal. Biopsy histology of the tumour deposit in the vagina was identical with the histology of the colon carcinoma.

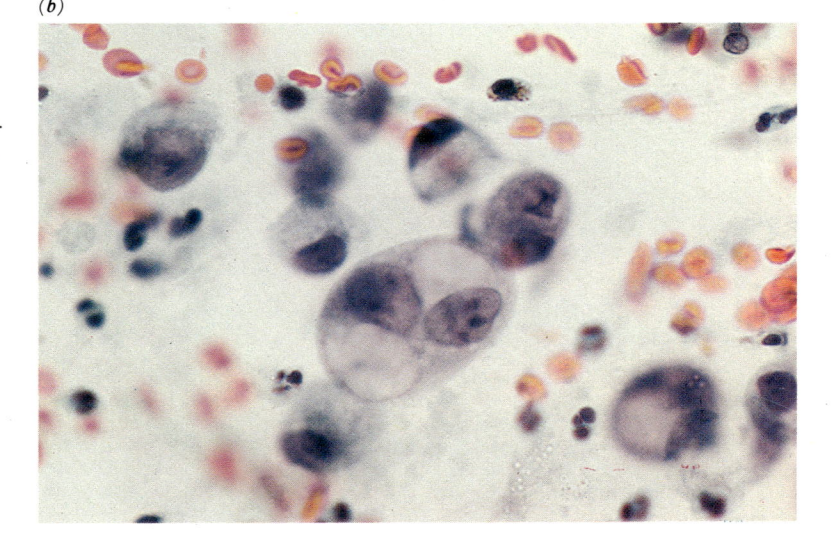

OVARY: FINE NEEDLE ASPIRATION

The ovary is the site of numerous lesions, inflammatory, tumour-like, neoplastic and others. The histological classification is extremely complex and refinement of precise definition is seldom possible in a cytological preparation. Within these limits, ovarian cytology has a useful role. The lesions that can be identified in a reasonable proportion of cases are pathophysiological functional cysts and some benign and malignant tumours, many of which are cystic.

Functional cysts

A functional cyst may develop at any stage in the maturation of a Graafian follicle (see p. 3) and is often a chance finding in the course of a laparoscopy or a laparotomy. It does not require surgical resection and as fine needle aspiration is without hazard, cytological confirmation of a clinical impression is of value.

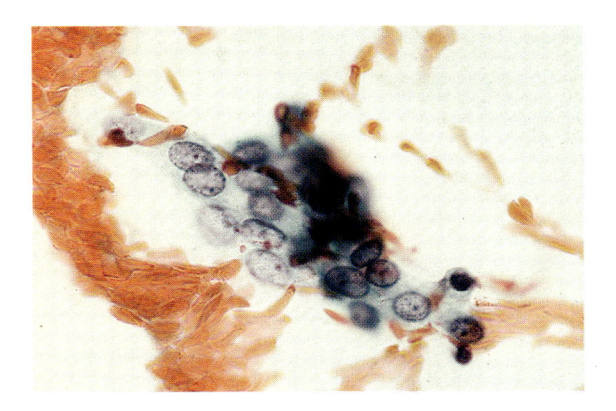

Fig. 1.46 Follicular cyst
Papanicolaou ×525

A follicular cyst occurs in the pre-menopausal years, may be single or multiple and varies in size from the microscopic to 10 cm or so in diameter; the average is 2–3 cm, and its size may be assessed in the laboratory by the volume of fluid aspirated. It develops in a follicle which, having reached a partial stage of maturation, undergoes regression and atresia. The cyst fluid is generally clear and colourless and contains a small number of follicle or granulosa cells from the lining. The cells are small with scanty cytoplasm and a high nuclear cytoplasmic ratio. The nuclei which appear hyperchromic in sections may be somewhat depleted of chromatin and hypochromic in free floating cells obtained from the cyst fluid.

(a)

(b)

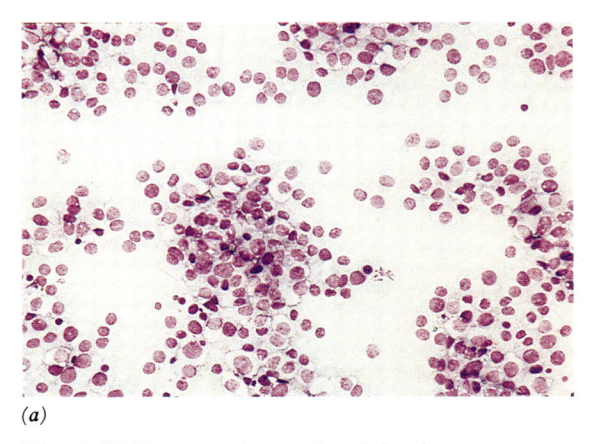

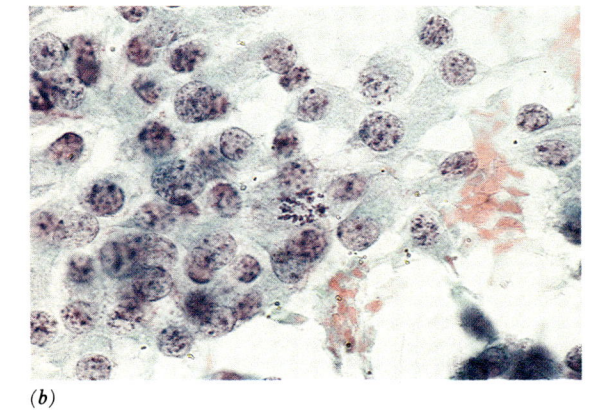

Fig. 1.47 Post-ovulatory luteinized cyst
(a) MGG ×133 (b) Papanicolaou ×525: another case

The cells surrounding an ovum in a maturing follicle multiply and become multi-layered; mitoses are frequently seen at this stage. After discharge of the ovum, they enlarge under the influence of LH and their cytoplasm is filled with a yellow pigment, hence they are referred to as granulosa lutein cells. Fluid from a cyst which develops at this stage is yellow in colour, occasionally blood-stained and contains numerous cells (a). Morphological detail of granulosa lutein cells is seen in (b). The cytoplasm is moderately abundant, the nuclei are monomorphic and the nuclear chromatin is granular and regularly distributed. A mitotic figure is seen in the centre of the field. On occasion, several mitotic figures are seen and this coupled with high cellular content may create a false impression of a benign neoplasm.

Fig. 1.48 Corpus luteum cyst
Papanicolaou ×720

As luteinization progresses, the granulosa lutein cells acquire more cytoplasm and the nuclear cytoplasmic ratio is reduced. The intracytoplasmic yellow pigment contains lipid which is dissolved by alcohol fixation and the cytoplasm appears thin and vacuolated. The nuclei are generally homogenous and hypochromic. The cyst fluid is yellow and the cell content moderate or low.

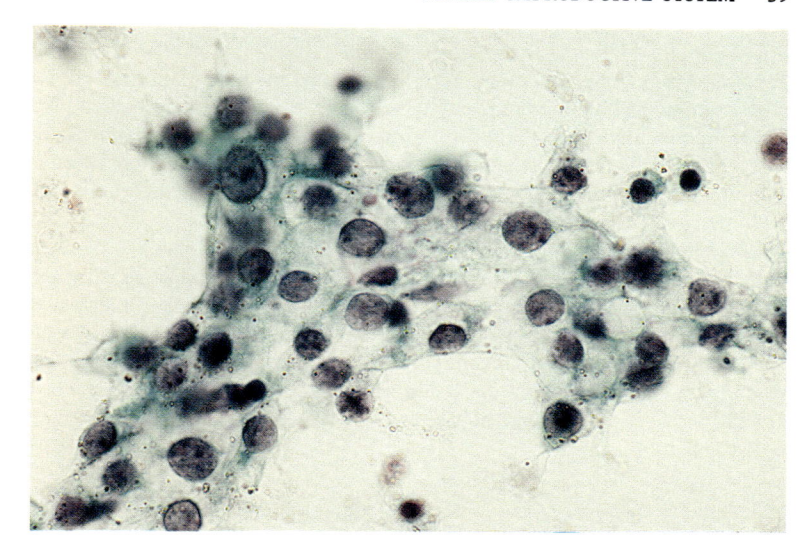

Fig. 1.49 Germinal inclusion cyst
Papanicolaou ×183

The external covering of the ovary is of mesothelial origin. It is referred to as germinal epithelium and consists of a single layer of cuboidal cells. These cells may invaginate the ovarian cortex, become separated from the external germinal layer, and form the lining of an inclusion cyst. The condition occurs most commonly in the perimenopausal years. The fluid is usually clear and colourless or straw coloured. The mesothelial cells are degenerate and appear as large foamy histiocytic cells. The appearance is similar to that of long standing cysts in other organs such as the breast or the kidney (see Figs. 2.7 and 8.17).

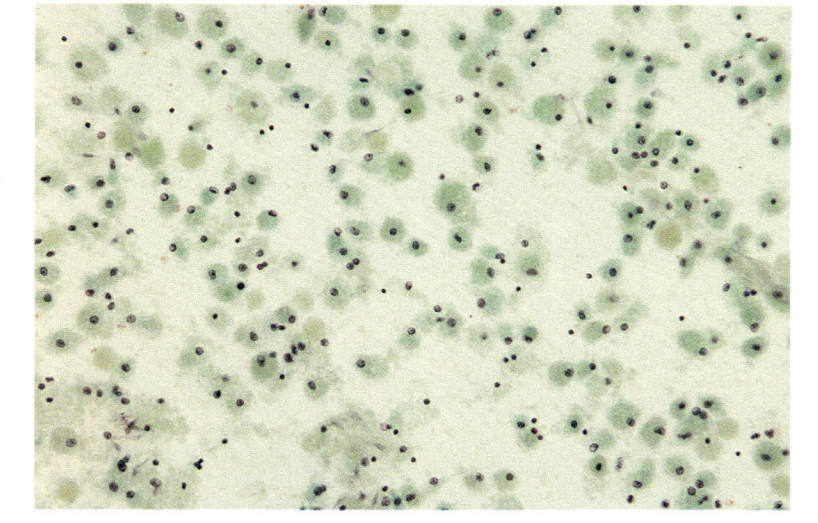

Fig. 1.50 Chocolate cyst
MGG ×183

This term is applied to cystic degeneration in an area of endometriosis in the ovary. The fluid is chocolate-coloured, and contains altered blood, a few leucocytes and many iron-laden macrophages. A few cuboidal epithelial cells may persist. The appearance of the cells is compatible with that of endometrial cells, but cannot be distinguished from endometrioid cells that occur in the ovary and from which tumours may develop. Degenerate follicle cells may be similar in size and a diagnosis of a chocolate cyst is essentially a clinical or/and a histological one.

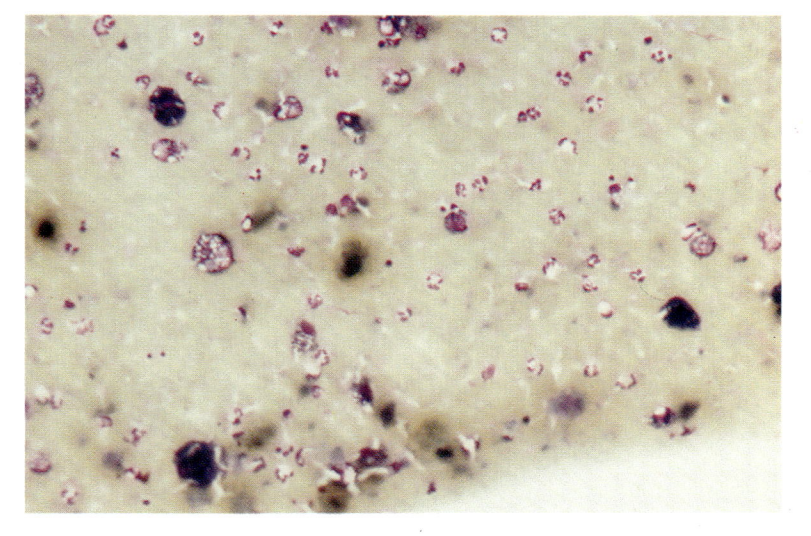

Neoplastic cysts

Epithelial tumours of the ovary, both benign and malignant are derived from cells of the germinal epithelium, either on the surface or in sequestrated foci included within the stroma. The epithelium, which is of Mullerian origin, retains the capacity for differentiation along the various pathways taken by the glandular mucous linings of the genital tract. Differentiation to tubal type epithelium is the most common and is seen in the serous group of tumours; endocervical type or occasionally intestinal type epithelium is found in the mucinous tumours; endometrioid cell tumours are relatively rare.

Fine needle aspiration of a suspected ovarian carcinoma needs to be undertaken with care, and spillage avoided as these tumours are believed quickly to form peritoneal seedlings. The aspiration is carried out under direct vision, usually during a laparotomy, but may be repeated through a laparoscope as part of an assessment procedure. Collection of peritoneal washings for cytological examination has been recommended as an essential part of the staging of ovarian carcinoma and to provide a basis for therapy and future management. The washings first performed during open operation may also be repeated at subsequent laparoscopy.

The cyst fluid and peritoneal washings are processed for cytological examination in the same manner as a serous effusion (Ch. 4).

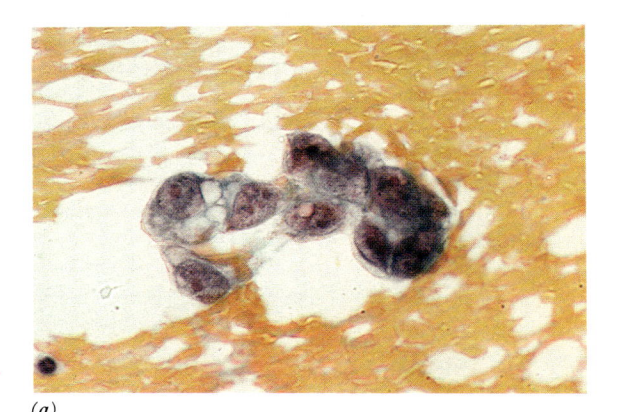

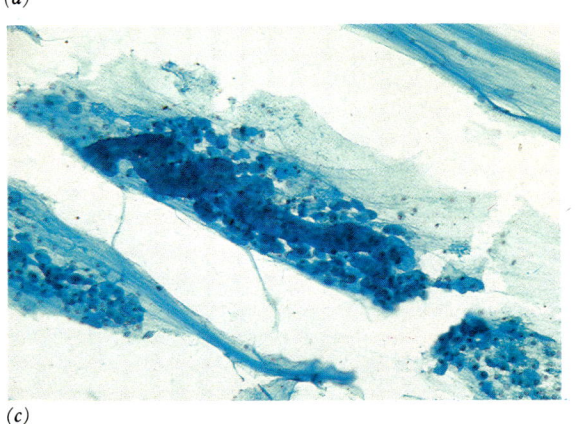

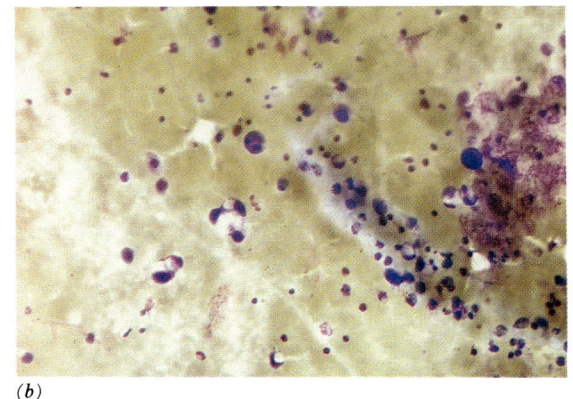

Fig. 1.51 Mucinous cystadenocarcinoma

(a) Papanicolaou ×525 (b) MGG ×133: same case; another smear (c) Alcian blue ×133: same case; another smear

Intracellular mucin vacuoles are evident in the cells in (a) which show stigmata of malignancy such as a variable chromatin pattern, anisonucleosis and disproportionately large nuclei. Note the hypochromasia of the nuclei, the prominent eosinophilic nucleoli and the smooth contours characteristic of a clump of exfoliated glandular cells. In the low power view of another smear from the same specimen, stained with May-Grünwald-Giemsa, a streak of cells is seen embedded in an amorphous violet stained deposit (b). This is free mucin and abundant intra- and extra-cellular mucin is confirmed in the alcian blue-stained smear (c).

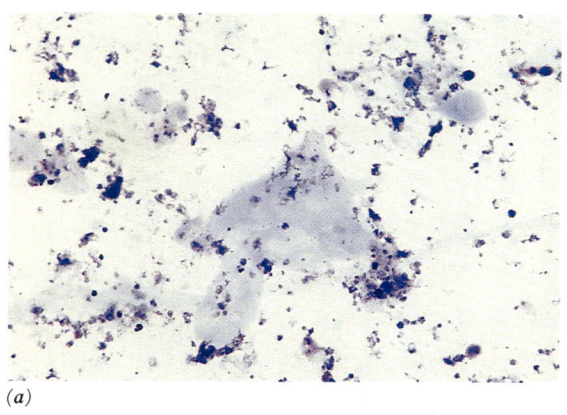

FEMALE REPRODUCTIVE SYSTEM   41

(a)

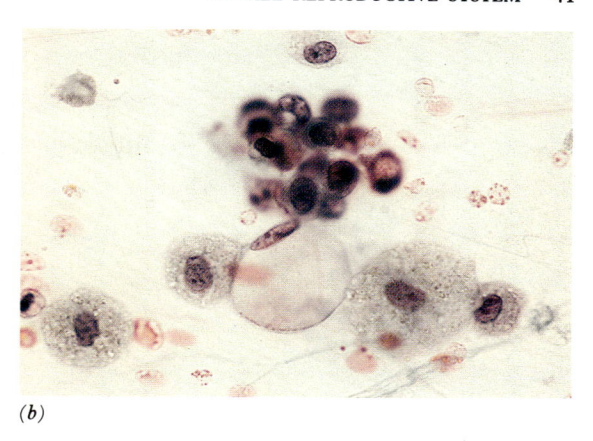

(b)

Fig. 1.52 Mucinous cystadenoma
(a) MGG ×133 (b) Papanicolaou ×525: another case

The consistency of the fluid aspirated from a mucinous tumour often provides a clue, whereas colour is non-contributory. The 15 ml of fluid from the case illustrated in (a) was yellow and the 20 ml from the case shown in (b) was chocolate coloured; however, both were described by the laboratory technician as thick and 'sticky', and both were difficult to spin and spread. The extra-cellular mucin responsible for the viscosity of the fluid may be seen in the stained smear as a homogenous translucent deposit which forms streaks or swathes in the background (a). The intracellular mucin which is also present, may push the nucleus to one pole of the cell which acquires a signet ring appearance. This is seen in one small cell in the cluster and the large discrete goblet cell flanked by foamy macrophages (b). The nuclei of the tumour cells are small, but the nuclear-cytoplasmic ratio varies with the degree of cytoplasmic vacuolization.

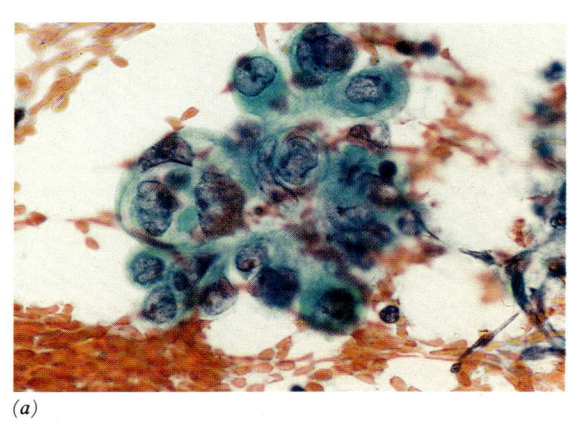

(a)

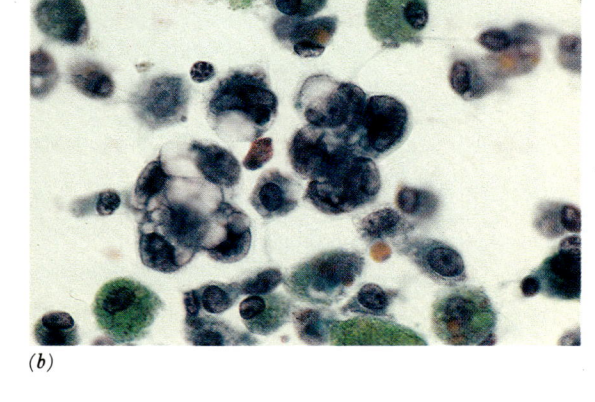

(b)

Fig. 1.53 Papillary serous cystadenocarcinoma
Papanicolaou ×525 (a) non-vacuolated adenocarcenoma cells (b) vacuolated adenocarcenoma cells; another case

Compare the cells from the two malignant serous tumours illustrated in these micrographs with the cells of the benign serous tumours (Fig. 1.54) and note that the carcinoma cells are larger and display variations in cell size, nuclear size and nuclear cytoplasmic ratios. The arrangement of the cell cluster is typically of an adenocarcinoma. The nuclei in (a) are distorted in shape by fairly advanced degeneration, the cytoplasm is firm and uniformly stained. The cells in (b) contain intracytoplasmic vacuoles with hard edges. The appearance is suggestive of mucous vacuoles and this was confirmed by staining with alcian blue. A serous cystadenocarcinoma may be heterogenous and contain foci of mucous metaplasia. Unlike true mucinous tumours which secrete large quantities of extracellular mucin, secretion in serous tumours is generally sparse and evidence of scattered intra-cellular mucin does not alter the classification of the tumour.

42 DIAGNOSTIC CYTOPATHOLOGY

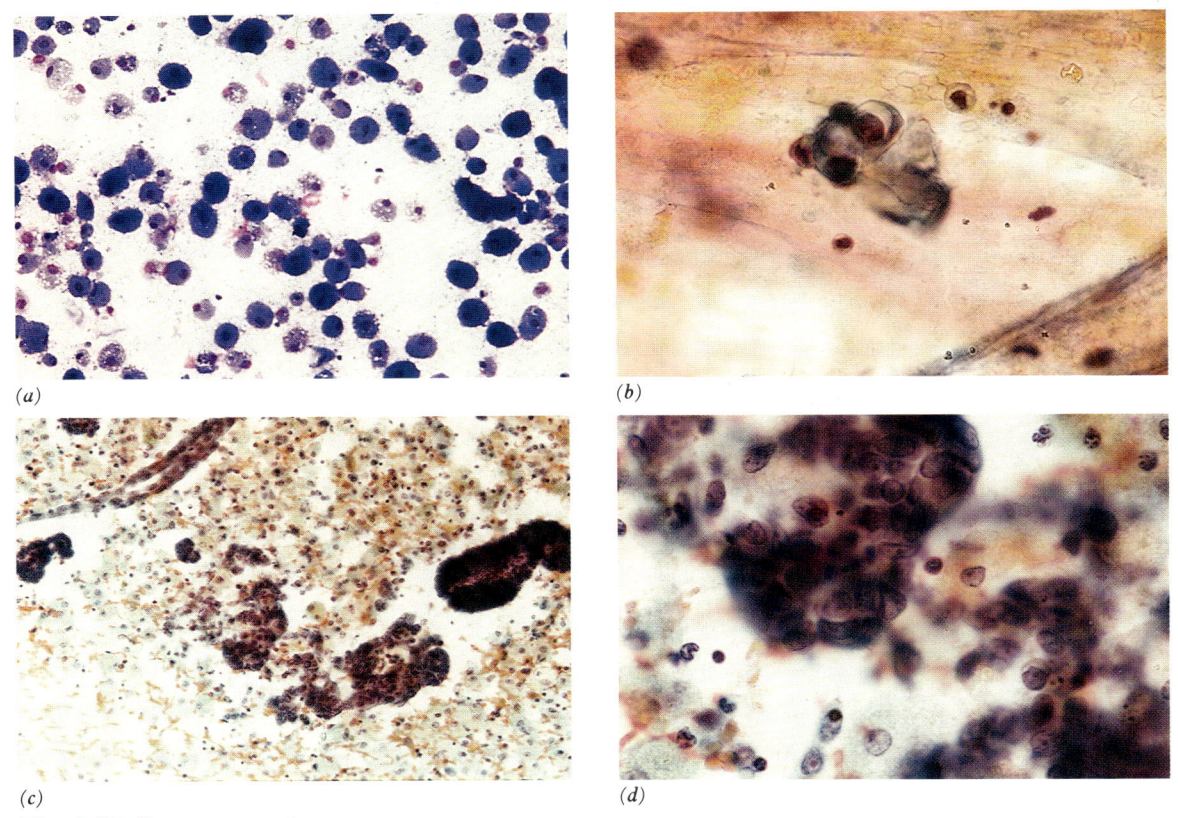

Fig. 1.54 Serous cystadenoma

(a) *MGG ×133: serous cystadenoma* (b) *Papanicolaou ×525: another case* (c) *Papanicolaou ×133: papillary serous cystadenoma; another case* (d) *×525: same case as (c)*

The cytological presentation of a benign serous tumour of the ovary is extremely variable. A papillary tumour may be immediately recognizable in some cases (c), the only problem remaining being to determine whether it is benign or malignant. In other cases, the appearance may be non-specific (a) and so closely resemble that of a functional cyst that the existence of the tumour may not be evident.

The volume, colour and consistency of the fluid may contribute to the diagnosis and should be noted. Whereas colour and consistency of the fluid from a serous tumour may be no different from that of a corpus luteum or a germinal inclusion cyst, the volume may be significant. An inclusion cyst is arbitrarily divided into non-neoplastic if 3 cm or less in diameter and neoplastic if it exceeds this size. The cell deposit in (a) consists of foamy cells and iron-laden macrophages and the appearance is similar to Figure 1.49. The fluid from which the cells were obtained was light green in colour, but the volume of 20 ml was consistent with a neoplasm; a serous cystadenoma was diagnosed by histology of the operation specimen.

In (b), small, cuboidal, uniform-sized cells are seen against a background of erythrocytes. The fluid was heavily blood-stained. This, however, is not a helpful factor as bleeding often occurs within a Graafian follicle at the moment of rupture and a luteal cyst may contain fresh or altered blood. Furthermore, a traumatic aspiration may contribute blood to the cyst fluid. A functional cyst was unlikely in the case illustrated on account of the patient's age of 62 years; in a pre-menopausal patient, the problem would remain unresolved. The three microspherites or psammoma bodies to the right of the benign cell cluster suggest a papillary tumour.

The numerous fronds of tissue in (c) are immediately diagnostic of a papillary tumour. At high magnification (d) the cells that line the fronds are seen to be regular and small. The nuclei resemble each other and contain the odd clump of chromatin.

2. Breast

In the adult female the breast, a modified sweat gland, consists of 15–25 lobes, each composed of several lobules. Each lobule consists of a system of compound ducts which drain into a large lactiferous duct, one per lobe, with its separate opening on the surface of the nipple. Secretory acini develop from the lobular ducts in pregnancy.

The ducts are lined by cuboidal to columnar epithelium. Between this and the basement membrane lies a discontinuous layer of myoepithelial cells. The lobes are separated from each other by dense connective tissue and adipose tissue; the connective tissue between the lobules is loose. The nipple is covered with stratified squamous epithelium.

SAMPLING TECHNIQUES

Four types of specimens may be obtained from the breast: nipple discharge, fine needle aspiration of cyst fluid, or of a solid lesion and imprint smears of the nipple or the cut surface of a resected mass.

Aspiration is generally carried out as an out-patient procedure and may be performed by one person, unaided, by using a special holder which stabilizes the syringe. A cyst is evacuated fully and the aspirated fluid processed in the laboratory in the same manner as a serous effusion (see Ch. 4). A solid lump is immobilized between the thumb and index finger of one hand, and punctured with a 21–23 gauge needle attached to a 20 ml syringe held in the other. The needle is moved in different directions as steady suction is applied until resistance is met. The piston is released to equalize pressure in the barrel and the needle and syringe are withdrawn in one movement. The aspirated material is transferred to pre-labelled, grease-free slides and fixed in 95% ethanol for Papanicolaou or H & E staining or air-dried for staining by the Romanowsky method. Imprint smears are processed in the same way.

The specimens illustrated in this chapter are fine needle aspiration smears except where otherwise stated.

BENIGN CONDITIONS

Normal tissue

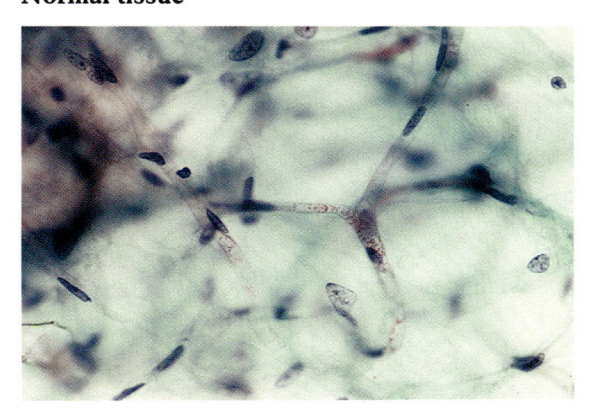

Fig. 2.1 Fibrofatty tissue: Capillaries
Papanicolaou ×333

Needle aspiration of a normal area of breast yields loose fibrofatty tissue and it is unusual to recover cells from a normal duct system. The breast has a rich blood supply and capillaries may occasionally be seen as ramifying channels in the fibrous tissue; red blood cells may be present in the channels.

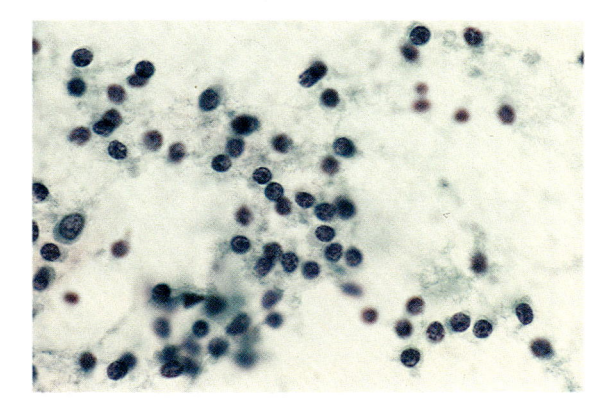

Fig. 2.2 Lymphocytes
Papanicolaou ×525

Lymphocytic infiltration occurs in some breast carcinomas and is an essential component of the variant, medullary carcinoma (see Figs. 2.27 and 2.28). The breast may harbour secondary lymphoma and is occasionally the primary site of a lymphoproliferative malignancy. On occasion, a focus of lymphocytes present in a normal breast may form a tiny palpable nodule as in the case illustrated in this micrograph. The needle aspirate smear shows small, mature lymphocytes with uniformly staining hyperchromatic nuclei with even granular chromatin and little or no visible cytoplasm (Compare with duct epithelial cells in Fig. 2.8).

Inflammatory disease

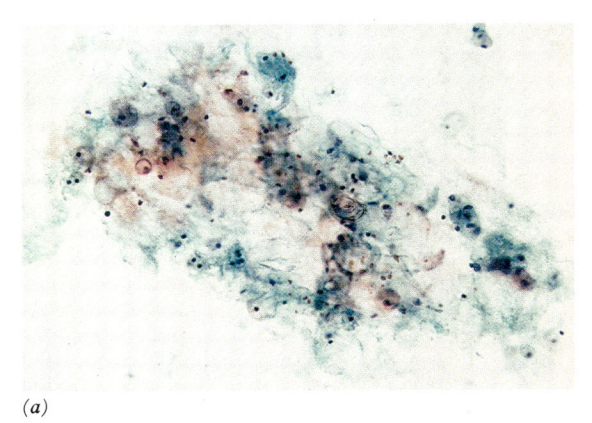

(a) 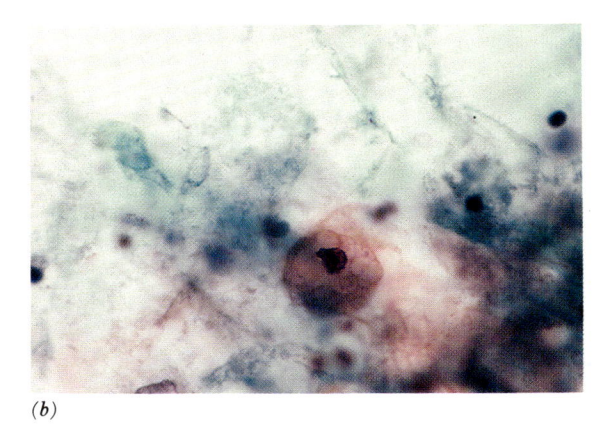 (b)

Fig. 2.3 Fat necrosis
Papanicolaou (a) ×133 (b) ×525

Inflammation of the breast is often preceded by a history of trauma which may cause a condition referred to as traumatic fat necrosis. The injured adipose tissue undergoes necrosis and excites an inflammatory response, which is initially acute but soon becomes chronic and is accompanied by fibrous proliferation at the edge of the necrotic zone. Fat necrosis may present as a hard mass attached to puckered skin and may resemble a carcinoma in appearance and feel. The cellular presentation consists of collapsed fat cells and the cytoplasmic debris of disintegrated fat cells (a), (b). Lymphocytes, plasma cells and macrophages with ingested lipid are usually present (a).

An acute abscess is uncommon; it occurs in a lactating breast and is due to pyogenic cocci. In the condition, known as inflammatory carcinoma, the breast is red, hot and swollen. This is caused by extensive permeation of the lymphatics by carcinoma cells and is not true inflammation.

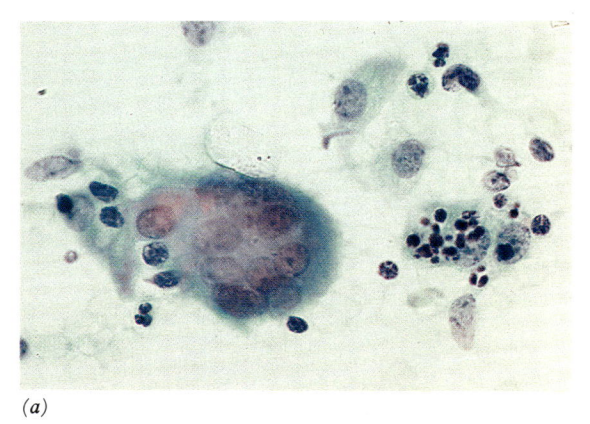

(a) 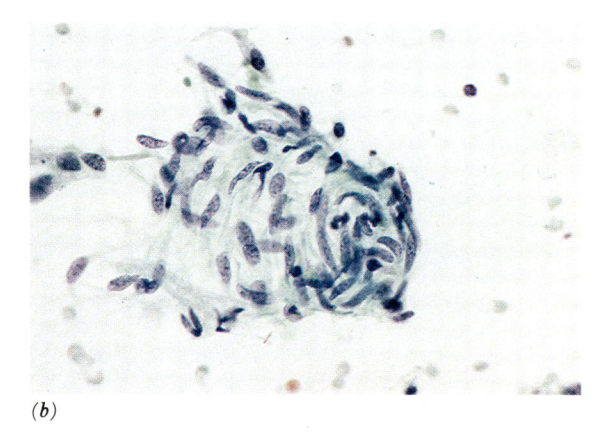 (b)

Fig. 2.4 Granuloma of breast
Papanicolaou (a) ×525: foreign body giant cell (b) ×333: cellular fibrous tissue

Inflammatory response to fat necrosis may progress to granuloma formation. Other provocations include talc from previous surgical intervention, intramammary injection of breast-enhancing substances, tuberculosis and fungal infections. The granuloma illustrated was clinically suspected to be a carcinoma. The cytological diagnosis of granuloma was confirmed by excision biopsy histology; the aetiology remained uncertain.

The diagnostic cell, a multinucleated giant epithelioid macrophage of the foreign body type is seen in (a). In a smear, the nuclei may fill the cell or show a random distribution in the cytoplasm and a neat alignment along the cell border is unusual. Other cells in (a) include duct epithelial cells, neutrophils, lymphocytes and a macrophage with ingested nuclear material. The fibroblastic proliferation of the granuloma is seen in (b) as a fragment of cellular fibrous tissue with many spindle-shaped nuclei in a translucent cyanophilic matrix.

Fibroadenosis

The normal female breast is dependent on a variety of hormones which affect its structure and function. While the most dramatic changes are seen at puberty, pregnancy, lactation and menopause, the breast also undergoes subtler alterations during each menstrual cycle.

Disturbances or imbalance of the hormones or an altered or uneven response of the different elements in breast tissue results in the condition known as fibroadenosis. The disorder is also variously referred to as cystic mammary dysplasia, benign mammary dysplasia, fibrocystic disease, and benign cystic mastopathy.

Fibroadenosis is the commonest disorder of the female breast. It simultaneously involves the ductal, lobular and stromal elements of the breast. The affected ducts show areas of dilatation (duct ectasia), which may appear as cysts containing fluid (cyst formation). The lobular ductules undergo hyperplastic proliferation (adenosis) and are surrounded by proliferating stroma (fibrosis). In one variant of fibroadenosis, the hyperplastic ductules are separated and compressed into tubular shapes by bands of dense fibrous tissue (sclerosing adenosis). Hypertrophy and multiplication of the lining epithelium may occur (epitheliosis).

A single component of fibroadenosis never occurs in isolation, but the term applied to the condition may be determined by the histological preponderance or the clinical presentation of one component. The disorder may produce a vaguely lumpy breast or present as a solitary mass. It occurs in the mature woman, particularly in the pre-menopausal years.

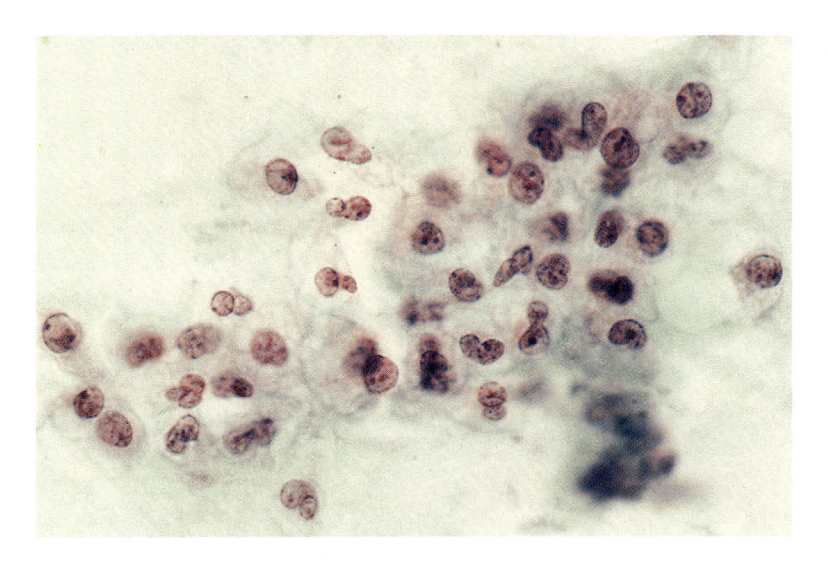

Fig. 2.5 Duct ectasia
Papanicolaou ×720: nipple discharge

Duct ectasia consists of dilatation of the mammary duct system and may be associated with a nipple discharge. This is usually clear, or may be slightly turbid. Duct epithelial cells are often seen although some secretions are acellular and consist only of amorphous debris and a few leucocytes. The epithelial cells are usually swollen and foamy, and may occur as small aggregates or single forms. The nuclei are degenerative and may be round or indented. The foamy cells with reniform nuclei closely resemble large histiocytes.

A nipple discharge may also be associated with galactorrhoea, papillary hyperplasia of ductal epithelium, benign papilloma, intraduct or invasive carcinoma with an intraduct component. The nipple discharge associated with benign or malignant tumours generally contains a fair number of red blood cells or fibrin. These therefore serve as useful signals and merit full investigation as to the cause and source of the blood.

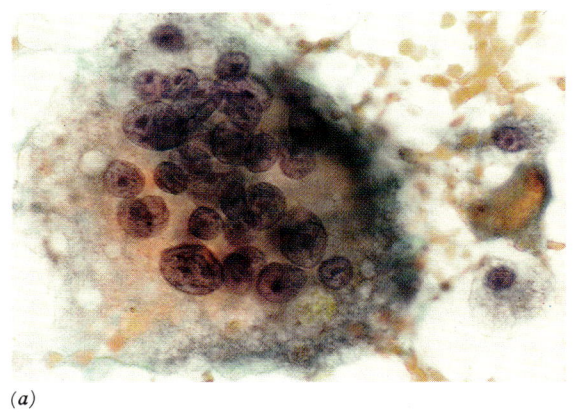

Fig. 2.6 Duct ectasia

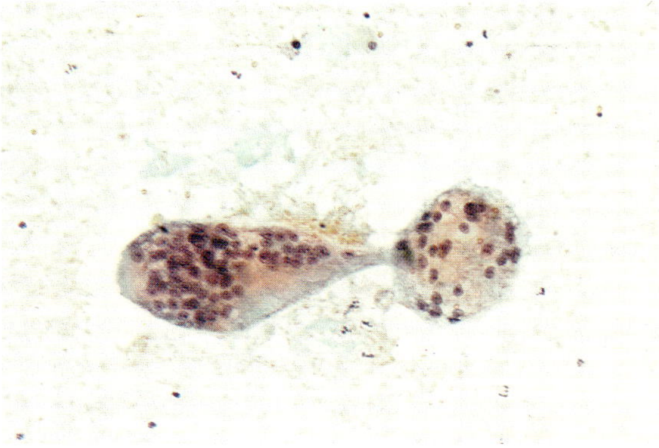

Papanicolaou (a) ×525: nipple discharge; foreign body giant cell (b) ×133: same smear as (a). Fibrous tissue: foamy epithelial cells

Duct ectasia may present as a sub-areolar mass. The duct lumen is filled with detritus and lipid; chronic inflammatory cells infiltrate the periductal tissue. The duct lining epithelium may become eroded and lipid enter the stroma and initiate a foreign body giant cell reaction (a). The illustration also shows small mononuclear macrophages and amorphous debris. Fragments of fibrous tissue and foamy epithelial cells may appear in the discharge (b).

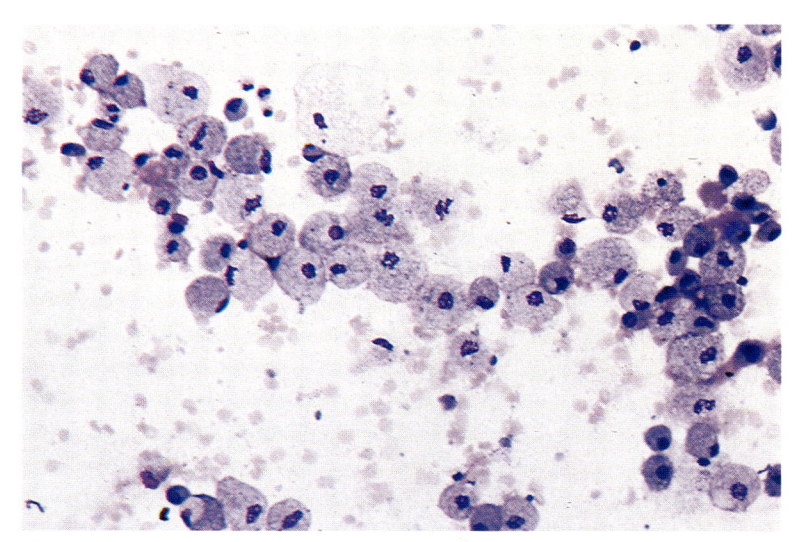

Fig. 2.7 Breast cyst

MGG ×183

A breast cyst may be small and microscopic or it may form a palpable tensile mass. A woman may present with one or more cysts in one or both breasts. The cyst collapses on aspiration of its contents and disappears altogether or recurs, or new cysts may appear. A solid lump overshadowed by the cyst may become apparent and it is customary to palpate the breast after the cyst has been aspirated and separately needle any residual lump.

In one type of cyst formation due to duct ectasia, the aspirated fluid contains mainly large foam cells, single or cohesive. The foam cells are considered to have several different origins. Some are histiocytic, others are degenerate duct epithelial cells (compare with Fig. 2.5), yet others have residual morphological characteristics which suggest degenerative forms of apocrine metaplasia cells. A periductal inflammatory response is a feature of duct ectasia. Neutrophils enter the cyst fluid and may be so numerous as to create an impression of pus.

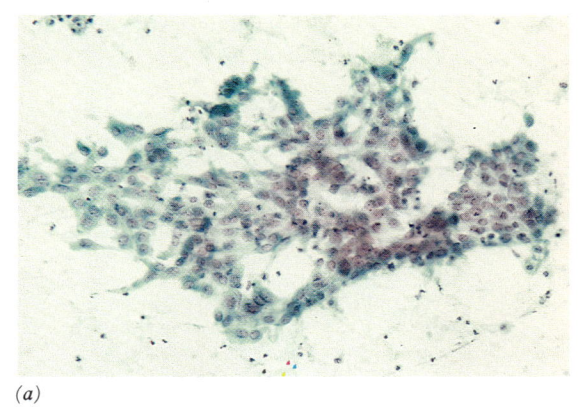

Fig. 2.8 Simple breast cyst

(a) Papanicolaou ×133 (b) MGG ×333

The lining of a breast cyst may consist of normal ductal epithelium which is shed into the fluid in loose aggregates; single forms are also seen. The cells are cuboidal or low columnar. If well preserved, they have cyanophilic cytoplasm with the Papanicolaou stain and vesicular nuclei with pinpoint nucleoli (a). Degenerative changes in exfoliated cells include shrinkage of nuclei, irregularity of nuclear shapes and an impression of anisonucleosis (b). A few neutrophils are usually present.

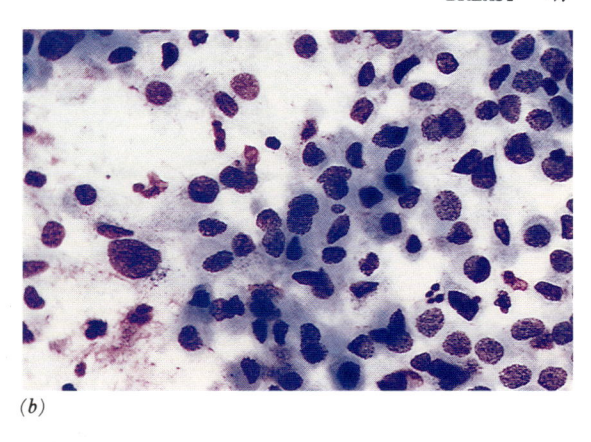

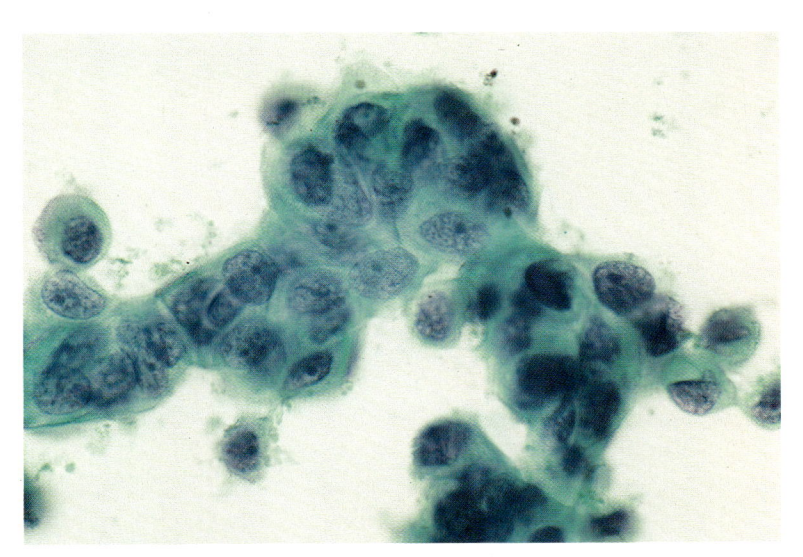

Fig. 2.9 Papillary cyst

Papanicolaou ×720

Occasionally, the epithelium lining a cystically dilated duct hypertrophies and forms papillary ingrowths into the cyst cavity. Branching fronds of epithelial tissue are seen in the cyst fluid. The cells show morphological features of proliferative activity. They are larger than their normal counterparts, basophilic and optically dense. The nuclei show some enlargement, but the nuclear cytoplasmic ratio remains within the limits of benign cells. Slight enlargement of the nucleolus is usually apparent. Hyperplastic epithelial cells in cysts may occasionally contain mucous vacuoles.

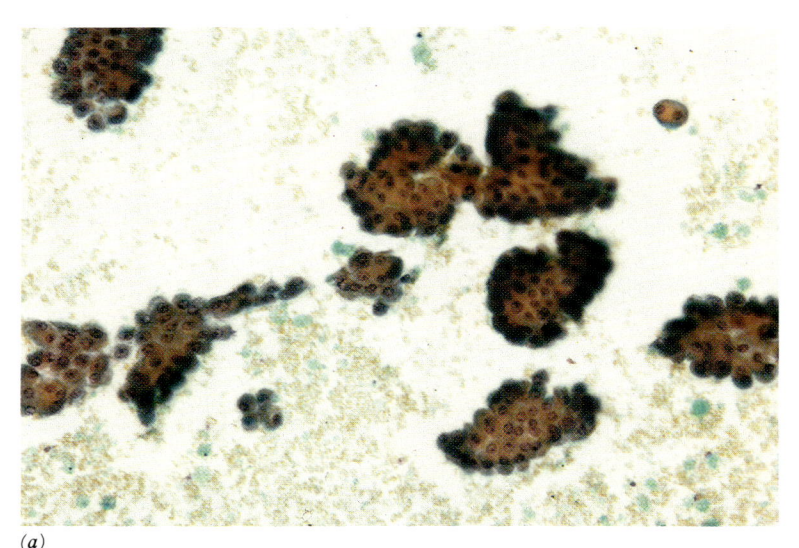

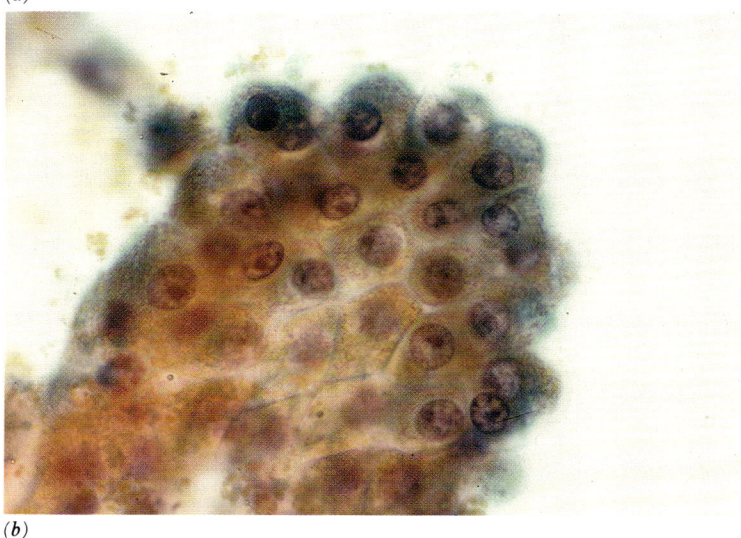

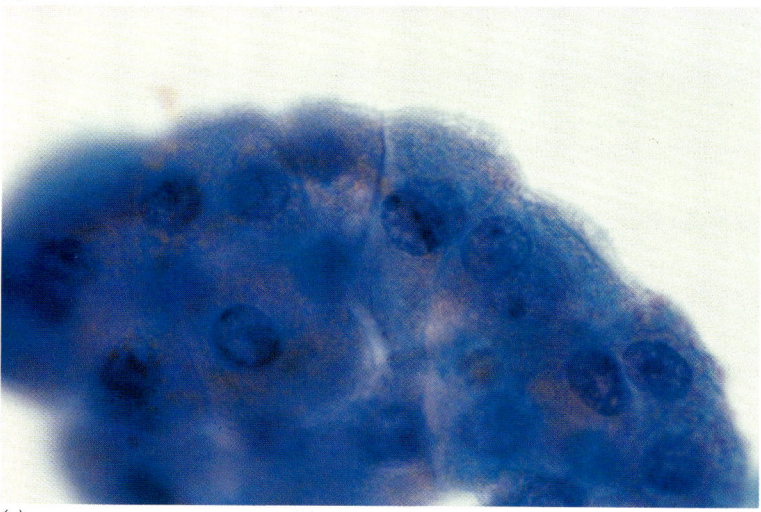

Fig. 2.10 Breast cyst: apocrine metaplasia

Papanicolaou (a) ×183 (b) ×720 (c) ×1144: another case

Approximately one-third of breast cysts are lined by large cells, referred to as apocrine metaplasia cells because of their resemblance to cells of apocrine sweat glands. Fully formed apocrine metaplasia cells have a distinctive and striking appearance. They are amongst the largest epithelial cells seen in breast specimens and appear in smears in aggregates; a few single cells are also usually present (a). Apocrine metaplasia cells contain numerous coarse granules which impart an eosinophilia to the cytoplasm (b). In a Papanicolaou-stained smear, the cell may be uniformly pink or a variable amount of green or blue cytoplasm may be seen between the granules (b), (c). The distal edge of the cell has a luminal fringe traversed by fine vertical lines (c). The fringe represents well developed microvilli seen by electron microscopy. The round vesicular nucleus occupies a small part of the cell and nuclear cytoplasmic ratio is low; binucleation is not uncommon (a), (b). Each nucleus has a prominent nucleolus.

Fig. 2.11 Breast cyst: transitional forms between ductal and apocrine cells

Papanicolaou ×720

The origin of the apocrine cell has been the subject of much interest and debate. Cytological preparations of cyst fluids often contain cells which show nuclear and nucleolar characteristics of apocrine cells and the cytoplasmic features of ductal cells or vice-versa. Work done in the author's laboratory has shown a continuous spectrum of morphological, biochemical and ultrastructural features between the small, non-granular ductal cell and the apocrine cell; this supports the theory of metaplastic transformation to account for the presence of an apocrine type cell in the breast.

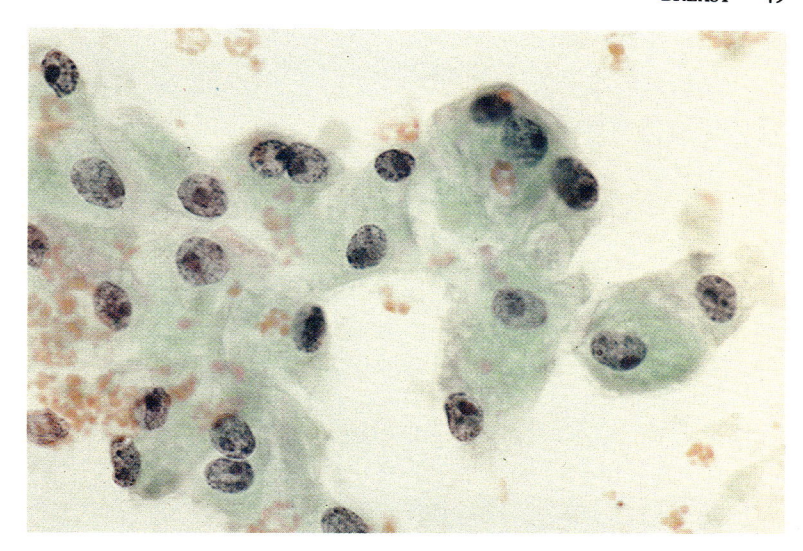

Fig. 2.12 Fibroadenosis

Papanicolaou ×183

The cellular presentation of fibroadenosis is variable. Dense fibrous tissue is resistant to aspiration and when fibrosis is the predominant component, the sample may be virtually acellular. In cases of marked adenosis, the smear may show only epithelial cells. The cytological diagnosis is therefore necessarily incomplete. In a few cases, fragments of hyperchromatic epithelial cells and cyanophilic connective tissue with few nuclei (lower right) may be recovered. The appearance is indistinguishable from that seen in fibroadenoma. However, samples from fibroadenosis may contain evidence of other components of the pathological complex, such as foam cells, apocrine metaplasia cells and neutrophils.

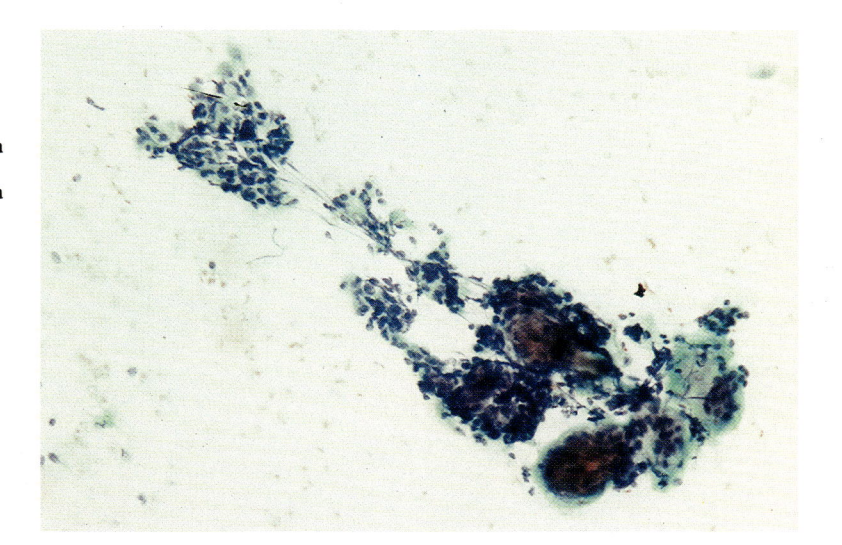

50 DIAGNOSTIC CYTOPATHOLOGY

Hormone-induced changes

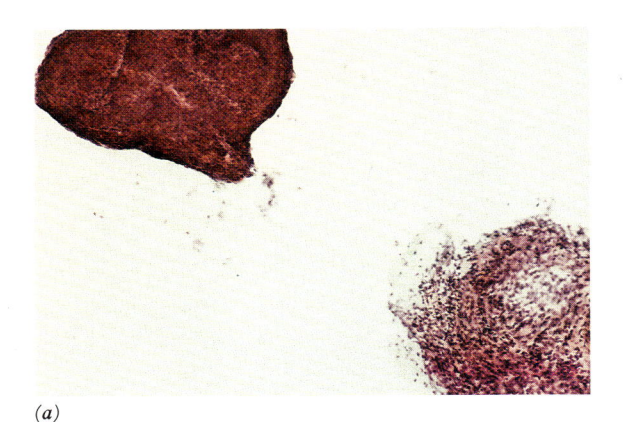

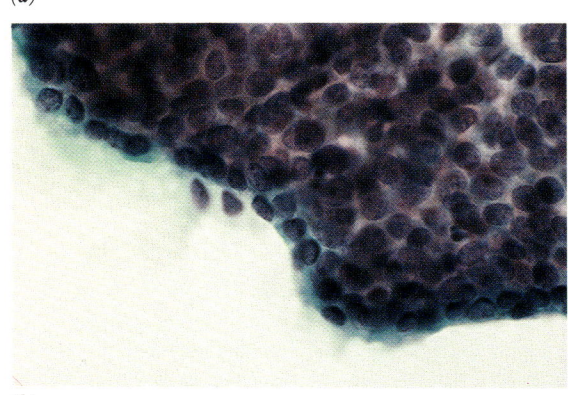

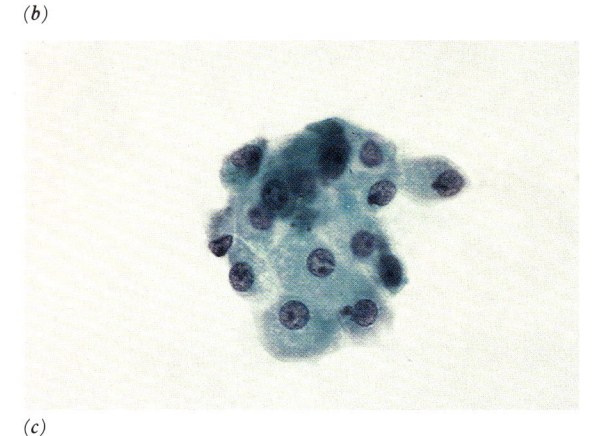

Fig. 2.13 Gynaecomastia

Papanicolaou (a) ×133 (b) ×525: another case (c) ×525: same smear as (b)

The normally rudimentary breast of the male may, under the effect of endogenous or exogenous hormones, undergo proliferative hyperplasia of ductal epithelium with a concomitant increase in periductal stroma. The condition is known as gynaecomastia. Certain therapeutic agents, notably cimetidine and spironolactone, oestrogens administered for carcinoma of the prostate, and ectopic hormone production by some neoplasms may induce hypertrophy of the male breast. Two cases of gynaecomastia are illustrated in these micrographs. Sample (a) shows a fragment of highly cellular fibrous tissue (lower right) and a large sheet of closely packed epithelial cells (top left). The epithelial component of another case is seen to consist of basophilic cuboidal ductal cells, enlarged hyperchromatic nuclei with granular chromatin and small nucleoli (b). A second population of cells (c) was present in the same smear. These cells are much larger, have abundant cyanophilic cytoplasm, a low nuclear cytoplasmic ratio and prominent nucleoli. Two cells have luminal fringes (top right and lower centre). The cells have several characteristics of apocrine metaplasia cells (compare with Fig. 2.11). Apocrine type cells occur in gynaecomastia but are extremely uncommon.

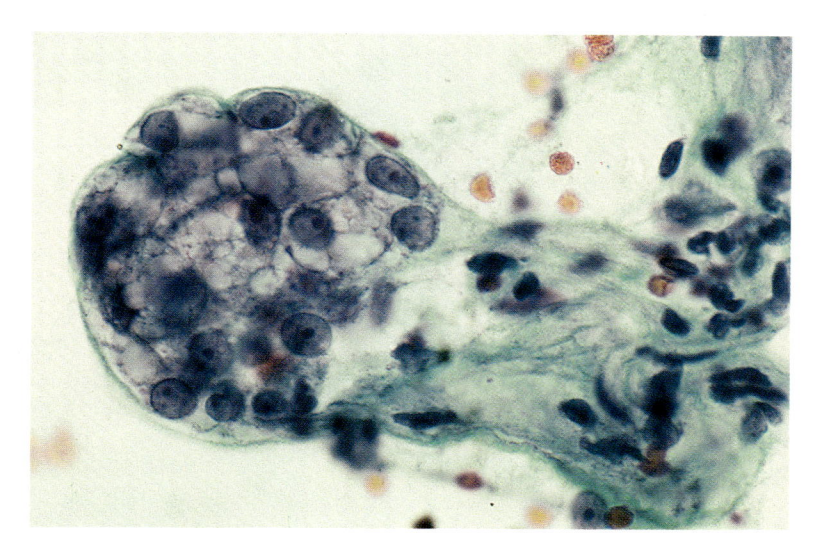

Fig. 2.14 Lactating breast

Papanicolaou ×720

A physiological response of the breast to hormones is illustrated in this micrograph. The specimen was a fine needle aspirate of a tiny nodule palpated in the breast of a young woman 1 week post-partum. A glandular structure and loose fibrous tissue are seen. The glandular cells are large and have abundant vacuolated cytoplasm. The nuclei are relatively small and contain prominent nucleoli. Excision biopsy showed fibrofatty tissue and normal lactating breast tissue.

During pregnancy, numerous secretory alveoli are formed from the alveolar ductules. As the pregnancy progresses, the acini begin to secrete protein-rich colostrum, low in fat content. The alveolar cells enlarge, and a distinct central nucleolus appears within a hypochromic nucleus. These cells are referred to in the Scandinavian literature as acinic cells. Soon after parturition, lipid rich milk secretion is stimulated by circulating prolactin. The lactating breast consists almost entirely of glandular tissue. The epithelial component of a fibroadenoma developing or persisting during pregnancy or lactation show the same features as physiologically altered cells.

Benign tumour

Fig. 2.15 Fibroadenoma

(a) MGG ×183 (b) Papanicolaou ×183: another case (c) Papanicolaou ×720: same smear as (b)

A fibroadenoma is generally accepted to be a benign mixed epithelial and connective tissue tumour. Foci of tissue proliferation in some cases of fibroadenosis are histologically identical with fibroadenoma; this has led to speculation that a fibroadenoma may be a localized manifestation of hormone-induced interplay of epithelial and stromal elements rather than a true tumour. The cytological presentation of fibroadenoma is indistinguishable from fibroadenosis in the absence of many foam cells and neutrophils. Apocrine metaplasia may occur in fibroadenoma and does not discriminate between the two lesions. The connective tissue of fibroadenoma is said to be made up of specialized substance rich in mucopolysaccharides. In a Romanowsky-stained smear, the connective tissue, occasionally shows the same fuschia coloured reaction (a) as mucin. With the Papanicolaou stain, the stromal element is often amphophilic (b). Unlike appearances seen in sections of fibroadenoma, the epithelial element dominates the cytological picture (b), and is not always accompanied by the stromal element. The epithelial cells in this example are cuboidal and regular and have uniform nuclei (c) with one to three small nucleoli.

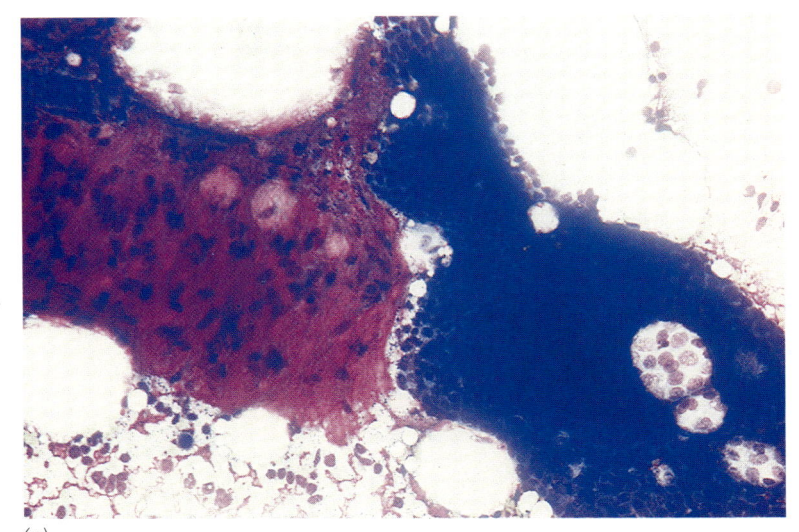

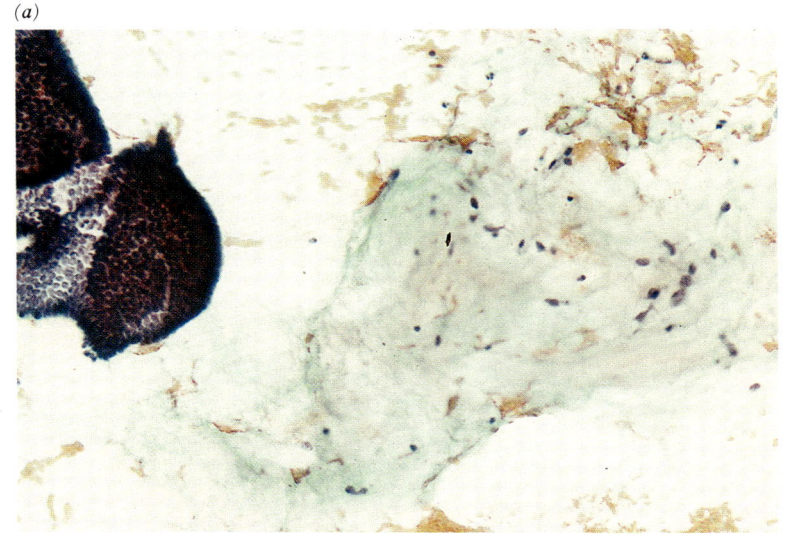

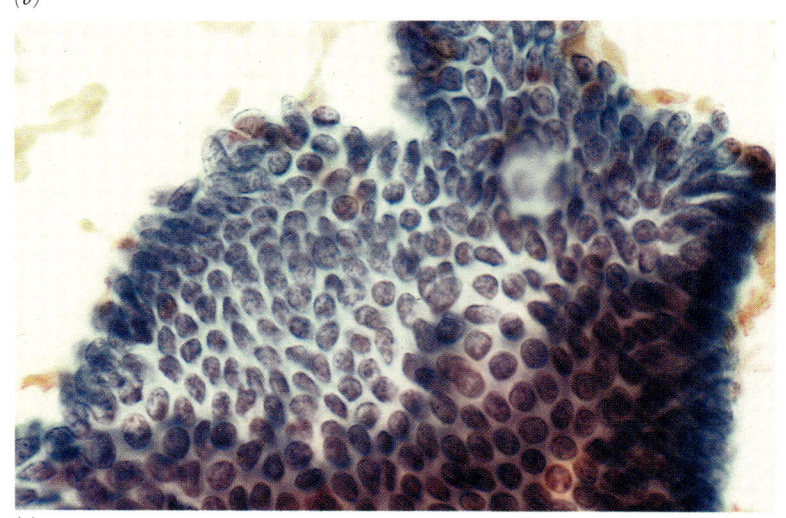

BREAST 53

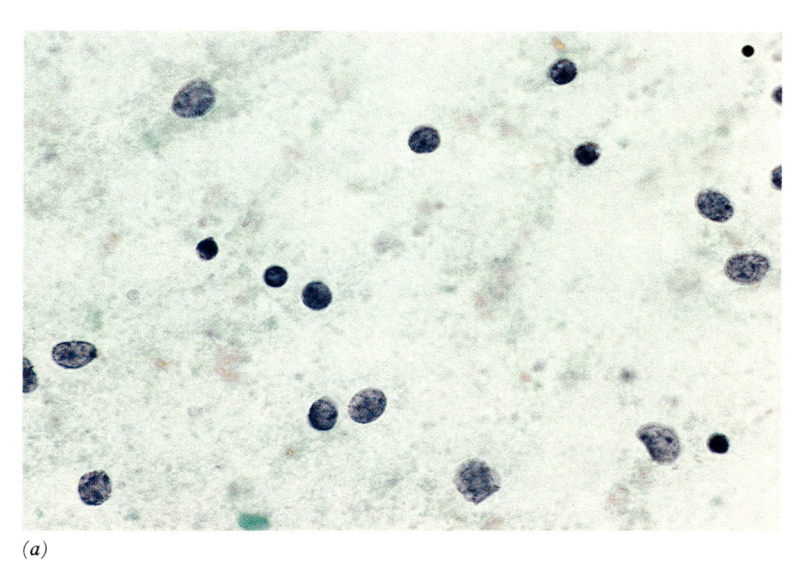

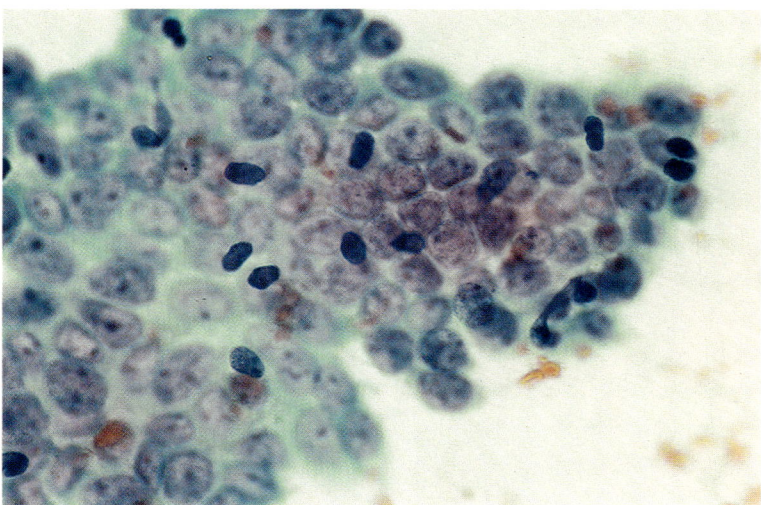

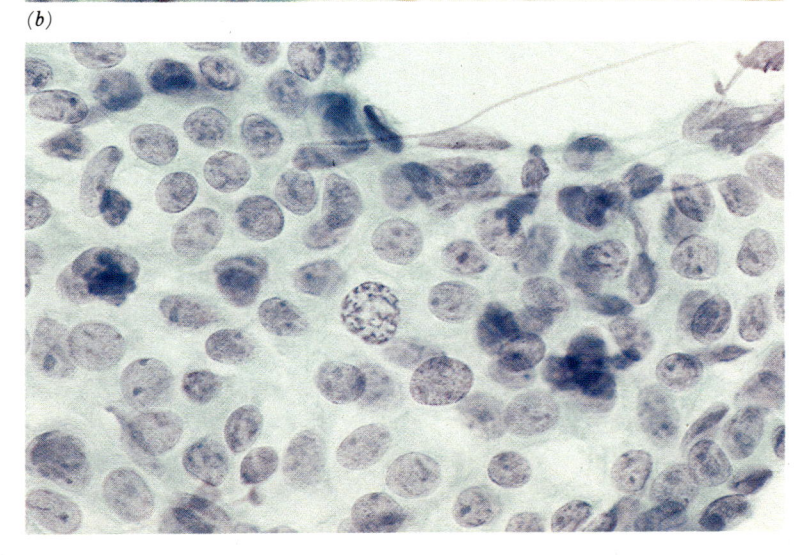

Fig. 2.16 Fibroadenoma
Papanicolaou ×720 (a) stripped nuclei (b) epithelial cell aggregates

Two types of stripped nuclei are shown in (a). The larger vesicular nuclei are of duct epithelial origin. The ones to note are the small dark ones, which are round and apical. These nuclei are released from disrupted myoepithelial cells which form a discontinuous layer between duct epithelial cells and the basement membrane. They are referred to as sentinel nuclei, as it is considered that their presence denotes the existence of an intact myoepithelial layer in the tissue under examination, and thereby excludes malignancy. While this is generally correct, exceptions occur; a needle may pick up myoepithelial cells from benign tissue on the way in or out of a breast with carcinoma. As a working rule, however, a cytodiagnosis of malignancy should not be made on a specimen in which myoepithelial cells or nuclei are present, unless pleomorphic unequivocal carcinoma cells can be identified.

The epithelial cells (b) in the same sample are somewhat larger than duct cells. The nuclei are finely granular and nucleoli more prominent. The slight variation in nuclear size is partly intrinsic, partly artefact. The hyperchromatic myoepithelial nuclei which overlie or are intermingled with the epithelial cells would exclude malignancy, even if the stripped nuclei were not present.

Fig. 2.17 Fibroadenoma
Papanicolaou ×720

A cell in prophase is seen in the centre of the field. The other cells in the cohesive sheet are identical with each other and have bland nuclei. Mitotic activity may be noted in epithelial cells in a fibroadenoma, albeit rarely, and does not indicate malignancy.

PRIMARY CARCINOMA

Most malignant tumours of the breast arise from ductal or lobular epithelium and are adenocarcinomas. They may be infiltrating or intraepithelial (intraductal carcinoma or lobular carcinoma in situ).

The greater majority by far are invasive ductal carcinomas (80%). Some variants of ductal carcinoma are classified separately; most are of no special type and are referred to as infiltrating duct carcinoma, not otherwise specified (NOS). A desmoplastic reaction is common and the tumour may be scirrhous; the cell yield in a needle aspirate is poor from tumours with extensive fibrosis.

Lobular carcinoma, both in situ and invasive, is frequently multicentric and may be bilateral. It may be preceded by lobular hyperplasia. Intralobular carcinoma may extend into ducts and replace the duct epithelium (pagetoid spread). Invasive lobular carcinoma infiltrates the surrounding stroma in a characteristic single or Indian file manner, a feature which is sometimes recognizable in fine needle aspiration cytology.

The phyllodes tumour (cystosarcoma phyllodes), a mixed connective tissue and epithelial tumour, is distinguished from an ordinary fibroadenoma by a greater cellularity of its connective tissue. The tumour may be entirely benign, or it may have an atypical or frankly malignant fibrous component, surrounding hyperplastic but benign epithelial cells. Local recurrence is common and distant metastases, when they occur, appear as fibrosarcomas. Primary stromal fibrosarcoma, lacking a benign epithelial component, is rare, as is a primary lymphoma.

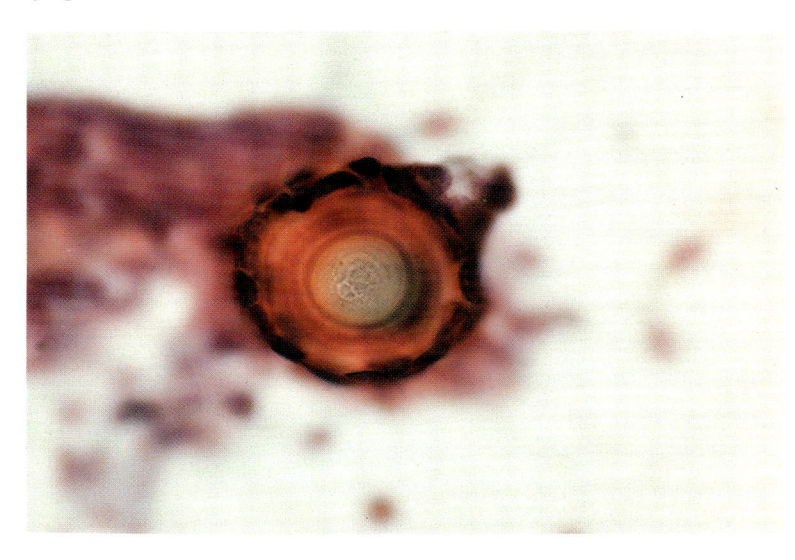

Fig. 2.18 Calcospherite (psammoma body)

Papanicolaou ×720

Microcalcification is often seen in benign and malignant lesions in mammographs. The calcific areas in carcinoma are generally finer. In cytological and histological material, the calcium may be seen as small, hyaline fragments or as an organised structure with concentric rings; a central glassy zone may be present. The structure is referred to as a calcospherite or psammoma body. See also Figures 1.43 and 1.44.

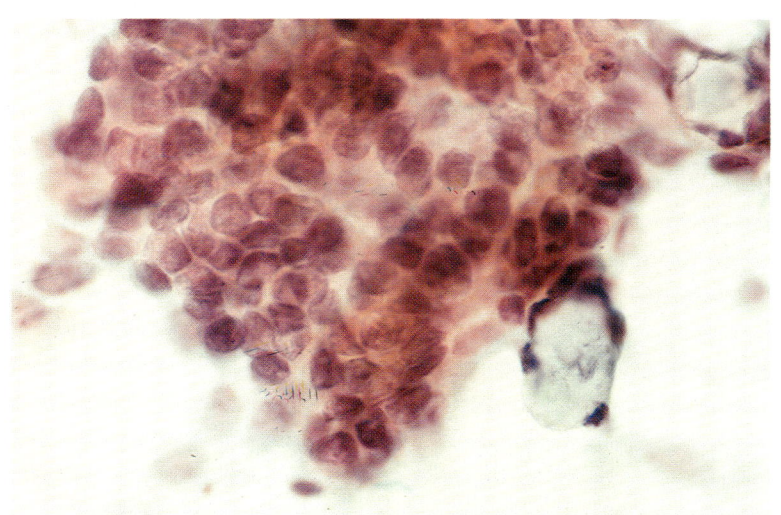

Fig. 2.19 Tubular carcinoma

Papanicolaou ×720: same case as Figure 2.18

Tubular carcinoma is a highly differentiated invasive carcinoma with uniform cells arranged in tubules. The illustrated cells from a case of tubular carcinoma, correctly identified as being malignant, are small. The nuclei are disproportionately large, and are compressed against one another with virtually no intervening cytoplasm. The nuclear chromatin is finely stippled. Note the amorphous calcium encircled by tumour cells.

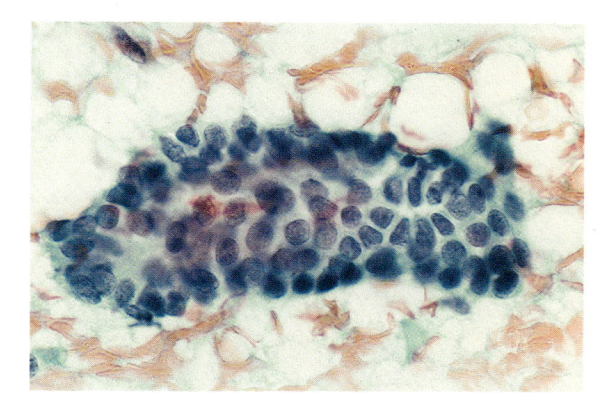

Fig. 2.20 Intraductal and tubular carcinoma
Papanicolaou ×525

Extremely well-differentiated carcinoma cells may be difficult to identify with certainty. The author's policy in such cases is to withhold a diagnosis of malignancy and recommend formal biopsy. The cells illustrated in this micrograph are more regular than in the preceding example and have more cytoplasm. The nuclei are finely reticulated and the arrangement of the cells is comparable to that seen in some fibroadenomas (see Fig. 2.15c) and in gynaecomastia (see Fig. 2.13b). A cytodiagnosis of marked epithelial hyperplasia, possibly benign, was submitted and a biopsy was advised. Cryostat section histology showed infiltrating carcinoma; invasive tubular carcinoma and extensive in situ carcinoma were identified in paraffin sections.

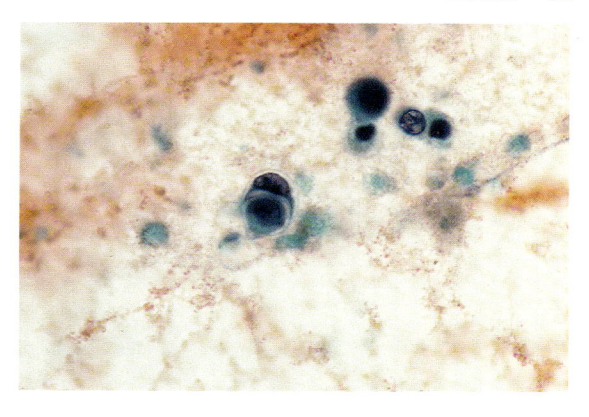

Fig. 2.21 Intracystic carcinoma
Papanicolaou ×525

Less than 3% of breast cysts are malignant; the fluid from these is generally tinged or heavily stained with blood. The cells in this micrograph, seen against a background of fibrin, are variable in size. Much of the intense hyperchromasia is due to nuclear pyknosis, but in the cells in the centre of the field, it is due to condensed coarsely granular chromatin. Palpation of the breast after aspiration of the fluid did not disclose a solid lump, and the carcinoma was found to be limited to the cyst lining epithelium. This type of tumour is classified as non-invasive intracystic carcinoma.

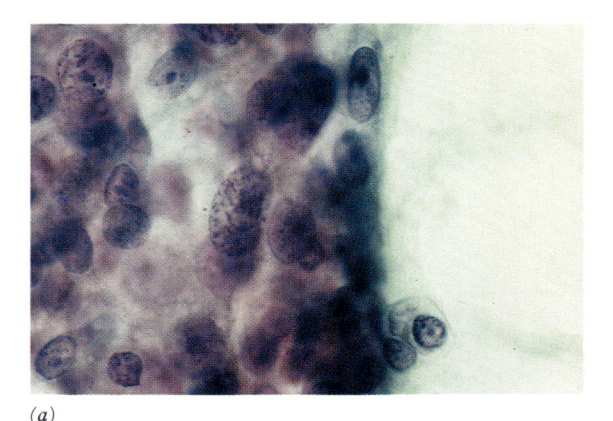

(a)

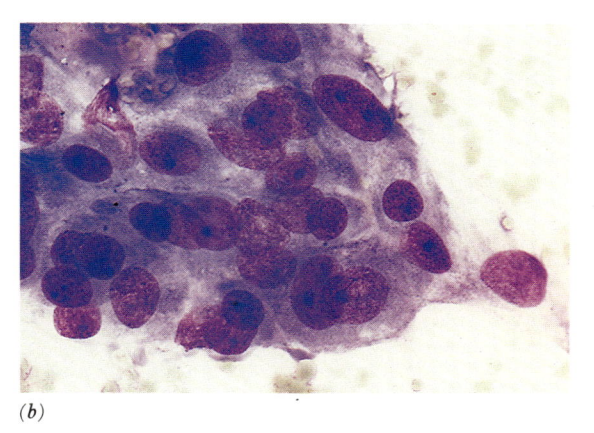

(b)

Fig. 2.22 Cystic and solid carcinoma
(a) Papanicolaou ×525: cyst (b) MGG ×525: solid mass

A malignant cyst is more likely to be an area of cystic degeneration in a solid carcinoma. In the case illustrated, a cystic and an adjacent hard solid mass were palpated; both were aspirated. Sheets of identical large carcinoma cells with a fair amount of cytoplasm, markedly variable granular nuclei and prominent nucleoli are seen in the cyst fluid (a) and in the solid lump (b).

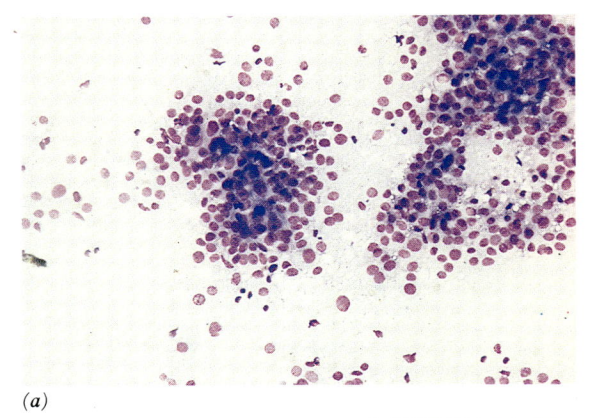

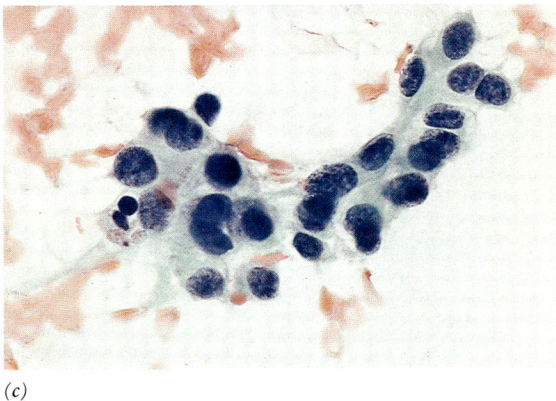

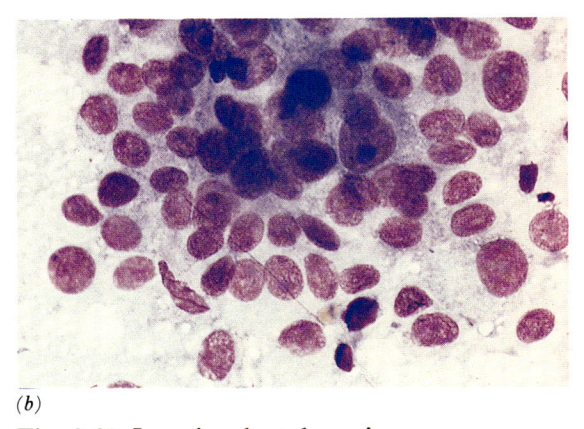

Fig. 2.23 Invasive ductal carcinoma

(a) MGG ×133 (b) MGG ×525: same field (c) Papanicolaou ×525: another case

Cancer cells often show reduced cohesiveness and dissociated carcinoma cells are often seen in aspiration smears. This characteristic of malignant cells has been somewhat overstressed in the literature on breast cytology. In a few cases, almost all the cells are discrete. The more usual finding is a combination of dissociated and cohesive carcinoma cell (a). In 25% of breast carcinomas, almost all the cells seen are in aggregates (c). Another feature to note in (b) and (c) are the small pear-shaped nuclei which superficially resemble sentinel nuclei. Unlike myoepithelial nuclei, the nuclei in (b) and (c) are surrounded by a sizable amount of cytoplasm; they are indicative of individual cell necrosis which is frequently observed in breast carcinoma cells.

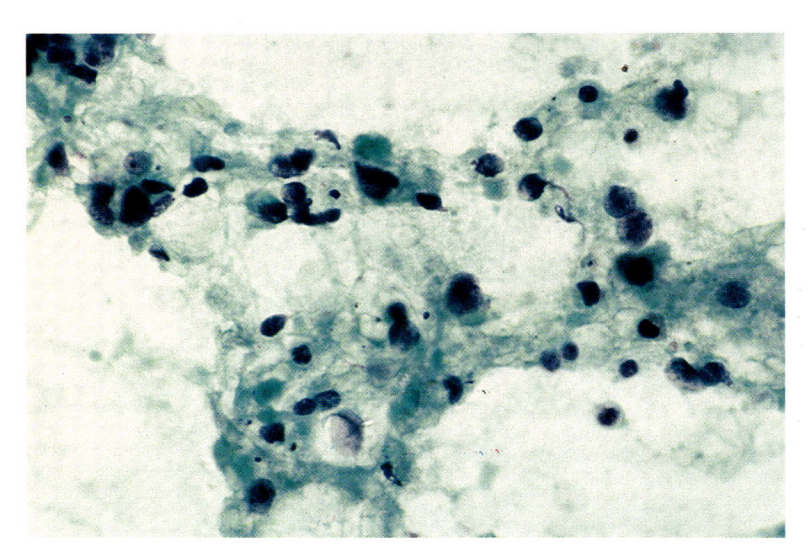

Fig. 2.24 Necrotic carcinoma cells

Papanicolaou ×720

In some cases, tumour necrosis may be extensive and more advanced. Fragments of cytoplasm without discernible borders or intercellular attachments may be seen overlaid by haphazardly disposed nuclei in various stages of degeneration. Cellular necrosis is not a feature of benign breast lesions and the appearance is highly suggestive of malignancy. However, for a firm diagnosis, carcinoma cells with well preserved morphology should be sought and identified as a heavy-handed spread of a smear may produce a picture of misleading disintegrated distorted cells.

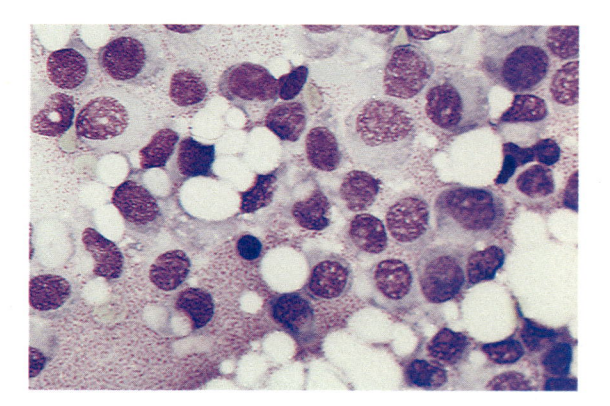

Fig. 2.25 Invasive ductal carcinoma
MGG ×525

Some tumours may be composed of moderately or wholly monomorphic cells. The cells in the example illustrated in this micrograph show minimal variation in size. They are seen against a background of fibrin and tissue fluid, are discrete, spheroidal in shape and about four times the lymphocyte to centre left.

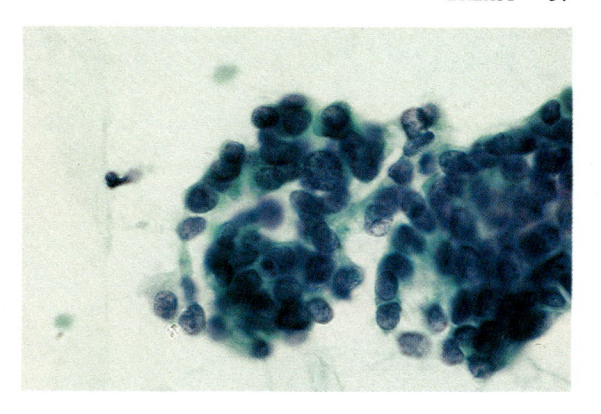

Fig. 2.26 Monomorphic invasive ductal carcinoma
Papanicolaou ×525

The monomorphic carcinoma cells in this example form a cohesive clump. Single cells were not in evidence in the specimen. The cells are small. In some small-celled, invasive carcinomas, it may not be possible, in histological sections, to establish whether the tumour is ductal or lobular. In cytological specimens, it is particularly difficult. The case illustrated was a ductal carcinoma.

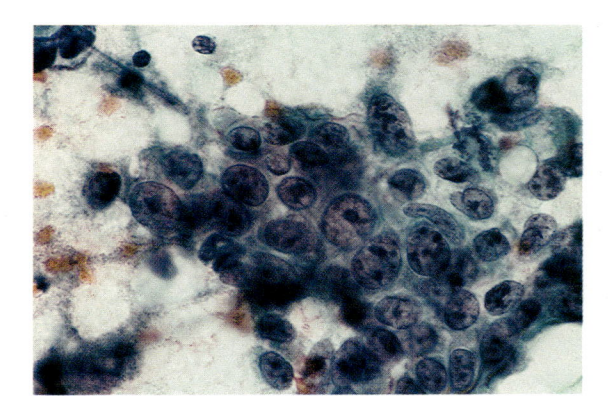

Fig. 2.27 Medullary carcinoma
Papanicolaou ×525

A medullary carcinoma has distinctive clinical, cytological and histological features. The tumour is soft to palpation and lacks the serpiginous hard edges of the usual infiltrating duct carcinoma. Macroscopically, it appears circumscribed; the cut surface tends to bulge outwards and the tumour is referred to by surgeons as encephaloid carcinoma. The histological pattern is of sheets and broad anastomosing cords of tumour cells without a discernible glandular structure or desmoplastic reaction. The cells are large, have mainly round, smooth bordered, vesicular nuclei with prominent nucleoli and resemble the cells of a seminoma. Infiltration by lymphoid cells is a feature of medullary carcinoma and was noted in other fields in the smear.

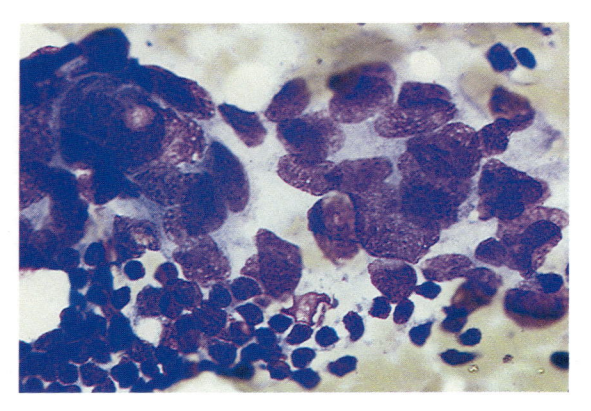

Fig. 2.28 Invasive ductal carcinoma: lymphocytic infiltration
MGG ×525

Prominent lymphoid infiltration may occur in invasive ductal carcinoma, not of the medullary type. Many lymphocytes are seen in the lower part of the field. The obviously malignant cells are large and pleomorphic. The nuclei are angular and nucleoli are inconspicuous. The cell morphology is not that of medullary carcinoma.

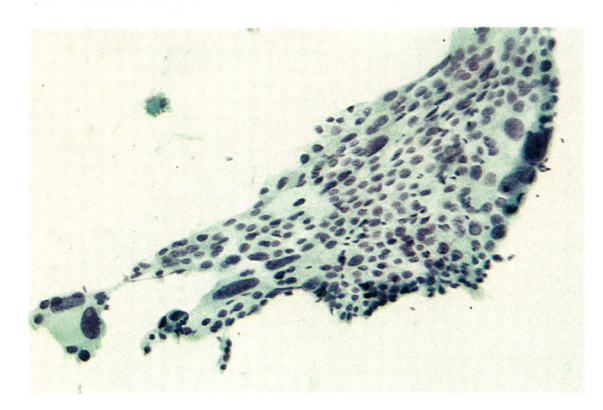

Fig. 2.29 Pleomorphic invasive ductal carcinoma

Papanicolaou ×133

The average ductal carcinoma, as seen in the preceding micrographs, is only moderately pleomorphic. A tumour showing exceptional variation in cell size is illustrated in this micrograph. The tumour cells have substantial amounts of cytoplasm. The majority of the nuclei are small and interspersed between these are bizarre giant nuclei. The aspirate smear contained many calcospherites. The appearance seen is more common in ovarian carcinoma (see Fig. 4.30). The tumour was found to be a primary ductal carcinoma of breast.

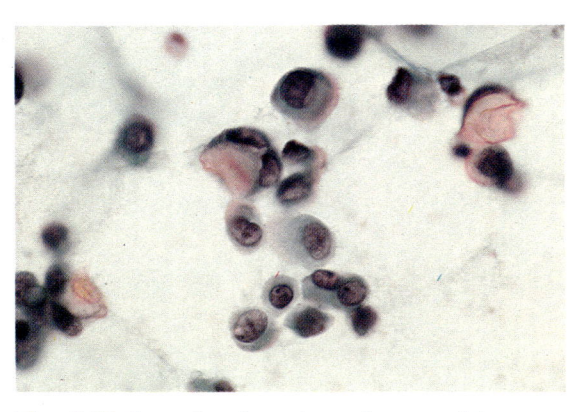

Fig. 2.30 Invasive ductal carcinoma with intracellular mucin

Papanicolaou ×525

A small amount of mucin can be demonstrated with special stains in most breast carcinomas. In some tumours, mucin-containing cells are more obvious. Four cells in this field show pink mucin diffused through the cytoplasm. One binucleate and one mononuclear carcinoma cell have assumed signet ring forms.

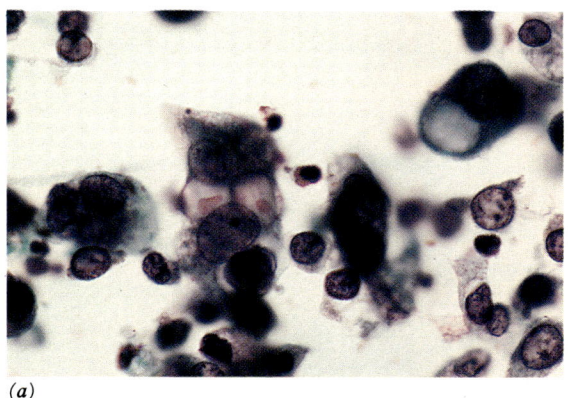

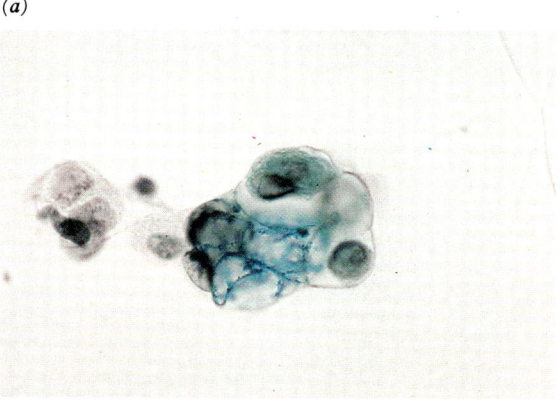

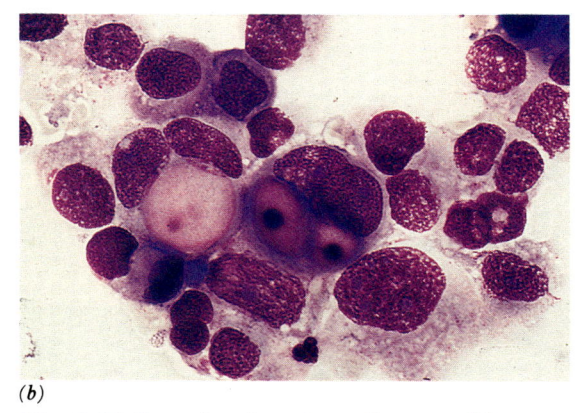

(a)

(b)

Fig. 2.31 Invasive ductal carcinoma with intracellular mucin

(a) Papanicolaou ×525 (b) MGG ×525 (c) Alcian blue ×525

Intracytoplasmic mucin may condense into a dense mass within the mucous vacuole (a), (b). The 'bird's eye' or 'bull's eye' appearance has been attributed to lobular carcinoma. While it may be seen in lobular carcinoma, the bird's eye mucous vacuole, which is not particularly common, occurs more often in ductal carcinoma and may be seen in benign and malignant cells in other organs (see Figs. 3.7, 3.67 and 4.33). Other cells in the same smears contain diffuse mucin which is positive with alcian blue (c).

(c)

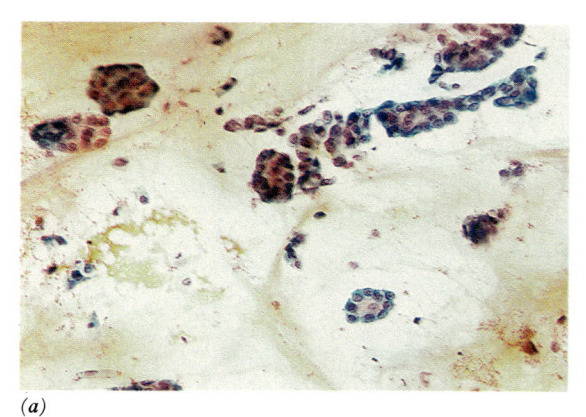

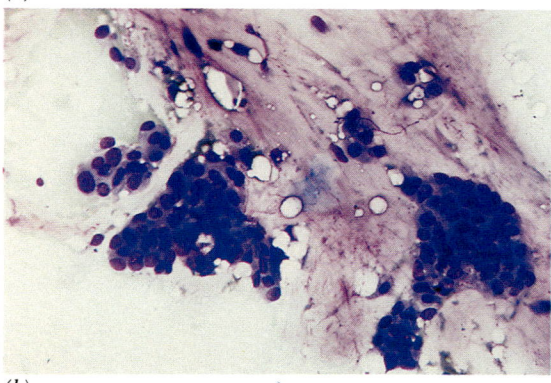

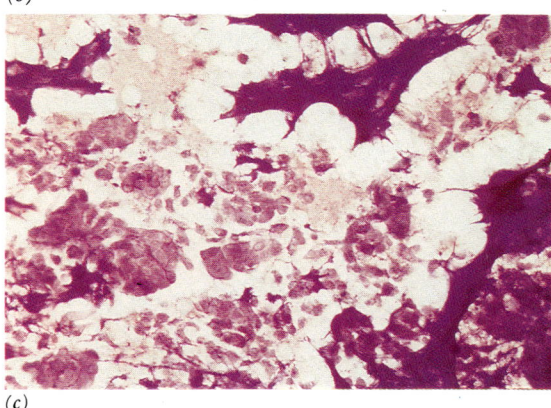

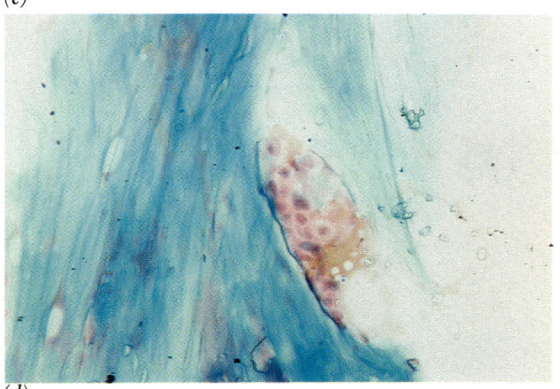

Fig. 2.32 Mucous carcinoma

(a) Papanicolaou ×133 (b) MGG ×133 (c) PAS ×133
(d) Alcian blue ×133: another case

Although small amounts of intracellular mucin can be found in most breast carcinomas, the term mucous carcinoma is applied to tumours which contain large amounts of extracellular mucin. In a typical appearance of mucous carcinoma, islands of well-differentiated carcinoma cells are seen in or near lakes of abundant free mucin. This forms swathes of amorphous material, pink or peach coloured in a Papanicolaou-stained smear (a), violet with MGG (b). The nature of the background material should be confirmed. The smear shown in (a) was re-stained with per-iodic acid Schiff reagent (PAS) which imparts a deep pink to both intracellular and extracellular mucin (c). In another case, the Papanicolaou smear was de-stained by immersion in 1% HCL for 30 seconds and re-stained with alcian blue. The extracellular mucin is alcian blue-positive, the nuclei of the malignant epithelial cells are stained pink with the counterstain (d).

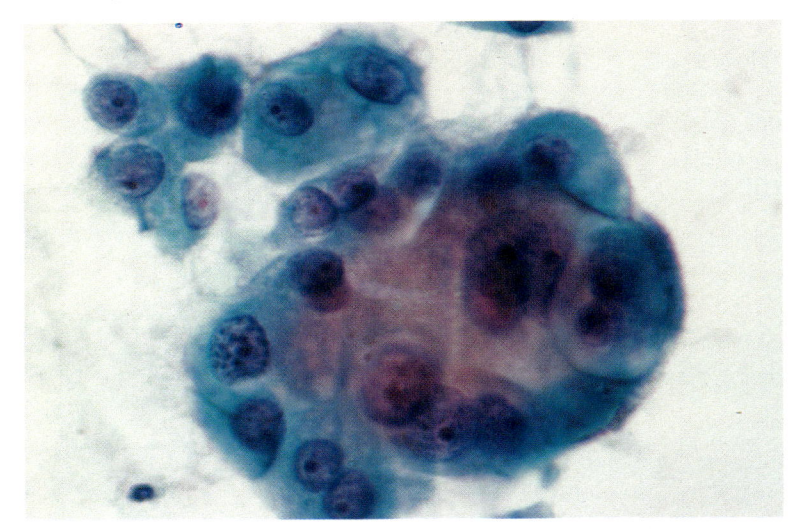

Fig. 2.33 Apocrine carcinoma

(a) *Papanicolaou* ×720 (b) *MGG* ×720: *another case*

An apocrine carcinoma is composed of large cells, eosinophilic with H & E, reminiscent of apocrine metaplasia cells. The variable-sized malignant cells in (a) are mainly large, the nuclear cytoplasmic ratio is low and nucleoli are prominent. The cytoplasm is amphophilic. Intracytoplasmic granules are not seen. The overall morphology is suggestive of apocrine carcinoma and was reflected exactly in sections of the mastectomy specimen. The cells in (b) are also devoid of granules but show all the other features of apocrine metaplasia cells. The histological diagnosis was apocrine carcinoma.

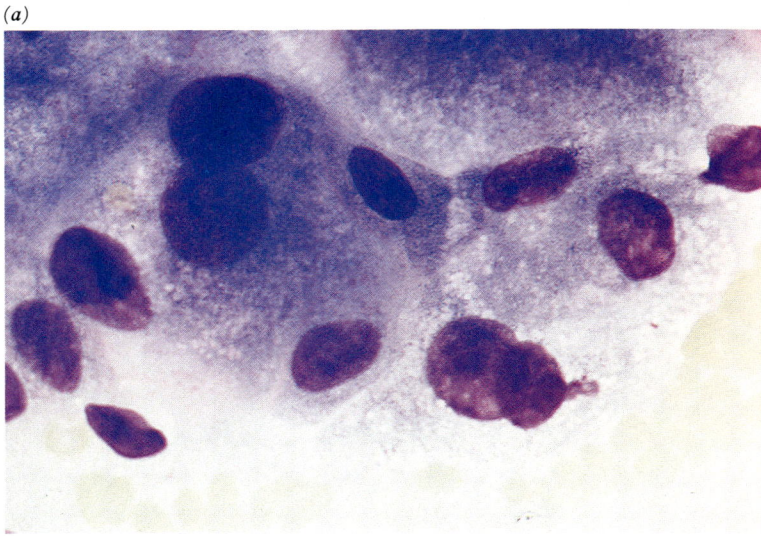

(a)

(b)

(a)

(b)

Fig. 2.34 Invasive lobular carcinoma

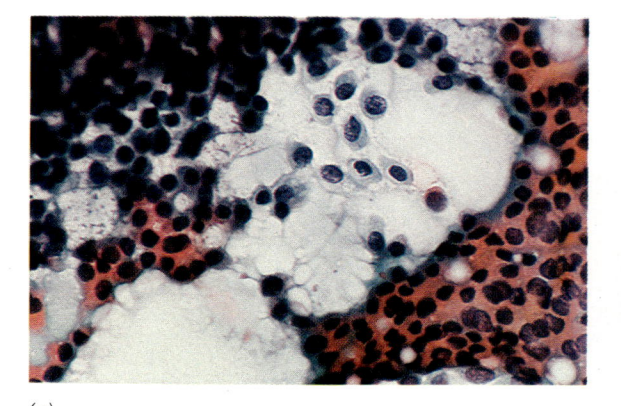

Papanicolaou (a) ×333 (b) ×832: same smear (c) ×832: imprint smear; same case

A case of infiltrating lobular carcinoma with a focus of intralobular carcinoma is illustrated. The cells of a lobular carcinoma are generally small and monomorphic, and display a distinctive pattern of infiltration of surrounding tissue in single file. Lobular carcinoma cannot be distinguished in cytological smears from small-celled ductal carcinoma on the basis of cell size only. The characteristic mode of invasion may occasionally be seen in an aspiration smear (a). The majority of tumour cells are uniform in size of cell and nucleus and nuclear cytoplasmic ratio. A very occasional gross, large nucleus may be present (b). The Indian file arrangement of the advancing cells is better appreciated in an imprint of the tumour (c).

(c)

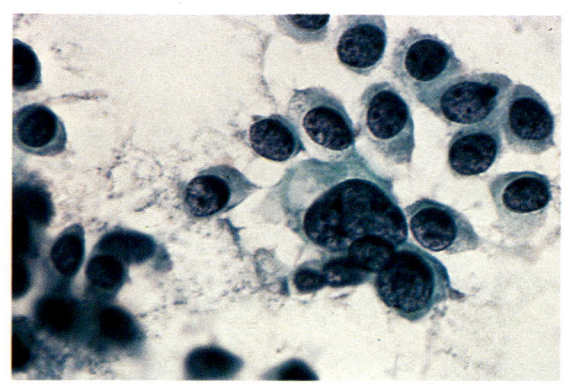

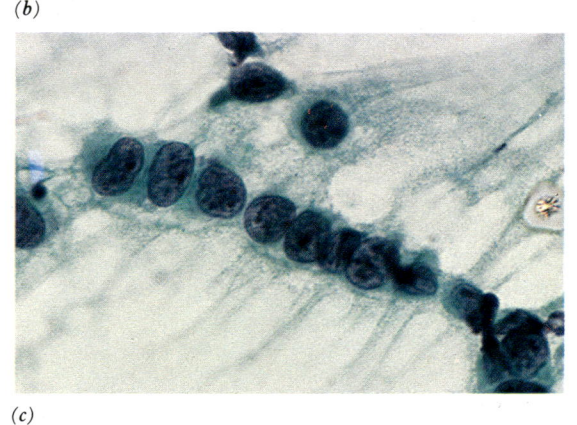

Fig. 2.35 Ductal carcinoma infiltrating adipose tissue

Papanicolaou ×458

Infiltration of fatty tissue by malignant ductal cells may also be encountered in breast aspiration or imprint cytology. Compare the cells in this micrograph with the lobular carcinoma in Figure 2.34 (a), and note the larger size and the prominent nucleoli of the ductal cells. Unequivocal evidence of infiltration of the septa between fat cells is confirmatory of malignancy but may not help to discriminate between lobular and small-celled ductal carcinoma.

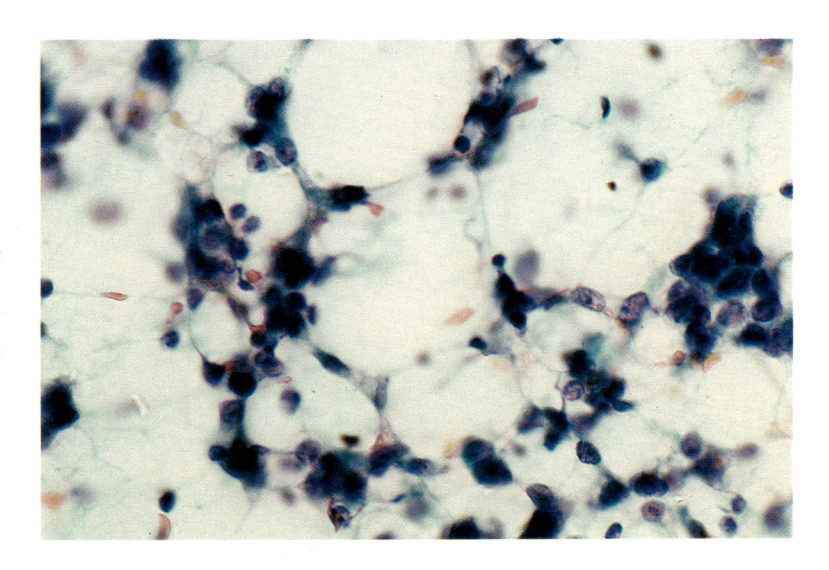

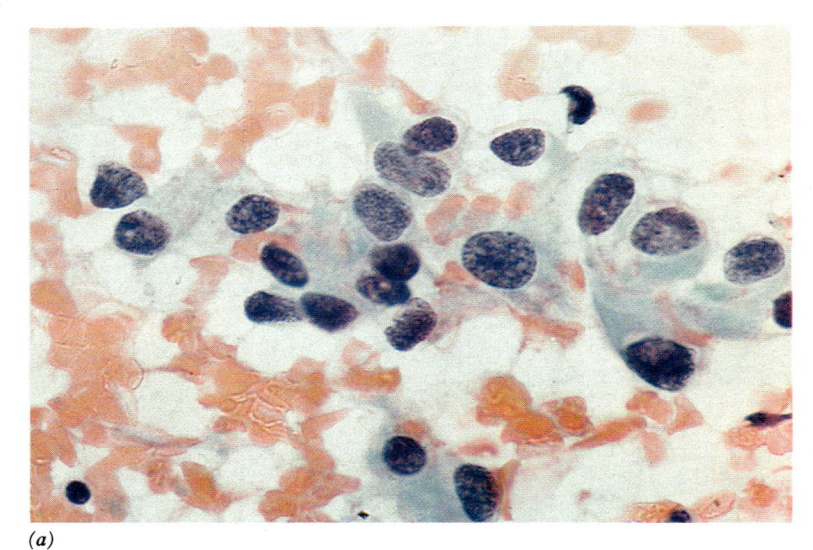

Fig. 2.36 Paget's disease of the nipple

Papanicolaou (a) ×720 (b) ×183: nipple scrape

In Paget's disease of the nipple, an underlying ductal carcinoma which may be invasive (but is more often intra-epithelial) spreads through the mammary ducts and infiltrates the squamous epithelium of the nipple. The areola is reddened and thickened, develops fissures and later usually ulcerates; it may appear eczematous. The carcinoma cells (a) are large and pleomorphic with abundant cytoplasm and granular nuclei. The squamous cells from the affected nipple and areola generally appear dyskaryotic and dyskeratotic in smears (b).

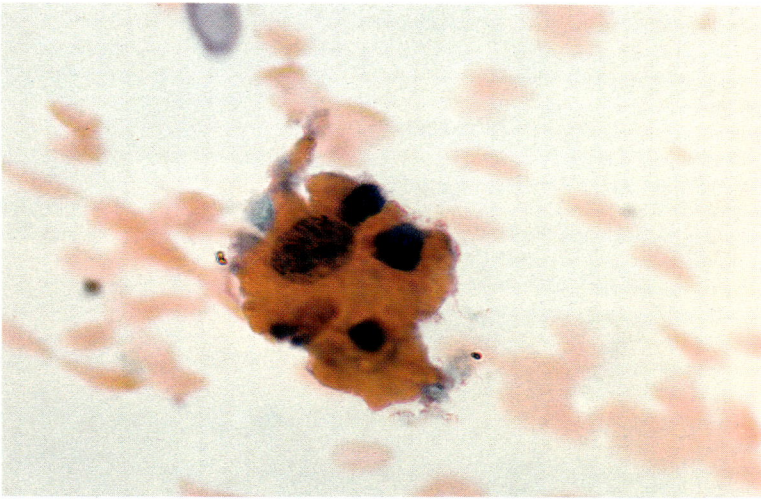

(a)

(b)

(a)

(b)

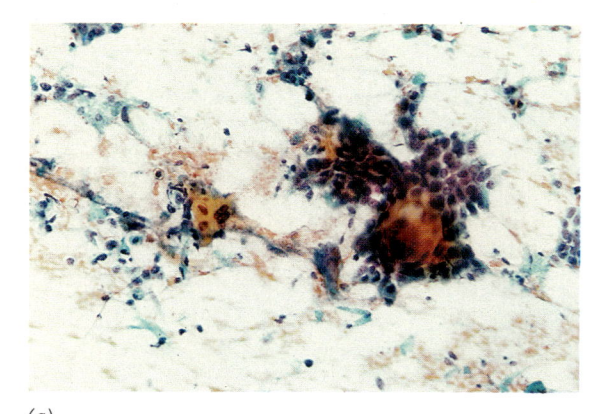

Fig. 2.37 Ductal carcinoma with squamous metaplasia

Papanicolaou (a) ×133 (b) ×525: same field (c) MGG ×525: same specimen; another smear

The World Health Organization classification of breast carcinoma includes the category 'carcinoma with metaplasia'. Foci of squamous cells, spindle cells, cartilage and osseous tissue may be seen in a recognizable ductal carcinoma. Small cyanophilic malignant ductal cells and a few large opaque orangeophilic cells are seen attached to each other in (a). At a higher magnification (b), the large cell with two giant nuclei and macronucleoli is seen to be of a different type from the surrounding ductal carcinoma cells. The squamous character of the cell is indicated by the size, texture and pale cytoplasm in the MGG smear (c).

(c)

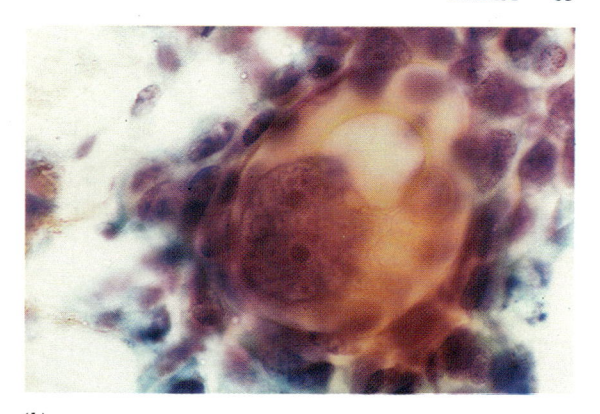

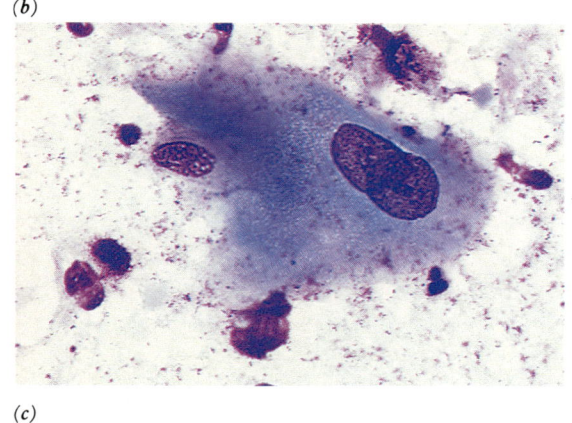

Fig. 2.38 Carcinoma of the male breast

Papanicolaou ×720

Carcinoma of the male breast is extremely uncommon. The malignant cells are of ductal origin, moderately large, moderately pleomorphic with hyperchromic granular nuclei and an occasional nucleolous.

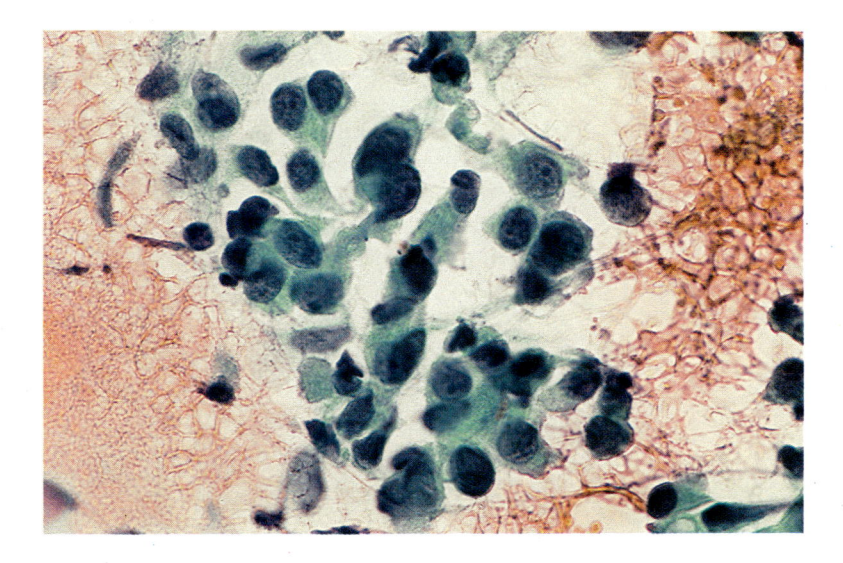

METASTATIC DISEASE

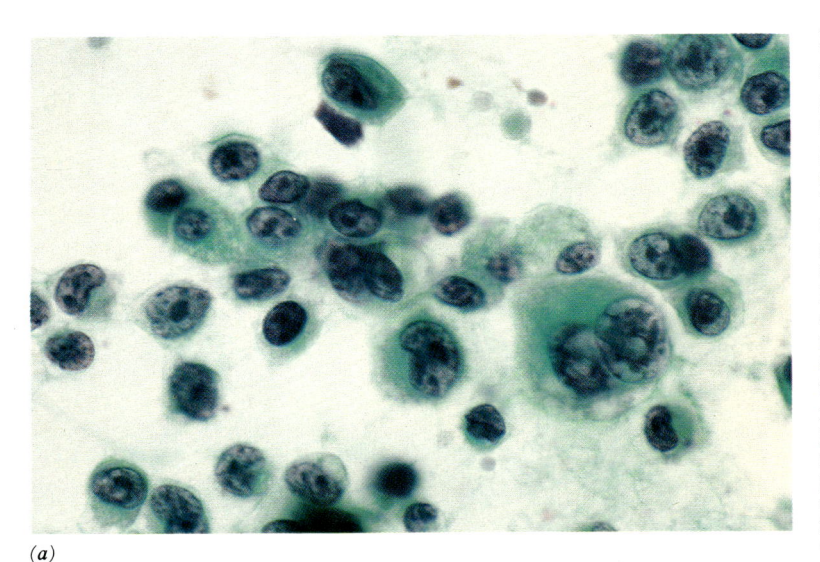

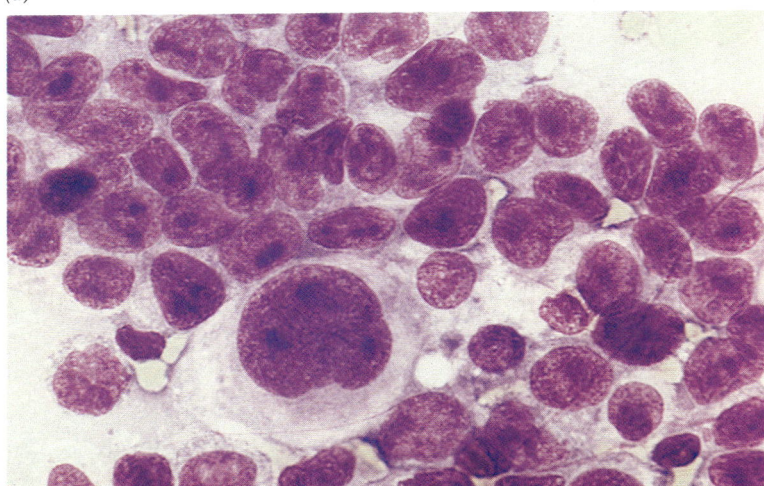

Fig. 2.39 Metastatic amelanotic melanoma

(a) Papanicolaou ×720 (b) MGG ×720: same specimen; another smear

Metastatic spread of extramammary cancer to the breast is exceedingly rare. The commonest source of metastatic deposits is primary carcinoma of the contralateral breast. Next most frequently seen is metastatic, non-Hodgkin's lymphoma, followed by oat cell carcinoma of the lung. A case of metastatic amelanotic melanoma is illustrated. Fluid aspirated from a fluctuant cystic mass in the breast of a young woman in the 28th week of pregnancy was found to contain pleomorphic malignant cells with prominent nucleoli and several mononuclear and binucleate large forms. The cells were unlike any of the usual variants of breast carcinoma generally seen. A history of an amelanotic melanoma on the back excised a year earlier was obtained. The solitary mass was resected and found to be a metastasis from the melanoma.

3. Respiratory tract

Exfoliative cytology of sputum and bronchial secretions for the diagnosis of bronchogenic carcinoma has a time-honoured history. Wider use of sophisticated interventional radiology and of the flexible fibre-optic bronchoscope which allows examination of the bronchial tree as far as the pulmonary parenchyma has increased the variety of diagnostic specimens obtainable and extended the scope of cytopathology.

The specimens selected and the sequence in which they are examined are determined by the presumptive pathology under investigation.

SAMPLING TECHNIQUES

Sputum

This *must* be an early morning 'deep cough' specimen from the lower respiratory tract, collected before food and drink, other than water, are taken and before the teeth are cleaned. As not every specimen is informative, it is common practice to examine three specimens, obtained on consecutive days; a persistent search may be indicated in cases in which invasive methods are contra-indicated. Sputum expectorated in the few days following bronchoscopy may contain diagnostic material, not previously identified.

The specimen is poured into a petri dish and examined for suggestive fragments such as opaque grey threads or blood-streaked strands. These are transferred to a glass slide, smeared and fixed.

Fibre-optic bronchoscopy specimens

Trap

Bronchopulmonary secretions are trapped in a tube interposed between the bronchoscope and a suction pump. The specimen is processed in the same manner as sputum.

Bronchial washings

10 ml of warm sterile buffered saline is introduced in small aliquots into the bronchi and reaspirated. Washings may be obtained from different bronchopulmonary segments. Smears are made from centrifugated deposit.

Broncho-alveolar lavage (BAL)

The tip of the bronchoscope is impacted in a peripheral bronchus. Two to three aliquots of 50–60 ml buffered saline are injected and reaspirated. Smears are made as from bronchial washings.

Bronchial brushings

These are collected following washings and biopsies. The brush can be extended beyond the tip of the scope and material obtained from a lesion not easily visualized or biopsied. Rapid fixation is essential to avoid dehydration and the smears are spread and fixed one at a time in the operating theatre.

Transbronchial biopsy

This is obtained at bronchoscopy with a fine needle introduced through the bronchial wall into adjacent lung tissue. The material obtained is usually sufficient for one or two smears.

Percutaneous fine needle aspiration (FNA)

The needle is introduced through locally anaesthetized skin and sub-cutaneous tissue into the lesion under imaging control. A syringe is attached to the needle which is moved in different directions whilst steady suction is applied. Resistance is met when tissue enters the needle lumen. At this point, the piston *must* be released to equalize pressure before the withdrawal of the needle. Smears are made immediately and may number up to ten or more. The syringe and needle are rinsed out in saline, or alcohol or a cell culture medium, this is held in reserve for analysis.

The recommendations laid down for the handling of class B pathogens should be observed in the processing of respiratory tract specimens.

Romanowsky stains are not satisfactory for sputum, trap and bronchial washings on account of their mucus content, and the Papanicolaou method is preferred by most cytopathologists. Both techniques are applicable to broncho-alveolar lavage and aspiration smears. In the author's laboratory, both methods are routinely employed and are found to be complementary.

Nasal secretions may be examined for eosinophils in allergic rhinitis and a maxillary sinus carcinoma may be identified in washings. Pharyngeal carcinoma may be scraped or brushed. Pathological lesions of the nasopharynx however are not commonly met with in routine diagnostic cytology and emphasis in this section has been laid on disorders of the lower respiratory tract.

RESPIRATORY TRACT 67

BENIGN CONDITIONS

Oral mucosa

Squamous cells from the upper respiratory tract are present in all respiratory trace specimens except transbronchial or percutaneous fine needle aspirations. In specimens from the lower respiratory tract, they are accompanied by macrophages and broncho-alveolar epithelial cells.

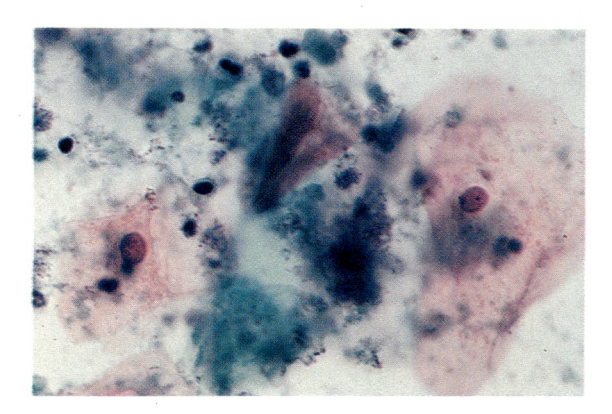

Fig. 3.1 Squamous cells
Papanicolaou ×525: saliva

A salivary specimen consists mainly of large polyhedral superficial squamous cells. Bacteria from the mouth and a few neutrophils are generally present; alveolar macrophages are conspicuous by their absence. Saliva is unsuitable for cytopathological assessment of diseases of the respiratory tract.

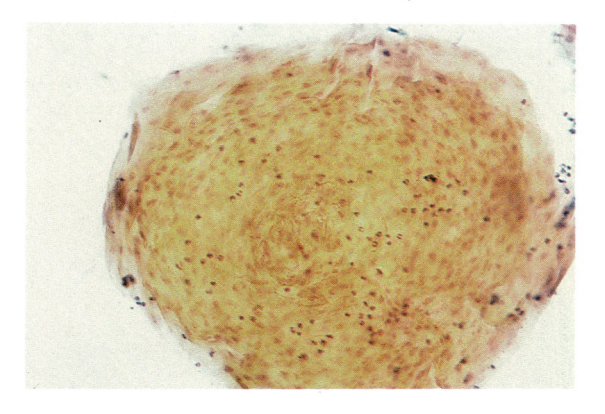

Fig. 3.2 Squamous cells
Papanicolaou ×133: bronchial washings

Instrumentation of the respiratory tract may dislodge a fragment of stratified squamous epithelium from the upper part of the tract. The tightly packed, normal squamous cells are identified by their large size, delicate translucent cytoplasm and the small regular nuclei.

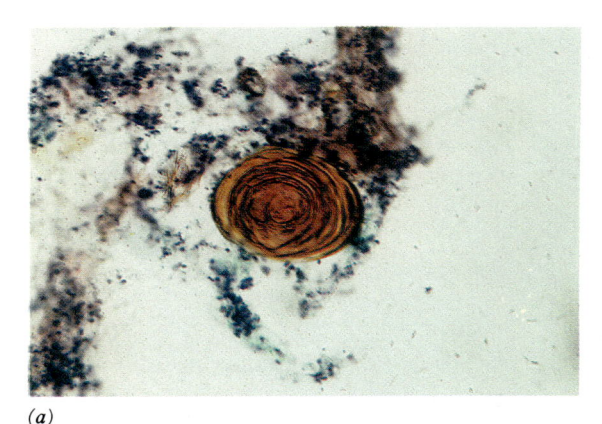

(a)

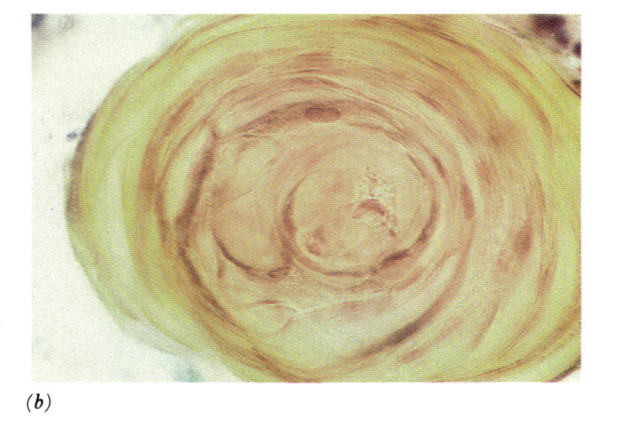

(b)

Fig. 3.3 Benign squamous pearl
Papanicolaou (a) ×133: bronchial washings (b) ×525: same field

Similarly dislodged hyperkeratotic epithelium may be arranged in a concentric manner and simulate a malignant epithelial pearl (a). At a higher magnification, the pearl is seen to consist of layers of anucleate keratinized cells rolled round intermediate squamous cells with bland nuclei and keratohyaline granules in the cytoplasm (b).

Respiratory epithelium

The respiratory epithelium lining the trachea and the major bronchi consists of ciliated columnar cells and mucus-secreting goblet cells. As the bronchi divide into smaller branches, the lining cells undergo a gradual transition into non-ciliated cuboidal cells; the goblet cells which are abundant in the trachea gradually diminish in number and are absent from the terminal bronchioles. A fourth type of cell which is non-ciliated and non-mucus secreting, the Clara cell, makes its appearance in the terminal bronchioles. It can be identified by its distinctive ultrastructure and is probably involved in the synthesis of surfactant. The aveolar epithelial lining has been shown by electron microscopy to consist of the type 1 pneumocyte which has an attenuated cytoplasm and which cannot be seen by light microscopy, and the type 2 pneumocyte, which is a rounded cell, the nucleus of which is visible by light microscopy. The type 2 pneumocyte may acquire phagocytic properties. Scattered through the bronchial mucosa is the endocrine Kultschitsky or Feyrter cell, characterised by neurosecretory dense core granules, derived from the APUD system.

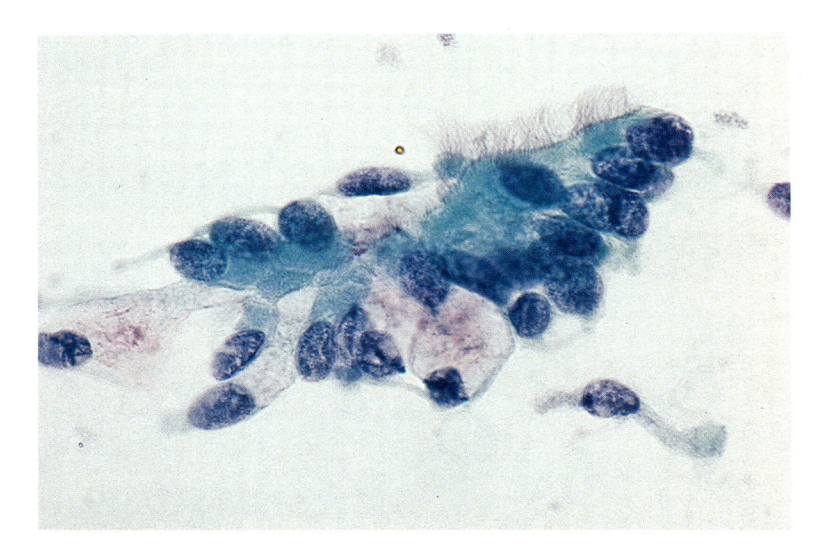

Fig. 3.4 Bronchial epithelial cells

Papanicolaou ×720: bronchial brush

This micrograph shows a sheet of normal bronchial mucosa. The ciliated broncho-epithelial cell is tall and slender. Its free luminal end has a clearly defined terminal bar or end plate to which the cilia are attached. The end anchored to the basement membrane tapers to a fine point or tail and gives the cell a pyramidal or triangular shape. The oval nucleus, nearer the apical end, is the same width as the cell and the lateral cell borders coincide with the lateral nuclear borders. The goblet cell is larger. Its cytoplasm is distended with secretory vacuoles and the nucleus lies at the base of the cell.

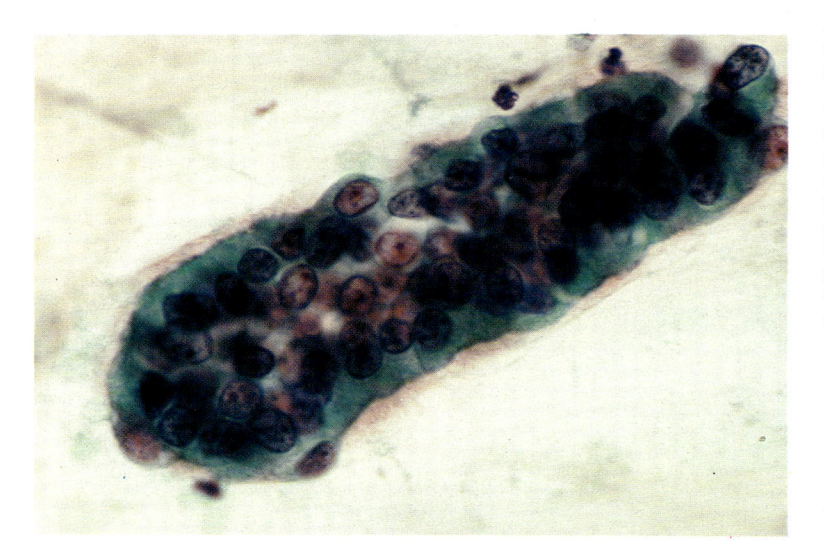

Fig. 3.5 Ciliated columnar cells

Papanicolaou ×720: sputum

Ciliated columnar cells may be shed in clusters, generally following mechanical or chemical irritation. The pseudopapillary arrangement seen here is due to a strip of bronchial epithelium being folded back on itself. Neither the arrangement nor the physiological variation in nuclear size is of significance.

RESPIRATORY TRACT 69

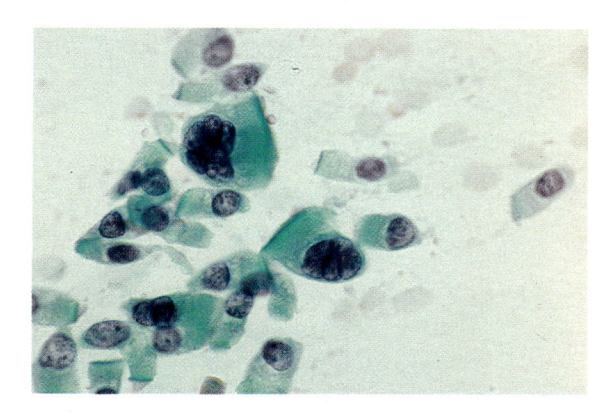

Fig. 3.6 Ciliated columnar cells
Papanicolaou ×525: bronchical brush

Multinucleated forms of ciliated bronchial cells are uncommon but normal. The cilia, being fragile, are easily lost; the cell type is nevertheless easily identified by the persistence of the end plate. Recognition of the end plate in a hypertrophic or otherwise morphologically abnormal cell can be of paramount diagnostic importance, as it is not elaborated by a malignant cell.

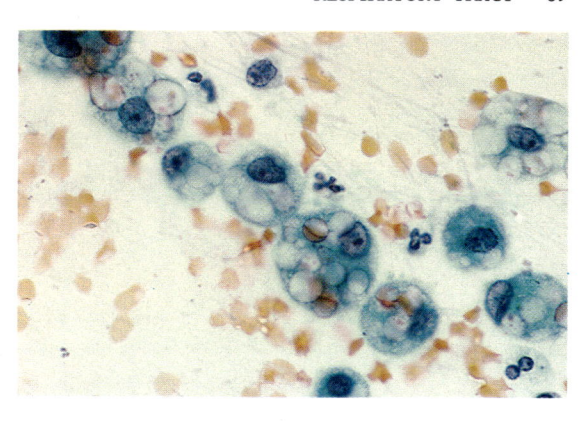

Fig. 3.7 Mucus-secreting goblet cells
Papanicolaou ×525: sputum

Goblet cells tend to become spheroidal when exfoliated into a fluid or semifluid secretion such as mucus. The cytoplasm is distended with single or multiple secretory mucous vacuoles. These are clearly outlined, often with a dark rim, have some depth of focus and not infrequently, indent the nucleus. Condensed mucus appears as an eosinophilic inclusion within the vacuole.

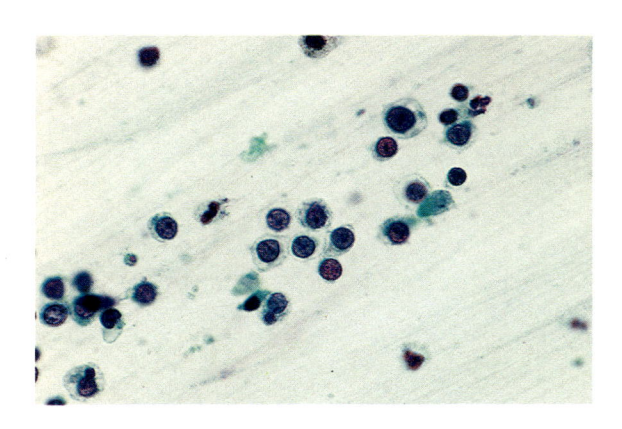

Fig. 3.8 Cuboidal bronchiolar cells
Papanicolaou ×525: sputum

The non-ciliated, non mucus-secreting cuboidal cells that line the smaller bronchi and bronchioles are not often exfoliated in sputum. They are a little larger than lymphocytes and have round nuclei surrounded by a narrow zone of transparent or translucent cytoplasm.

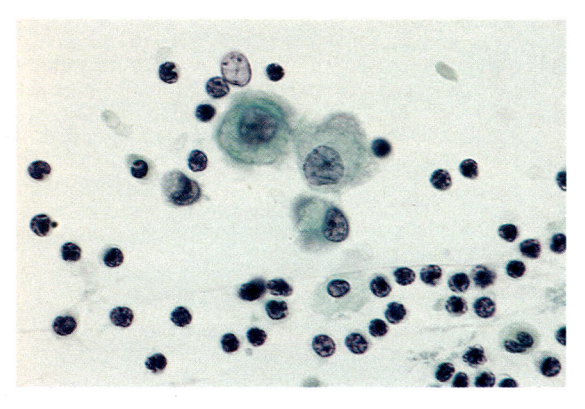

Fig. 3.9 Broncho-alveolar cells: Lymphocytes
Papanicolaou ×525: broncho-alveolar lavage

Moderately large cells with hypochromic nuclei and a fair amount of translucent cytoplasm are a feature of broncho-alveolar lavage specimens. The cells may be discrete or they may be attached to each other in the manner of epithelial lining cells. They also frequently contain phagocytosed inclusions and are probably the source of alveolar macrophages. The small cells are mature lymphocytes. The lavage specimen was from a patient with pulmonary sarcoidosis, a disease in which lymphocytes constitute a high proportion of cells in the alveoli.

Macrophages

The presence of alveolar macrophages is mandatory for the identification of a deep cough sputum suitable for cytology. Microscopic examination is necessary to establish this fact as not every mucoid specimen is derived from the lower respiratory tract, nor every thin watery specimen merely saliva. Indeed, small cell carcinoma of the lung is occasionally associated with thin, clear secretions. Alveolar macrophages are frequently present in bronchial brush and fine needle aspiration smears, but their presence in these specimens is not essential.

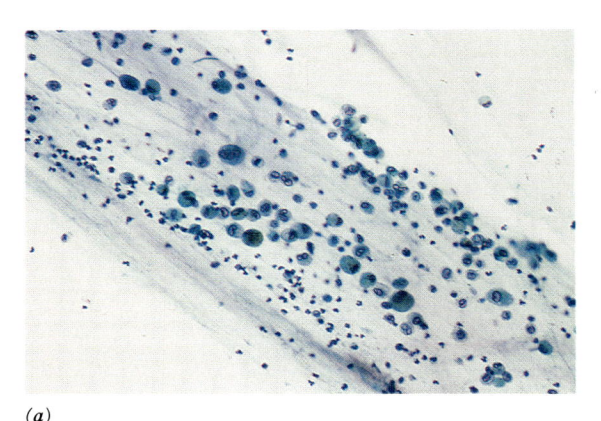

(a) (b)

Fig. 3.10 Pulmonary alveolar macrophages: anthracotic macrophages

Papanicolaou (a) ×133: sputum (b) ×525: same field

Macrophages are usually seen in streaks against a background of mucus, accompanied by neutrophils. As a rule, they are round and the average size approximates to that of a rounded goblet cell. The nuclei, usually eccentric, are remarkable for wide variations in shape and size; they may be round, oval, indented or lobulated. Each nucleus has one or more small nucleoli. The cytoplasm is finely vacuolated and foamy. Phagocytosed material, most notably, black carbon is a common feature (anthracotic macrophage). However, not all macrophages contain inclusions.

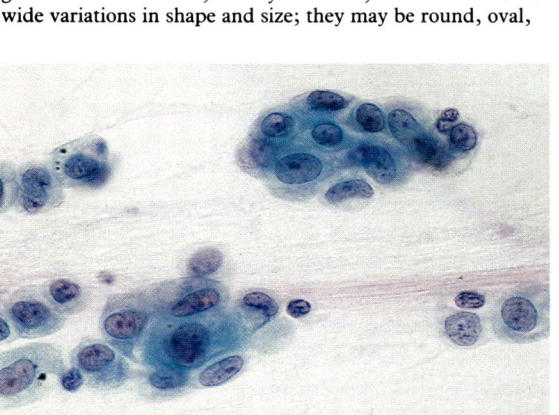

Fig. 3.11 Cohesive alveolar macrophages

Papanicolaou ×525: sputum

Whereas macrophages derived from blood monocytes are always discrete and generally smaller, pulmonary macrophages often appear in cohesive sheets and resemble epithelial cells. The presence of phagocytosed particles identifies the histiocytic nature of the cells illustrated. Compare these with the broncho-alveolar cells in Figure 3.9. The similarities in cytoplasmic texture and nuclear characteristics support the hypothesis that some of the pulmonary macrophages are derived from the type 2 alveolar cell.

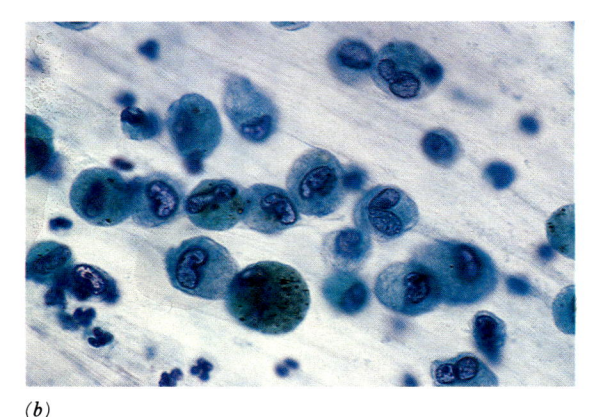

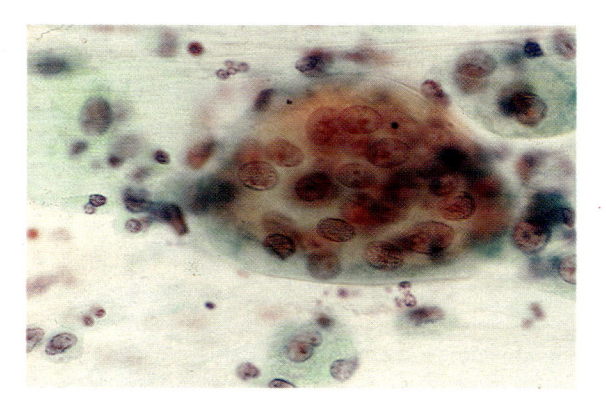

Fig. 3.12 Multinucleated macrophages

Papanicolaou ×525: sputum

Giant multinucleated epithelioid macrophages are present in a wide variety of benign pulmonary disorders, particularly granulomatous lesions. Since they also occur in the absence of such diseases, their presence in a respiratory tract cytology specimen is non-contributory to any consistently reliable diagnosis.

RESPIRATORY TRACT 71

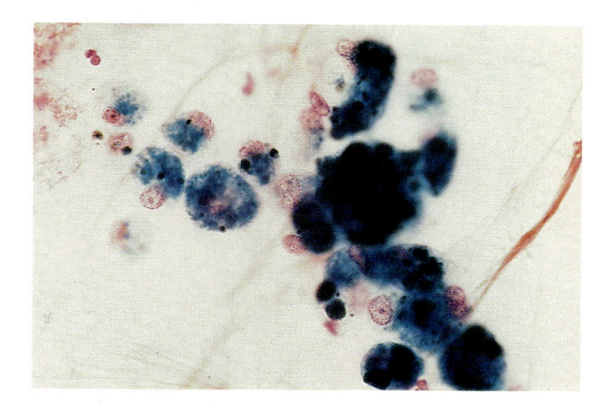

Fig. 3.13 Iron-laden macrophages: siderophages
Perl's Prussian blue ×525: sputum

Macrophages which have ingested haemosiderin released by the lysis of erythrocytes (siderophages) contain iron pigment which can be correctly identified with an appropriate stain, such as Prussian blue. Their presence in a respiratory tract specimen is indicative of either past intrathoracic bleeding or extravasation of red blood cells into the alveoli due to a sluggish blood flow as in congestive cardiac failure; hence they are referred to as heart failure cells. Large numbers of siderophages are seen in Goodpasture's syndrome, a condition in which anti-glomerular membrane nephritis is associated with pulmonary haemorrhage. The presence of siderophages together with considerable extra-cellular haemosiderin is of considerable value in establishing a diagnosis of the rare disorder, idiopathic pulmonary haemosiderosis.

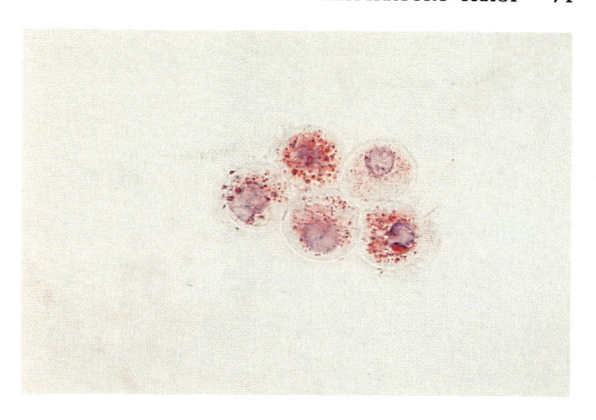

Fig. 3.14 Fat-laden macrophages: lipophages
Sudan III (oil scarlet) ×525: tracheal suckings

Macrophages containing many fat globules have been reported in lipoid pneumonia. Their presence in carefully collected bronchial suckings from neonates suspected to have aspiration pneumonia has proved useful in the author's laboratory. Once again, in order to establish the true nature of the diagnostic inclusions, the use of specific stains such as oil scarlet or Sudan black is mandatory. A duplicate smear from which the fat has been extracted by exposure to a lipid solvent such as chloroform acts as a control.

Obstructive airway disease

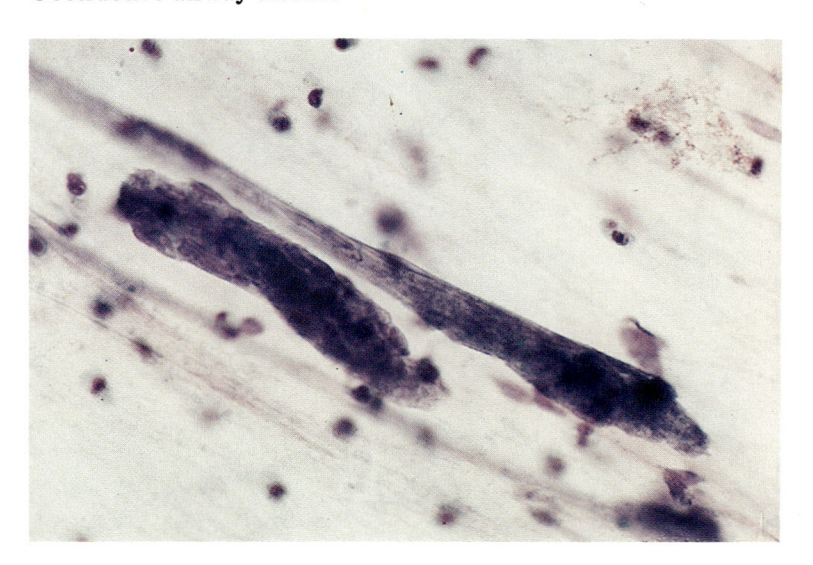

Fig. 3.15 Mucus
Papanicolaou ×720: sputum

Mucus derived from goblet cells is present in every respiratory tract specimen, as a thin film or in small streaks. Mucosal oedema in acute asthma and marked mucous gland hyperplasia in chronic bronchitis and asthma result in excess mucus production; the problem is compounded by loss of ciliary activity. The sputum of such subjects generally has few cells and consists mainly of thick irregular masses of viscid mucus showing varying degrees of inspissation.

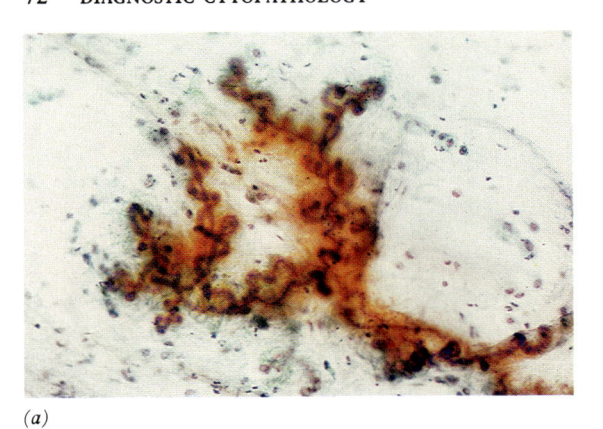

72 DIAGNOSTIC CYTOPATHOLOGY

(a)

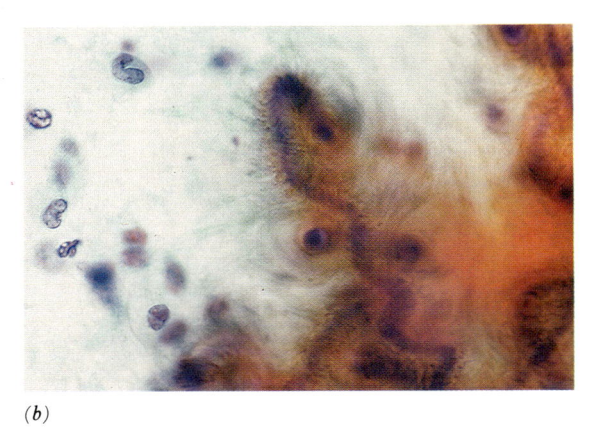

(b)

Fig. 3.16 Curschmann spiral

Papanicolaou (a) ×133: sputum (b) ×525: same field

Inspissated mucus plugging the smaller bronchi forms a complex branching spiral or corkscrew-shaped cast known as the Curschmann spiral; such a structure is diagnostic of bronchial obstruction and is very common in sputum from cases of obstructive airway disease. Malignant cells should be looked for in the more feathery part of the mucus that fans out from the dense central axis of a Curshmann spiral when a neoplasm is the suspected cause of bronchial occlusion.

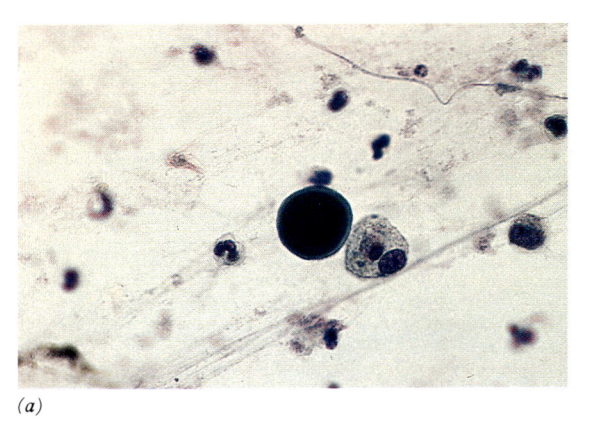

(a)

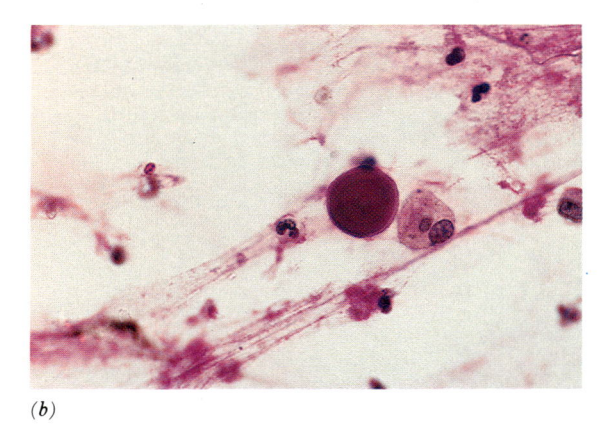

(b)

Fig. 3.17 Corpora amylacea

(a) Papanicolaou ×525: bronchial washing (b) PAS ×525: same field

Small structures composed of concentric rings of varying density may be formed in the broncho-pulmonary passages (a). One of these, the corpora amylacea, is composed mainly of glycoproteins which give a positive reaction with PAS (b). There is some uncertainty about the origin of this structure. In view of its positive reaction with PAS, it seems likely that it is an organised form of inspissated mucus.

RESPIRATORY TRACT 73

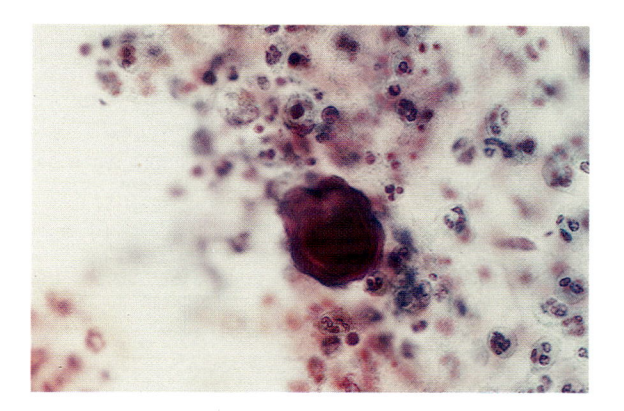

Fig. 3.18 Calcospherite (psammoma body)
Papanicolaou ×525: sputum

The terms calcospherite and psammoma body are considered to be synonymous. Somewhat similar in structure to the corpora amylacea but dissimilar in its chemical composition, the calcospherite consists of various minerals. These bodies are commonly formed when the minerals, mainly calcium, are deposited in degenerating tips of tumour tissue. They are also seen in large numbers in the extremely rare condition, pulmonary alveolar microlithiasis. The structure illustrated was non-reactive with PAS

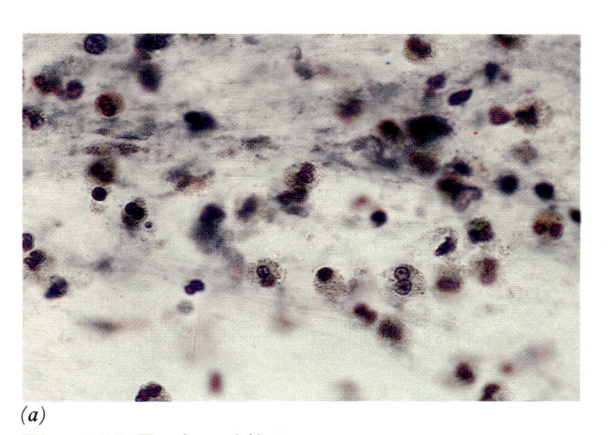

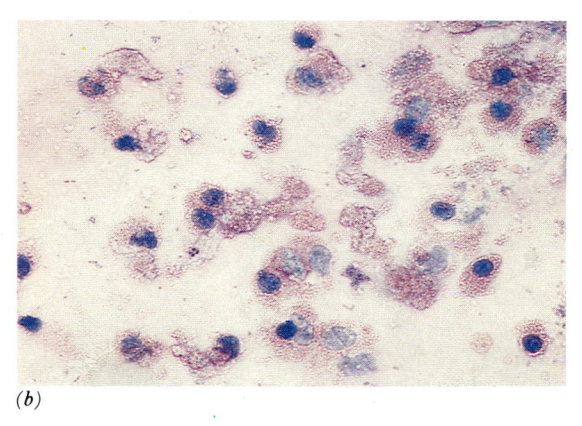

(a) (b)

Fig. 3.19 Eosinophils
(a) Papanicolaou ×525: sputum (b) Hansel's stain ×525: sputum; another specimen

Eosinophils in respiratory tract specimens are usually associated with a component of hypersensitivity. These include chronic bronchitis with or without wheezing, Wegner's granuloma, primary pulmonary eosinophilia, helminthic infections, some types of interstitial airway disease and, occasionally, malignant tumours. However, by far the commonest cause of pulmonary eosinophilia is bronchial asthma. A high percentage of eosinophils in sputum is of considerable value in discriminating bronchial asthma which causes reversible airway disease from the irreversible type caused by chronic bronchitis.

The characteristic bi-lobed 'pair of spectacles' nucleus of the eosinophil is easily recognised, but the less mature mononuclear eosinophil, often seen in sputum in asthma, is difficult to identify in a smear stained by the Papanicolaou method (a). Correct identification is facilitated by the use of special stains such as a Romanowsky stain, carbol chromatrobe, and Hansel's stain (composed of methylene blue and eosin) which highlight the specific granules of this polymorphonuclear leucocyte (b).

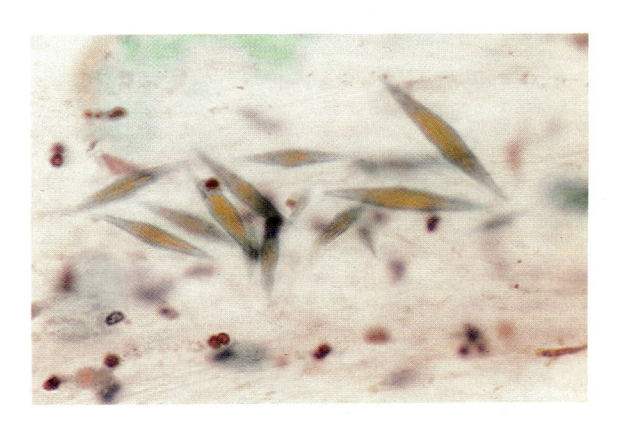

Fig. 3.20 Charcot-Leyden crystals
Papanicolaou ×525: sputum

The cell membrane of the eosinophil contains several enzymes. One of these, lysolecithinase (together with phospholipase A and D) spontaneously forms rhomboid-shaped structures termed Charcot-Leyden crystals. Often associated with intact eosinophils, the crystals may persist when the eosinophils have disintegrated, and remain the only clear indication of an allergic condition. With the Papanicolaou stain, they are bright orange and sometimes have green borders and apices.

Pneumoconioses

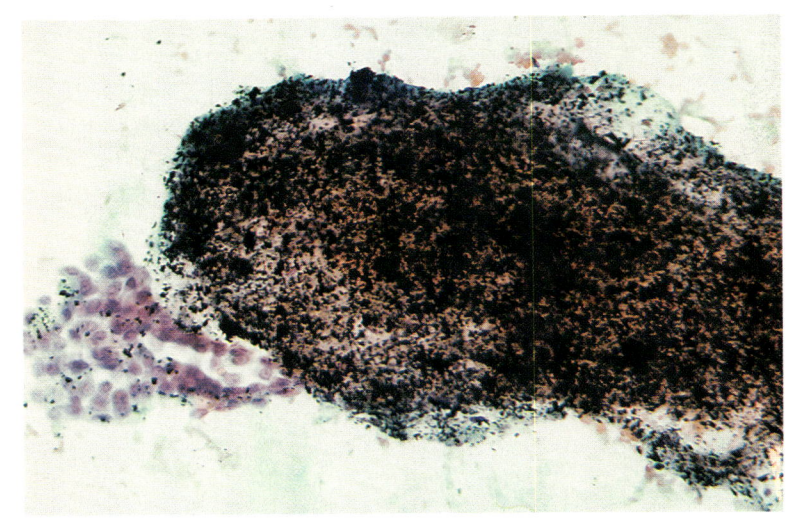

Fig. 3.21 Coal miner's lung
Papanicolaou ×183: FNA; lung

Exposure to silica dust which cannot be seen in routine cytological and histological preparations is an occupational hazard of miners. Chronic irritation by the inhalant provokes a multifocal fibrotic reaction; the alveoli and the aveolar macrophages are filled with black-staining carbon.

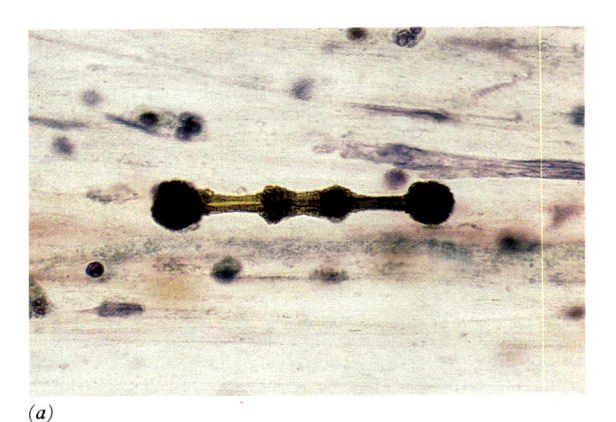

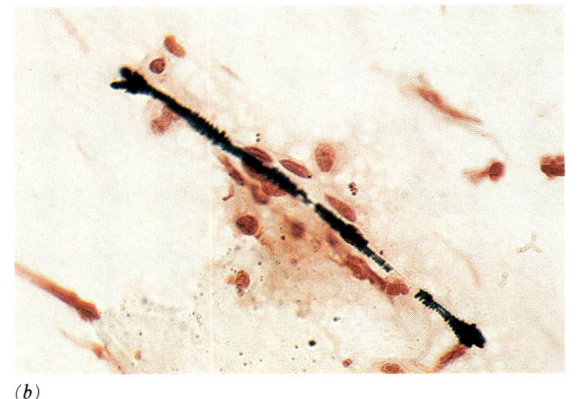

(a) (b)

Fig. 3.22 Ferruginous body: asbestos body
(a) Papanicolaou ×525: sputum (b) Perl's Prussian blue ×525: same specimen; another smear

A variety of long, needle-like mineral fibres inhaled into the lung become coated with proteinaceous material derived from bronchial secretions. Contraction of the bronchial muscles as the coated fibre is propelled forward is believed to produce the curious coiled structure with transverse corrugations and club-shaped ends. Haemosiderin is gradually incorporated into the coat and gives the ferruginous body a typical golden brown colour (a). The iron in the haemosiderin is specifically stained by Perl's method (b). Note that the fibre is clearly visible where it has not yet acquired the proteinaceous coat (b). Ferruginous bodies were formerly known as asbestos bodies in the belief that the reaction was specific to asbestos, a complex silicate. While this is now known not to be the case, asbestos remains the most significant source of the fibres to result in the formation of these structures. Exposure to the uncommon blue asbestos is the main aetiological factor in the causation of mesothelioma, and exposure to the common white asbestos when coupled with cigarette smoking plays a major role in the development of bronchogenic carcinoma.

Flora and fauna

Investigation and confirmation of the common bacterial and viral infections of the respiratory tract generally lie within the province of a microbiologist. Some parasitic infestations and primary mycoses of the lung have, however, been successfully diagnosed by sputum, bronchoscopic and aspiration cytology.

The immunosuppressed host is particularly prone to pulmonary complications with high morbidity and mortality rates. Accurate diagnosis and prompt treatment are essential in such a life-threatening situation, and in recent years, identification of several of the opportunistic infective agents has been added to the cytopathologist's more traditional role of diagnosing malignant disease. Some of the pathogenic fungi, such as Histoplasma, Coccidioides, and Blastomyces are common in the Americas, but virtually unknown in Europe. The reader is referred to specialist literature on these. The pathogenic and opportunist infective agents met with in the author's laboratory are illustrated below.

Fig. 3.23 Mycobacterium tuberculosis
Ziehl-Neelsen ×1144: FNA; lung

The acid-fast bacilli shown in this micrograph were recovered from a patient with a lung mass; the differential diagnosis included pulmonary tuberculosis and primary carcinoma. The organism was subsequently identified as *M. tuberculosis* by culture studies. Since saprophytic varieties of mycobacterium found in water and soil and the avian type may act as opportunists in man, laboratory investigation of pulmonary complications in an immunodeficient subject should include a search for acid-fast bacilli. The tubercle bacillus may appear as a slender rod or it may be finely beaded.

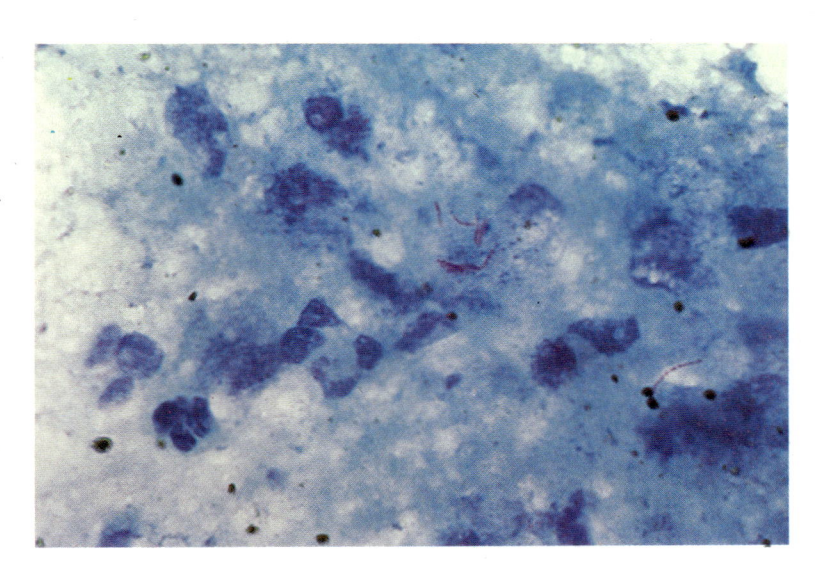

Fig. 3.24 Nocardia
Papanicolaou ×720: FNA; lung

Nocardia is an aerobic member of the actinomyces family which has a filamentous appearance, but is, in fact, a bacterium. The two strains responsible for human nocardiosis are *N. asteroides* and *N. brasiliensis*. The disease may, rarely, be primary, but is more frequently an opportunistic infection. Actinomycetes-like organisms may colonize the mouth and their presence in a sputum or bronchoscopic specimen is of no significance. The lung aspirate illustrated was obtained from a middle-aged man with an immunodeficiency state consequent on alcohol abuse.

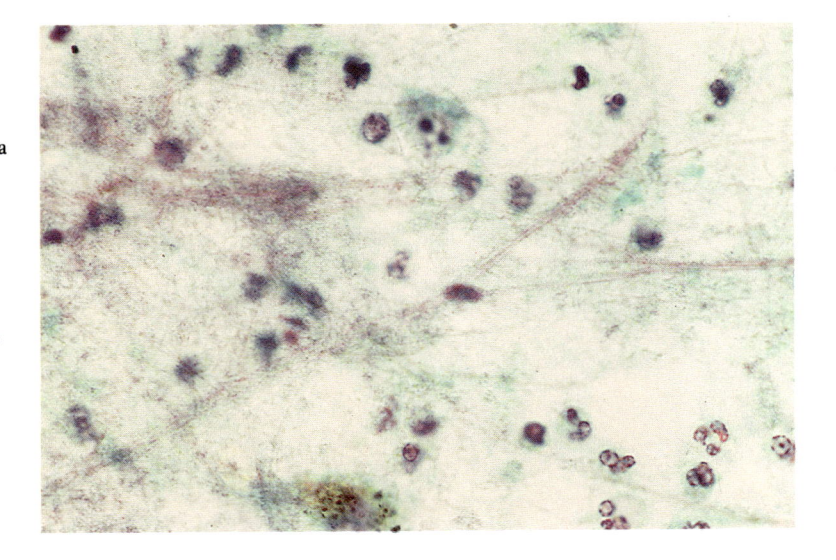

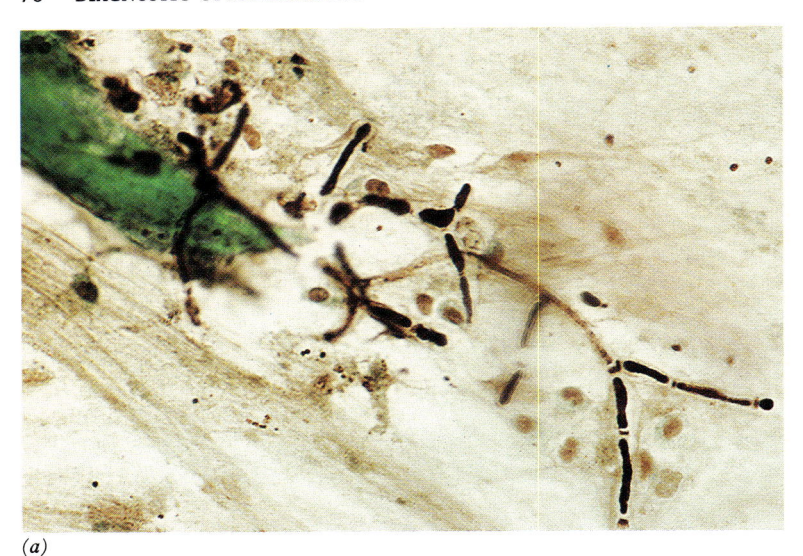

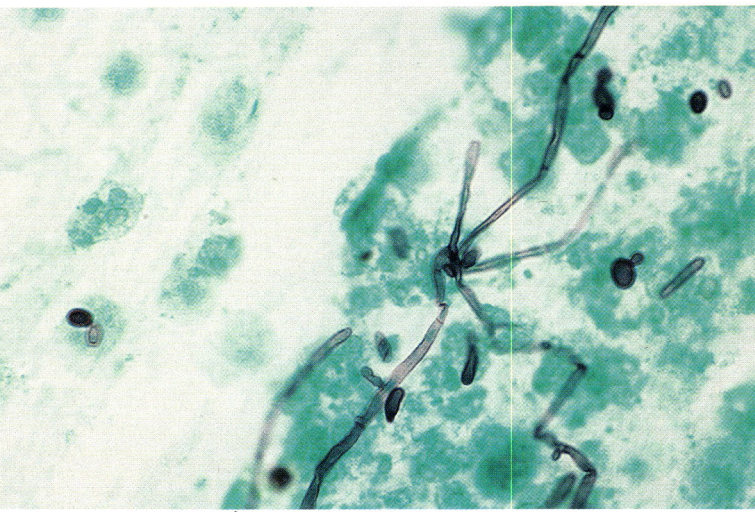

Fig. 3.25 Candida spp.

Grocott's silver methanamine (a) ×720: sputum; C. albicans (b) ×720: broncho-alveolar lavage; C. parapsilosis

Candidiasis is the most wide-spread of mycotic diseases. Muco-cutaneous and cutaneous infections are common, systemic infections less so. Primary pulmonary candidiasis is rare, but secondary infections of the lower respiratory tract are frequent in immunocompromised subjects and in patients with some other primary lung disease such as neoplasm, tuberculosis, bacterial or viral pnuemonia.

The most common pathogenic species is *Candida albicans*, one of the natural flora of the body. The other species are essentially saprophytes, but opportunistic infections are caused by *C. glabrata, C. guilliermondi, C. krusei, C. parapsilosis* and *C. tropicalis*.

C. glabrata consists only of yeast forms. All the other species form blastospores, pseudohyphae and true hyphae. A blastospore is a round or oval asexual spore, 3–5 mm in diameter, produced by budding of the yeast cell or along a hypha. A psuedohypha is a filament like chain of successive blastospores that elongate, but do not separate. The hypha is the vegetative filament that makes up the body of the fungus. The hyphae of the Candida species are septate and branch freely in various directions.

The clinical significance of Candida in a respiratory tract specimen requires fine judgement. Candida seen in sputum frequently comes from the mouth and must on no account be taken to indicate bronchopulmonary infection. The sputum sample shown in (a) came from a young woman with Legionnaire's disease and oral and vulvovaginal Candidiasis acquired prior to the respiratory tract infection.

In the case illustrated in (b), the Candida sp. present in the broncho-alveolar lavage of an immunodeficient patient treated for leukaemia with a bone marrow transplant indicates opportunistic Candidiasis. Culture of the lavage specimen yielded a growth of *C. parapsilosis*.

Fig. 3.26 Aspergillus fumigatus

*Papanicolaou (a) ×183: sputum
(b) ×720: same field*

Four types of pulmonic infections are caused by the Aspergillus species, three are invasive, one is non-invasive. Primary invasive infection is rare, but may occur in a normal individual subjected to a massive exposure of the fungus. A sensitized individual may develop primary allergic broncho-pulmonary aspergillosis. Secondary invasive infection is common in a immunodeficient or debilitated host. Non-invasive colonization of a pre-existing cavity results in an Aspergilloma or fungus-ball. Most cases of aspergillosis are caused by *A. fumigatus*, some are due to *A. flavus*, *A. niger* and *A. terreus*.

Colonization of the upper respiratory tract by this fungus can occur but is extremely rare. The presence of Aspergillus in a sample of sputum is consequently of clinical significance.

The fungus is seen as a tangled mycelium formed by hyphae which show characteristic dichotomous branching at about 45°. Secondary and tertiary branches radiating in one direction create the typical sun-burst pattern or the actinomycetoid form. The hyphae are septate, fairly uniform and between 4–6 μm wide. Variable staining of the hyphae is due to alterations of rapid and slow growth phases.

The diagnostic feature that absolutely identifies Aspergillus is the fruiting head from which the fungus derives its name (Aspergillus: a kind of brush used to sprinkle holy water). A stalk arises from a specialised cell, the foot cell, of the mycelium, the stalk expands at its upper end to form a club-shaped vesicle; peg-like structures develop from fertile areas of the vesicle to give rise to unbranched chains of conidia. The vesicle and the conidia constitute the fruiting head or conidiophore, which requires air for its development. It may be seen in an Aspergilloma in an aerated cavity, but does not develop in invasive aspergillosis. Calcium oxalate crystals, which are birefrigent by polarised light, may be formed from oxalic acid produced by the fungus.

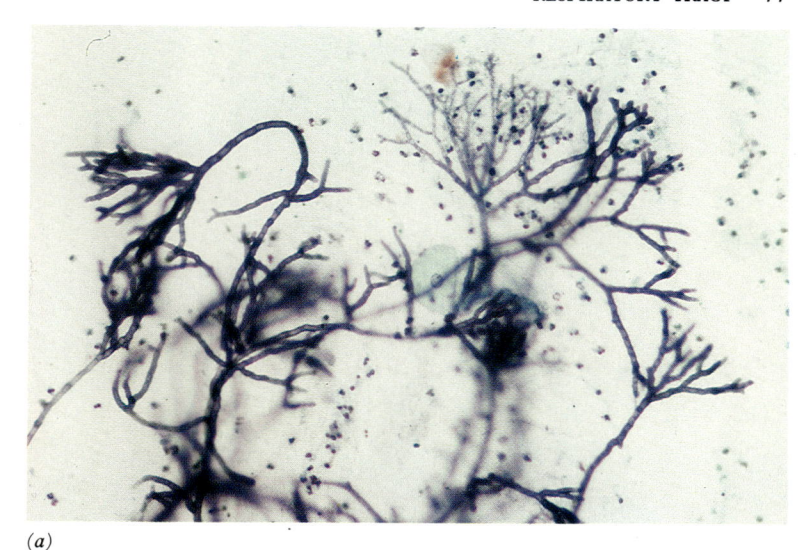

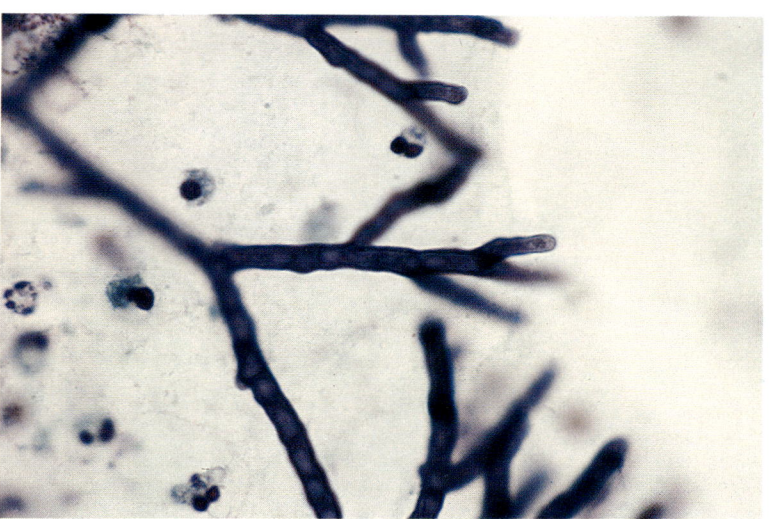

78 DIAGNOSTIC CYTOPATHOLOGY

(a)

(b)

(c)

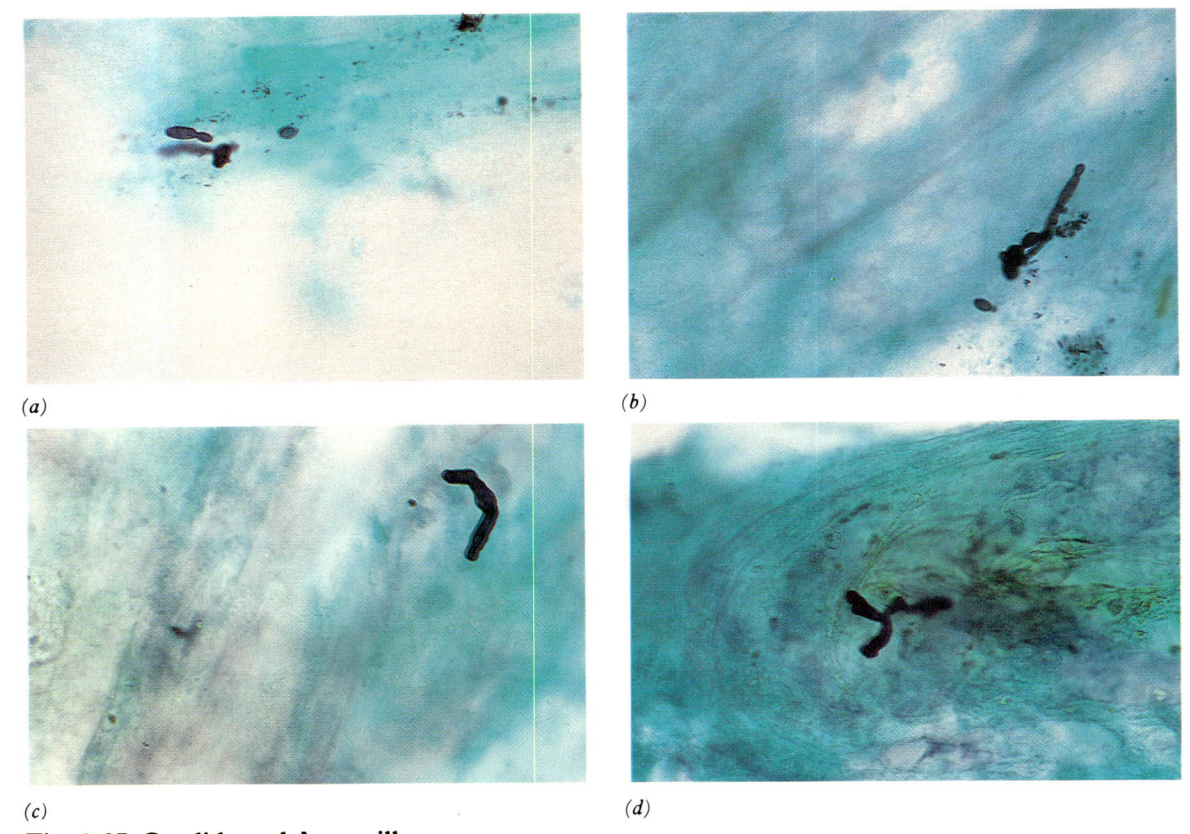

(d)

Fig. 3.27 Candida and Aspergillus

Grocott's silver methanamine (a) ×525: sputum; Candida albicans (b) same smear as (a) (c) ×525: sputum; Aspergillus (d) same smear as (c)

Aspergillus is, as a rule, easily recognized by its dichotomous branching, but may, on occasion, be confused with other fungi that form hyphae, one of which is Candida. Both fungi were present in the sputum of a patient who developed an allergic broncho-pulmonary condition of sudden and rapid onset.

Candida albicans was isolated from the sputum and although there was no clinical evidence of oral Candidiasis, its pathogenicity could not be assumed. The serum IgE was markedly elevated and precipitins to Aspergillus were present.

Compare the Candida in (a) and (b) with the Aspergillus (c) and (d). The Candida is seen in the form of blastospores (a) and (b) and pseudohyphae (b), neither of which is formed by the Aspergillus spp. Note also the budding blastospore at the segmental line of the hypha (b); this is another characteristic of Candida and is never seen in Aspergillus. The latter consists of a thicker septate hypha (c) and shows dichotomous branching (d).

RESPIRATORY TRACT 79

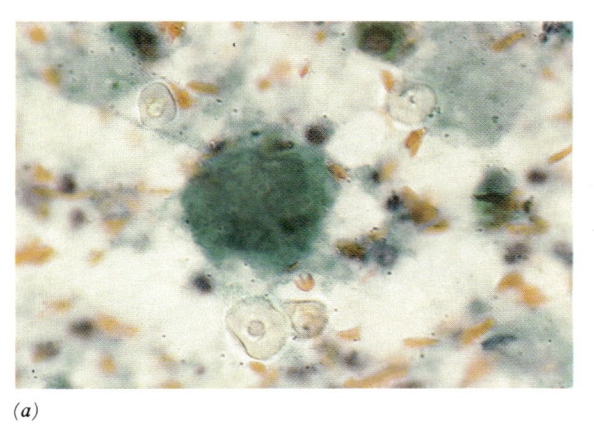

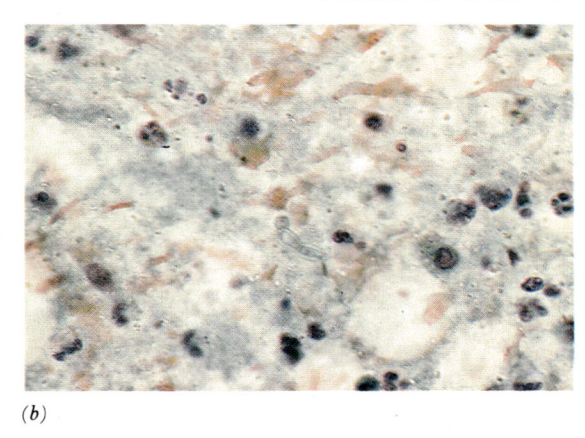

(a) (b)

Fig. 3.28 Cryptococcus neoformans
Papanicolaou ×525 (a) FNA: lung; capsulated budding yeasts (b) same smear; another field; pseudo-hypha

The lung is the principal portal of entry for the yeast *C. neoformans* found in the excreta of birds, particularly the pigeon. The primary lesion may consist of sub-pleural fibrotic nodules, a single large solid granulomatous lesion known as cryptococcoma, or a cavitating lesion. Occasionally, the yeast causes miliary disease with blood-borne dissemination. Cryptococcal meningitis is frequently the first manifestation of infection.

In the case of a cryptococcoma such as the one shown, large numbers of the yeasts are seen in extra-cellular collections or within giant cells. The individual yeast is round or has a single bud and is surrounded by a capsule which does not stain with the Papanicolaou stain or H & E (a). The capsule contains mucopolysaccharides and can be demonstrated by mucin stains (see Fig. 5.9). *C. neoformans* does not form hyphae in tissues or culture but pseudohyphal forms consisting of short chains of elongated buds occur (b).

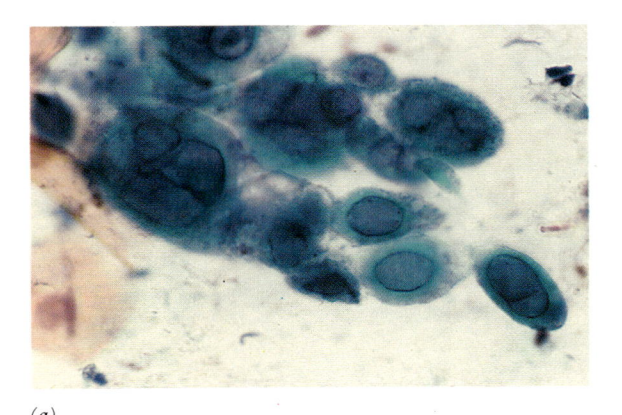

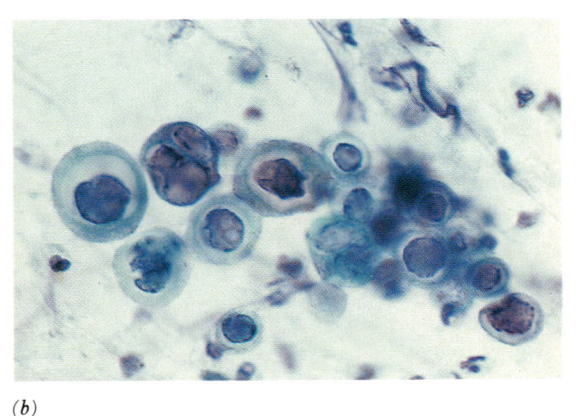

(a) (b)

Fig. 3.29 Herpesvirus simplex (HVS)
Papanicolaou ×525 (a) sputum (b) bronchial washings; another case

The cytopathic effects of herpesvirus simplex, a DNA virus, are seen characteristically in the nucleus; the cytoplasm shows non-specific degenerative changes. The nucleus is filled with homogenous inclusions and acquires a 'ground glass' appearance; a heavy deposit of chromatin on the margin sharply defines its outline. A dense intranuclear inclusion, seen in the occasional cell (a) or not at all (b) in the early stages of infection, is usually present in the majority of cells in later stages or in recurrent infections. The number of nuclei varies from one to several; in the multinucleated cells, the nuclei adjoin and typically mould one another (a).

The diagnostic relevance of herpesvirus cytopathia has to be assessed with reference to the clinical status of the patient and the type of specimen. Superficial muco-cutaneous lesions are not uncommon in susceptible subjects and are of little clinical significance. The sputum specimen illustrated in (a) came from a man with bronchopneumonia and herpetic vesicles round the lip margin. There was no evidence of viral involvement of the lower respiratory tract.

Immuno-compromised and debilitated individuals, on the other hand, are more susceptible to tracheo-bronchial and pulmonary infections. A bronchial wash specimen from an elderly woman with bilateral pneumonia and respiratory failure which required intensive therapy is shown in (b). There were no vesicles on the lips or the oropharyngeal mucosa; herpetic infection of the tracheo-bronchial mucosa was suggested by the cytopathic effects seen in sheets of bronchial mucosal cells.

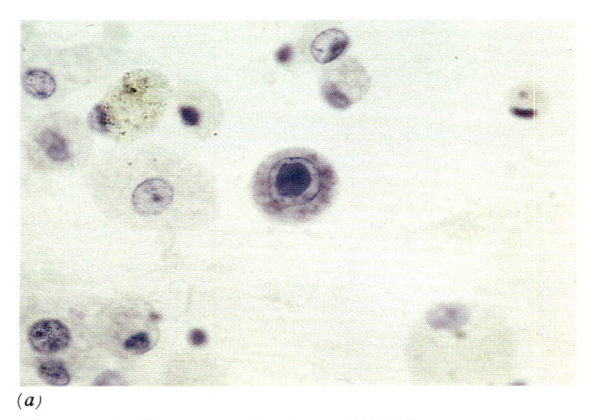

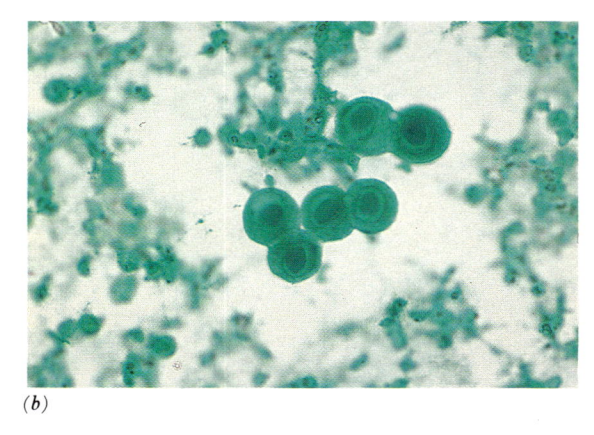

Fig. 3.30 Cytomegalovirus (CMV)

(a) Papanicolaou ×525: broncho-alveolar lovage (b) Grocott's silver methanamine ×525: broncho-alveolar lavage; another case

The diagnostic feature of infection with the cytomegalovirus, a member of the Herpes family of viruses, is the presence of a large intranuclear inclusion surrounded by a clear halo. A punctate deposit of chromatin marks the outline of the ghost nucleus. The fine intracytoplasmic inclusions seen in (a) are not always evident. The intranuclear inclusion is basophilic with the Papanicolaou stain (a), green or black with silver methanamine (b). It is neither necessary nor customary to use a silver stain to demonstrate CMV. However, familiarity with this appearance is useful, as CMV is often associated with pneumocystis carinii which is best demonstrated by the Grocott method. This broncho-alveolar lavage was from a 21-year-old woman with leukaemia, who had received a bone marrow transplant.

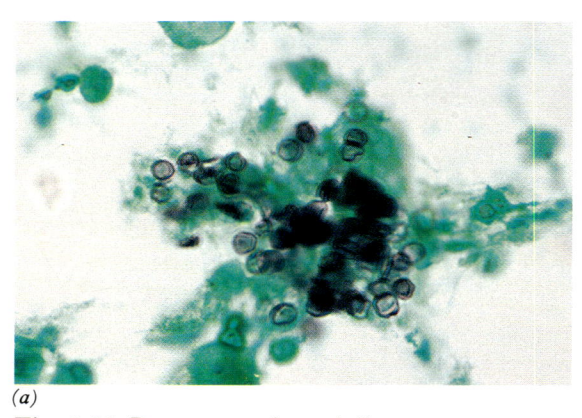

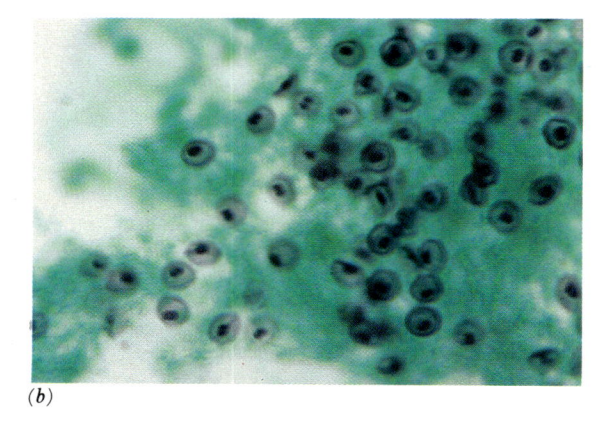

Fig. 3.31 Pneumocystis carinii

Grocott's silver methanamine (a) ×525: broncho-alveolar lavage; same case as in Fig. 3.30 (b) ×832: broncho-alveolar lavage; another case

The parasite, Pneumocystis carinii, has long been known to cause chronic interstitial pneumonia in premature and malnourished infants. It has become increasingly important in recent years, as a common opportunistic pathogen in subjects of all ages whose immune mechanism is deficient. The deficiency may be due to congenital causes, acquired immune deficiency syndrome (AIDS), malignant disease particularly that of lymphoid cells, or it may be iatrogenic for purposes of organ transplant or cytotoxic therapy.

The parasite is difficult to discern in sputum and by the Papanicolaou, H & E and PAS methods. It is more often recovered from transbronchial and percutaneous needle aspirations and is more easily identified by Grocott's method. The specimen of first choice, due to its negligible morbidity, is broncho-alveolar lavage.

Pneumocystis has not been completely classified but is considered to be a protozoon, Class Sporozoa. By the Grocott method, it is seen as a thin-walled black cyst, round or crescentic. Within the cyst are the trophozoites, 1–6 in number; these may be close to or applied to the cyst wall, when they resemble Barr bodies (a). In some preparations, the trophozoites are close together in the centre of the cyst and resemble a very small safety pin (b). The cyst wall collapses when the trophozoites are extruded (a).

The parasites illustrated in (a) are from the same case with CMV shown in Figure 3.30. The lavage specimen show in (b) came from a male who presented with atypical pneumonia and was found to have serum antibodies to HTLV III.

RESPIRATORY TRACT 81

Fig. 3.32 Pneumocystis carinii and Candida spp.

Grocott's silver methanamine ×720: broncho-alveolar lavage

Multiple opportunistic infections are by no means rare. *P. carinii*, as shown above, is often associated with CMV. In the case of AIDS illustrated here, large numbers of parasites were seen side by side with equally large numbers of budding yeasts and pseudohyphae. The many amorphous black irregular structures are contaminants, mainly talc granules.

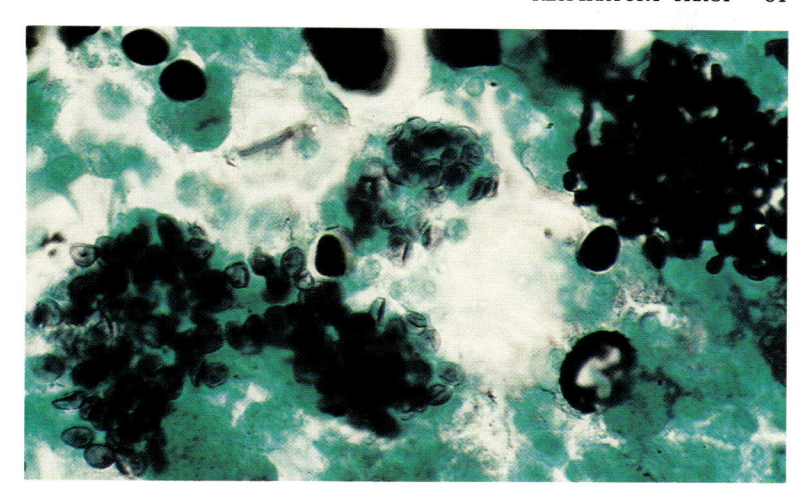

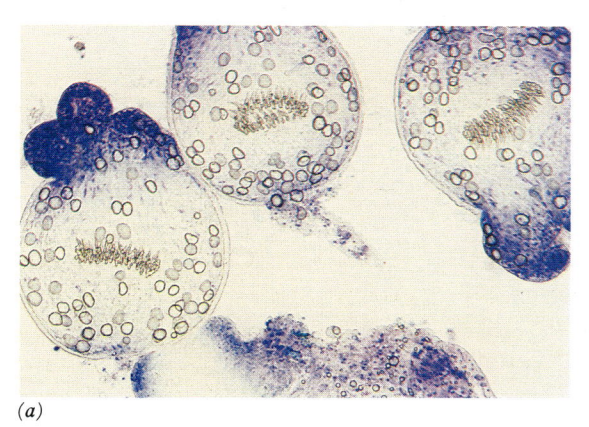

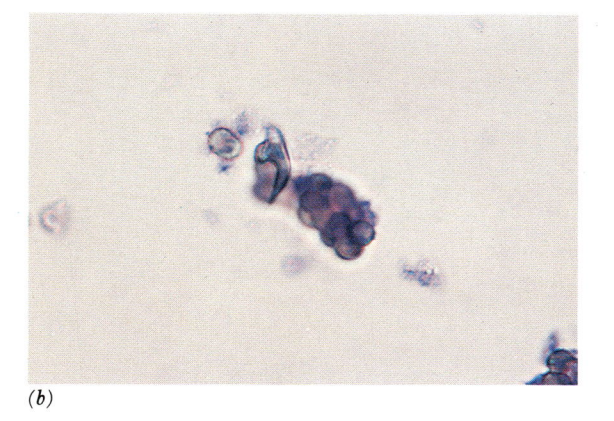

(a) (b)

Fig. 3.33 Echinococcus granulosus (Hydatid)

Methylene blue (a) ×133: hydatid cyst fluid; scolices (b) ×525: same specimen; another preparation; hooklets

The causative agent of hydatid disease is Echinococcus granulosus, a 5 mm long tapeworm which has a head, a neck and three proglottides. The dog and other canines act as definitive hosts, harbour the adult worm in the jejunum and excrete numerous eggs. The usual intermediate hosts are sheep, cattle and camels. Man becomes an intermediate host, usually in childhood, by ingesting eggs present in contaminated food and water, or in faecal dust on the coats of dogs. The embryo (onchosphere) is liberated in the stomach and upper small intestine, penetrates the bowel mucosa and enters the portal circulation. From here it is carried to the liver (50%), lung (25%) and bone, brain, kidney and other organs. The larva forms a typical cystic structure with an external laminated wall and an inner nucleated germinal layer. Brood capsules and second and third generation daughter cysts develop from the germinal layer and in turn give rise to the scolex or head. This has a distinctive structure with four sucking discs and a circlet of hooklets. Hydatid sand found in cyst fluid consists of scolices from ruptured brood capsules.

Leakage of hydatid cyst fluid into tissues and body cavities is likely to induce anaphylactic shock and aspiration of a suspected hydatid cyst is contra-indicated. The case illustrated was aspirated with care at thoracotomy.

Micrograph (a) shows typical scolices. In the absence of these, a firm diagnosis can be made by finding the flanged, sickle-shaped hooklet (b). The round or oval hyaline structures which stud the scolices in (a) and are seen in an aggregate next to the hooklet in (b) are known as calcareous corpuscles, and characterise cysticercus larvae.

Squamous metaplasia and cell atypia

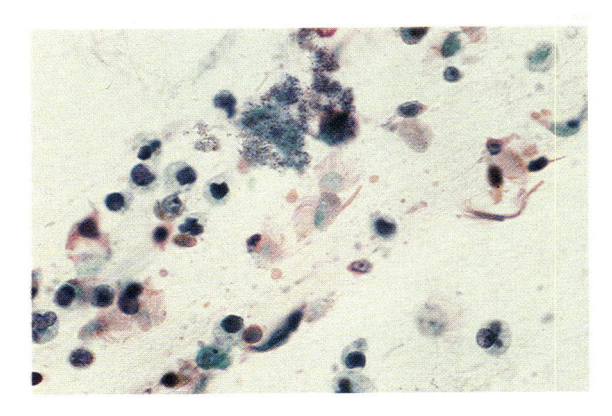

Fig. 3.34 Ciliocytophthoria (CCP)
Papanicolaou ×525: sputum

The fanciful term, ciliocytophthoria, was applied by Papanicolaou to a particular form of cell disintegration in which a distal tuft of cytoplasm with intact cilia is nipped off and lies free. Cytoplasmic fragmentation, karyopyknosis or karyorrhexis of the remaining part of the cell completes the picture. Papanicoloau observed an association of this form of cell destruction with viral pneumonias and some cases of bronchogenic carcinomas. The appearance is neither specific to these conditions, nor restricted to the lower respiratory tract and has been observed by the author in peritoneal fluid from the Pouch of Douglas in cases of salpingitis and in cervical smears.

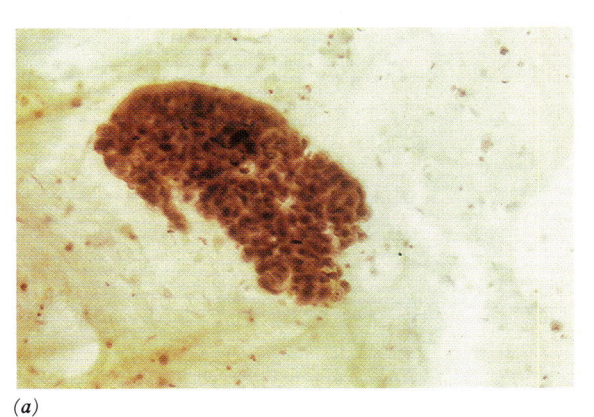

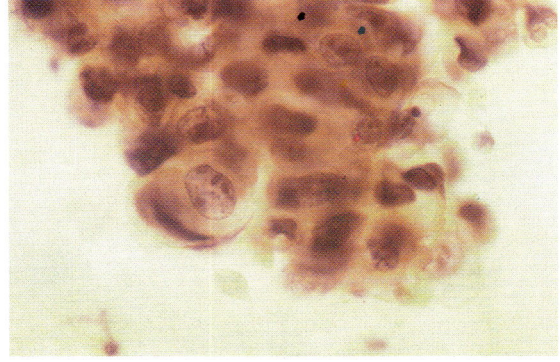

(a)

(b)

Fig. 3.35 Reserve cell hyperplasia
Papanicolaou (a) ×133: sputum (b) ×525: same field

Hyperplasia of reserve cells which lie between the surface bronchial cells and the basement membrane occurs in response to a variety of exogenous toxic agents, particularly cigarettes, and in some long-standing lung diseases. The columnar cells (a) which initially cover the hyperplastic reserve cells eventually degenerate and desquamate. The reserve cells proliferate to form a multilayered epithelium. At this stage, they have scant cytoplasm and hyperchromatic nuclei; exfoliated in sheets, they may mimic oat cell carcinoma. The cells gradually enlarge, acquire squamoid characteristics (b) and differentiate into metaplastic squamous cells.

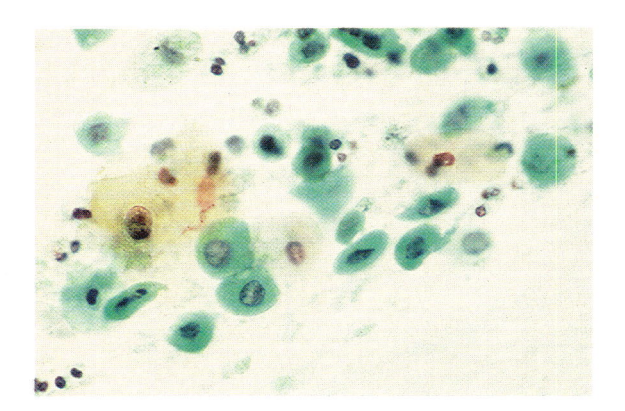

Fig. 3.36 Squamous metaplasia
Papanicolaou ×525: sputum

Metaplastic squamous cells tend to dissociate from each other and have the morphological features of the Malphigian layer cells. They may be round or roughly ovoid, some retain the angular projections characteristic of prickle cells. The cytoplasm is generally cyanophilic and firm in texture.

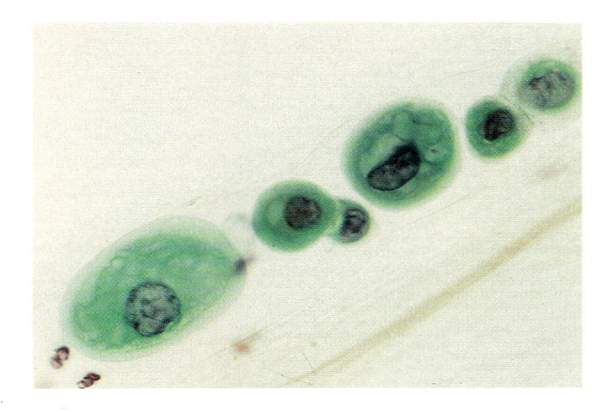

Fig. 3.37 Squamous metaplasia
Papanicolaou ×525: sputum

Degenerative changes are common in metaplastic cells and the cytoplasm frequently contains autolytic vacuoles which vary in number and size. The better preserved nucleus occupies a small part of the cell and is round and reticular. The degenerating nucleus may be hypochromic and blurred; more frequently it tends to pyknosis and intense hyperchromasia (Fig. 3.36). A heavy deposit of chromatin on the membrane which appears thick, and crenation of the margin are two common and significant indications of early degenerative changes in the nucleus. Both characteristics are often seen in malignant cells which have a marked propensity to degeneration, but they are not criteria of malignancy per se.

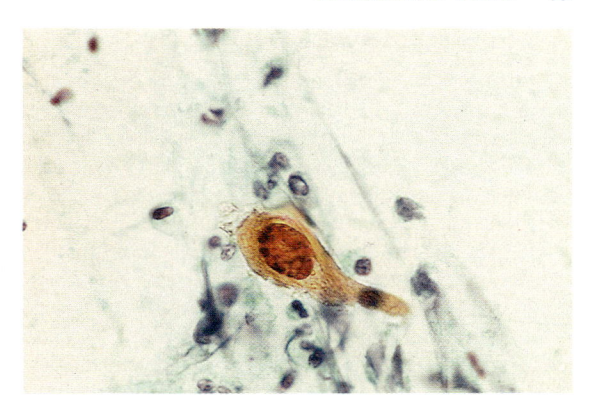

Fig. 3.38 Atypical squamous metaplasia
Papanicolaou ×525: sputum

Foci of squamous metaplasia may undergo progressive atypia in the continued presence of the initial or another irritant. The most significant change is seen in the irregular distribution and size of the chromatin particles, some of which are fine, others coarse. Associated degenerative changes tend to exaggerate the degree of abnormality.

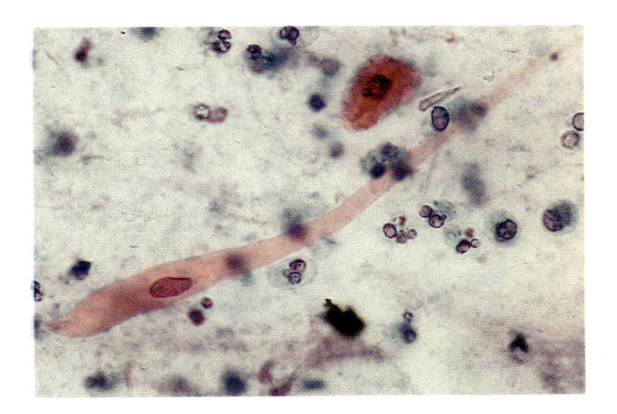

Fig. 3.39 Atypical squamous metaplasia: caudate cell
Papanicolaou ×525: sputum

A disturbing aspect of an atypical metaplastic squamous cell is alteration of cell shape. Caudate forms with short or long tails (tadpole cell) occur. The nucleus of a benign caudate cell is very small relative to the cytoplasm and some of its structure is preserved. Compare the benign cell illustrated with the malignate caudate cells in Figure 3.47 (e) (f).

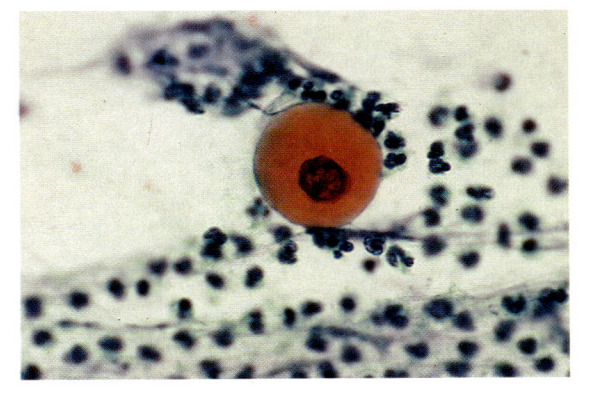

Fig. 3.40 Atypical squamous metaplasia: dyskeratotic cell
Papanicolaou ×525: sputum

Dyskeratosis is a common feature of the atypical metaplastic squamous cell. The cell which still retains its nucleus becomes partially or fully keratinized. Grossly atypical metaplastic squamous cells, suspicious of malignancy, may occur in the bronchial tree in the absence of squamous carcinoma or may co-exist with bronchogenic carcinomas of all cell types. A diligent search for confirmatory evidence in further specimens is indicated, but a firm diagnosis of carcinoma should be made only when unequivocal malignant cells are identified.

Hyperplasia of bronchial mucosa

Reactive cells from hyperplastic bronchial mucosa are met with in a variety of pulmonary disorders, notably asthma, chronic bronchitis, slowly resolving pneumonia, bronchiectasis, and occasionally viral pneumonia.

Benign cells lining the bronchi are one layer deep or pseudostratified and may be expected to exfoliate in flat monolayers. While this is often the case, it is by no means universally true and this aspect of benign mucosal cells has been overstressed in some literature. The appearance seen is influenced to some extent by the nature of the specimen and the functional state of the cell. In sputum and bronchial secretions, hyperplastic mucosal cells (especially distended goblet cells) are not infrequently spheroidal and shed in clusters which have a considerable depth of focus. The overall appearance may resemble that seen in adenocarcinoma cells and pose a major diagnostic problem. In brush and aspiration smears, both types of cells tend to be flat. Unlike keratinized squamous carcinoma and small cell carcinoma, which are often recognizable at a glance, close attention to morphological detail is necessary to avoid a misdiagnosis of adenocarcinoma.

More often than not, benign clumps contain both goblet and ciliated cells. The most helpful feature in the identification of a group of hyperplastic cells is the presence of cilia, or, since these being fragile, are easily lost, the persistence of the terminal bar.

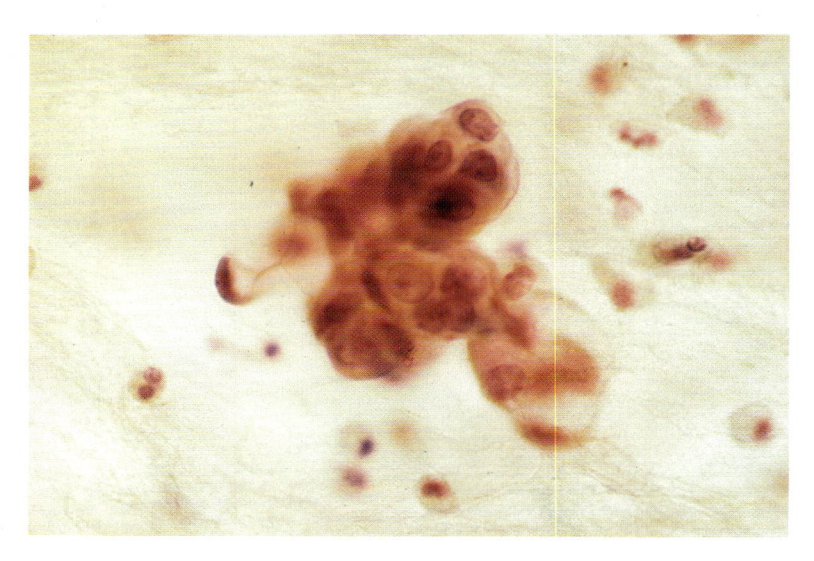

Fig. 3.41 Bronchial asthma. Hyperplasia of bronchial mucosa

Papanicolaou ×720: sputum

Clumps of mixed ciliated and mucous cells, known as Creola bodies, after the patient in whom they were first noted, are seen in sputum in bronchial asthma. The columnar cells opposite 1 o'clock have clearly defined terminal plates. The intracytoplasmic mucous globules of the goblet cells have made characteristic cup shaped depressions in some of the nuclei. The slight variation in cell and nuclear size is due mainly to compression and an impression of orderly palisading and normal polarity is maintained. The nucleoli are small.

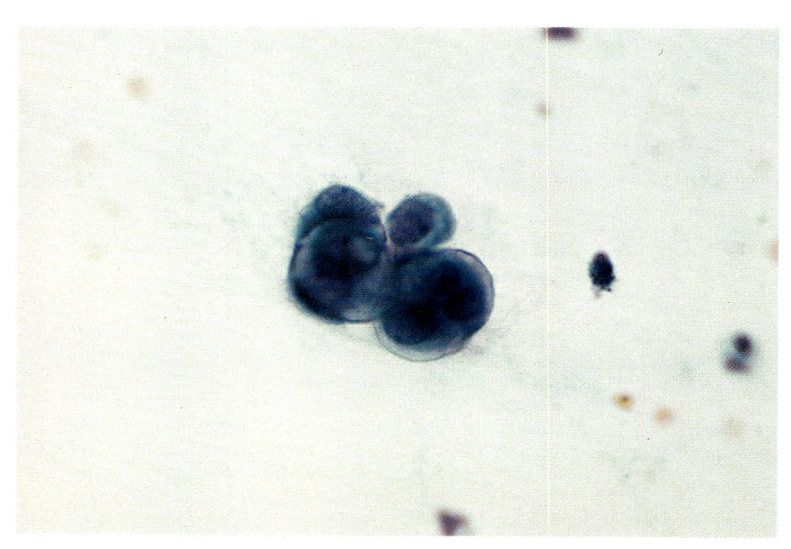

Fig. 3.42 Slowly resolving pneumonia. Hyperplasia of bronchial mucosa

Papanicolaou ×720: sputum

This and the two following fields were seen in the sputum of a 26-year-old woman who suffered from homozygous sickle cell disease and who developed a bronchopneumonia which was slow to resolve but eventually cleared completely. The variation in cell size is minimal. End plates are visible on the luminal surfaces of two cells. The circumscribed intracytoplasmic vacuole of the goblet cell lies on top of the nucleus. The impression it gives of being intranuclear is not uncommon in mucous cells, and has also been observed by electron microscopy.

RESPIRATORY TRACT 85

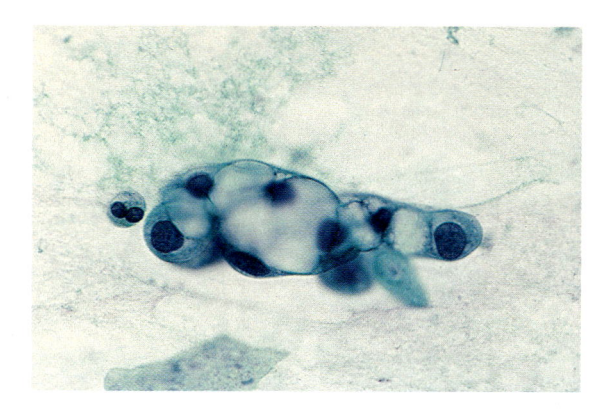

Fig. 3.43 Hyperplasia of bronchial mucosa

Papanicolaou ×525: sputum; same specimen as in Figure 3.42

Two features may be seen in both benign mucous hyperplasia and in adenocarcinoma. Firstly, the nuclear cytoplasmic ratio varies inversely with the degree of distension of the cytoplasm by the secretory product. Secondly, one of the nuclei is pushed to the periphery of the cell which has thereby acquired a signet ring appearance.

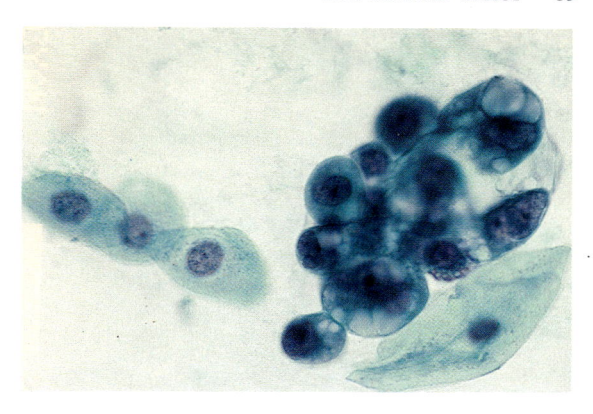

Fig. 3.44 Hyperplasia of bronchial mucosa

Papanicolaou ×525: sputum; same case as in Figures 3.42 and 3.43; another specimen

The prominent large nucleoli are indication of proliferative activity of these cells from hyperplastic bronchial epithelium. There is considerably variation in the size of the nuclei and in their relation to the periphery of the cluster. Several lie on the outer edge and there is loss of polarity and of an orderly surface configuration. The terminal plate on the one columnar cell within the group identifies the benign character of the entire group.

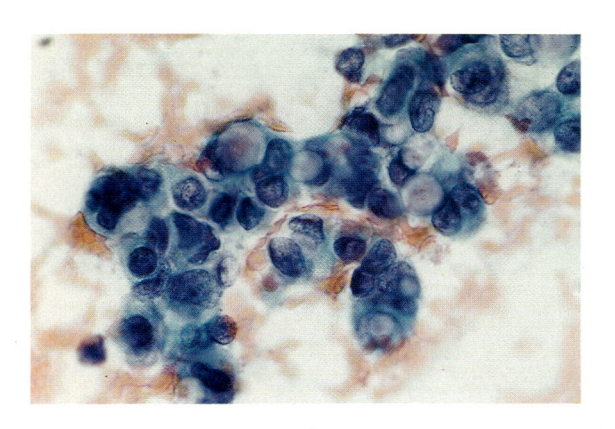

Fig. 3.45 Hyperplasia of bronchial mucosa

Papanicolaou ×525: bronchial brush; unresolved pneumonia

In brush smears, even large fragments of mucosa tend to spread flat. The sheet in this micrograph is composed of ciliated and goblet cells. Note the terminal plate at one edge and the scattered mucous globules. The variation in the shape and size of the cells and the nuclei is enhanced by intracytoplasmic vacuoles and compression of the cells. A suggestion of reticulation is evident in the chromatin.

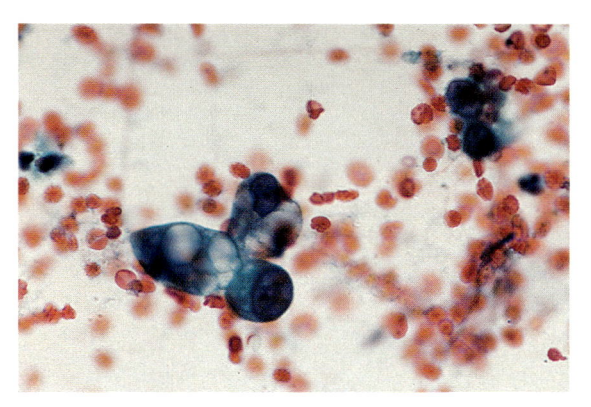

Fig. 3.46 Hyperplasia of bronchial mucosa

Papanicolaou ×525: bronchial washings; same case as in Figure 3.45

In bronchial washings, clumps of cells are likely to become rounded and three-dimensional. The nuclei are more liable to distortion and examination of the chromatin pattern may be unrewarding. A diagnosis of carcinoma should not be submitted unless single cells with unequivocal malignant features are identified.

PRIMARY BRONCHOGENIC CARCINOMA

The three main types of primary bronchogenic carcinomas are squamous cell carcinoma, small cell carcinoma and adenocarcinoma. A sub-type of adenocarcinoma which arises either from cells of the terminal bronchioles including the Clara cells, or less commonly from the type 2 pneumocyte, and forms either a localized mass or spreads laterally along the scaffolding provided by the alveolar walls is designated by the World Health Organization as broncho-alveolar carcinoma. The very poorly differentiated adenocarcinoma or squamous cell carcinoma is sometimes difficult to classify by light microscopy; vestigial features which provide a clue to the cell type being identifiable only by electron microscopy. Such a tumour is classified as a large cell undifferentiated carcinoma. In a cytological specimen, the material available for analysis is relatively sparse and the pattern of cell arrangement less informative than in a histological specimen. The cytodiagnostic rate for large cell undifferentiated carcinoma tends to be higher than in histological series.

Squamous cell carcinoma

Squamous cell carcinoma is the commonest primary tumour of the lung. The majority develop in the main bronchi or their major divisions close to the hilum and most are visible through the bronchoscope. The small number of peripherally located squamous carcinomas not accessible to the biopsy forceps may, sometimes, be reached and sampled by the bronchial brush.

In histological preparations, the well differentiated squamous cell carcinoma is characterized by a basic stratified pattern, distinct intercellular bridges and keratinization, progressing in several areas to epithelial pearl formation. The moderately differentiated tumour has features intermediate between the well differentiated and the poorly differentiated squamous carcinoma, in which the intercellular bridges are barely discernible.

In cytological material, architectural structure is not evident. The diagnosis of malignancy is based on analysis of cell morphology.

Fig. 3.47 Well differentiated squamous cell carcinoma (illustrations opposite)

(a) Papanicolaou ×525: bronchial washings (b) MGG ×525: FNA; lung; another case (c) Papanicolaou ×525: same smear as (a) (d) Papanicolaou ×525: sputum; another case (e) Papanicolaou ×525: same specimen as (b); another smear (f) Papanicolaou ×525: sputum; another case (g) Papanicolaou ×525: sputum; another case (h) Papanicolaou ×133: FNA; lung; another case

A good proportion of the cells from a well differentiated squamous cell carcinoma contain keratin, or more often, prekeratin. This imparts a number of distinctive characteristics to the cell. In consequence, the cytoplasmic features are of particular importance in this type of carcinoma and contribute more to the correct diagnosis than does the nucleus.

Papanicolaou included the cytoplasmic counterstain Orange G to the compound stain he devised because of its affinity for keratin. The dyskeratotic cell, stained by his method is strongly orangeophilic and conspicuous against the background of mucus, macrophages and bronchial mucosa (a), (c), (d), (e), (f). In a Romanowsky-stained smear, cytoplasm containing keratin is pale, has a bluish or violet tinge (b) or may be unstained and almost white.

The texture of the keratinized cell is sometimes hard, homogenous and matt. This gives a sculptured look to the cell which will have a sharply defined outline (a), (b). More often, the cytoplasm in a Papanicolaou stained smear is bright and refractile; lowering the condenser enhances the refractility (c), (d). Focal collections of smooth, glistening droplets are often present (c), (d). Whether refractile or dull, the cell does not transmit light.

Variations of shape are another striking feature, and cells from a squamous carcinoma may have the most bizarre appearance (d). The cell often has cytoplasmic processes which may be short or long, single or multiple (e), (f). The tail-like process may end sharply (e) or in a bulbous expansion (e), (f). Forms with cytoplasmic tails are referred to as caudate or tadpole shaped cells.

The number of nuclei and the nuclear cytoplasmic ratio vary considerably in this type of tumour. The single nucleus or the total mass of the multiple nuclei is often disproportionately great, but small pyknotic nuclei may also be seen (d), (e), (f). Dyskeratosis of the cytoplasm is invariably associated with nuclear degeneration. The perinuclear membrane is crenated (a), (b), (c) and may be thick with a heavy deposit of chromatin. Progressive condensation of the chromatin results in marked hyperchromasia; eventually the nucleus shrinks into a small opaque smooth or jagged mass, with a black 'India-ink' staining reaction (e), (f). Finally, the remains of the nucleus may be indicated only by a faint outline (d), (g) or it may be altogether absent (d). Anucleate orange 'cell ghosts' are particularly abundant in cytological material from a squamous carcinoma which has undergone central necrosis (h). The high nuclear cytoplasmic ratio characteristic of most malignant cells is irrelevant to the diagnosis of a keratinizing carcinoma cell.

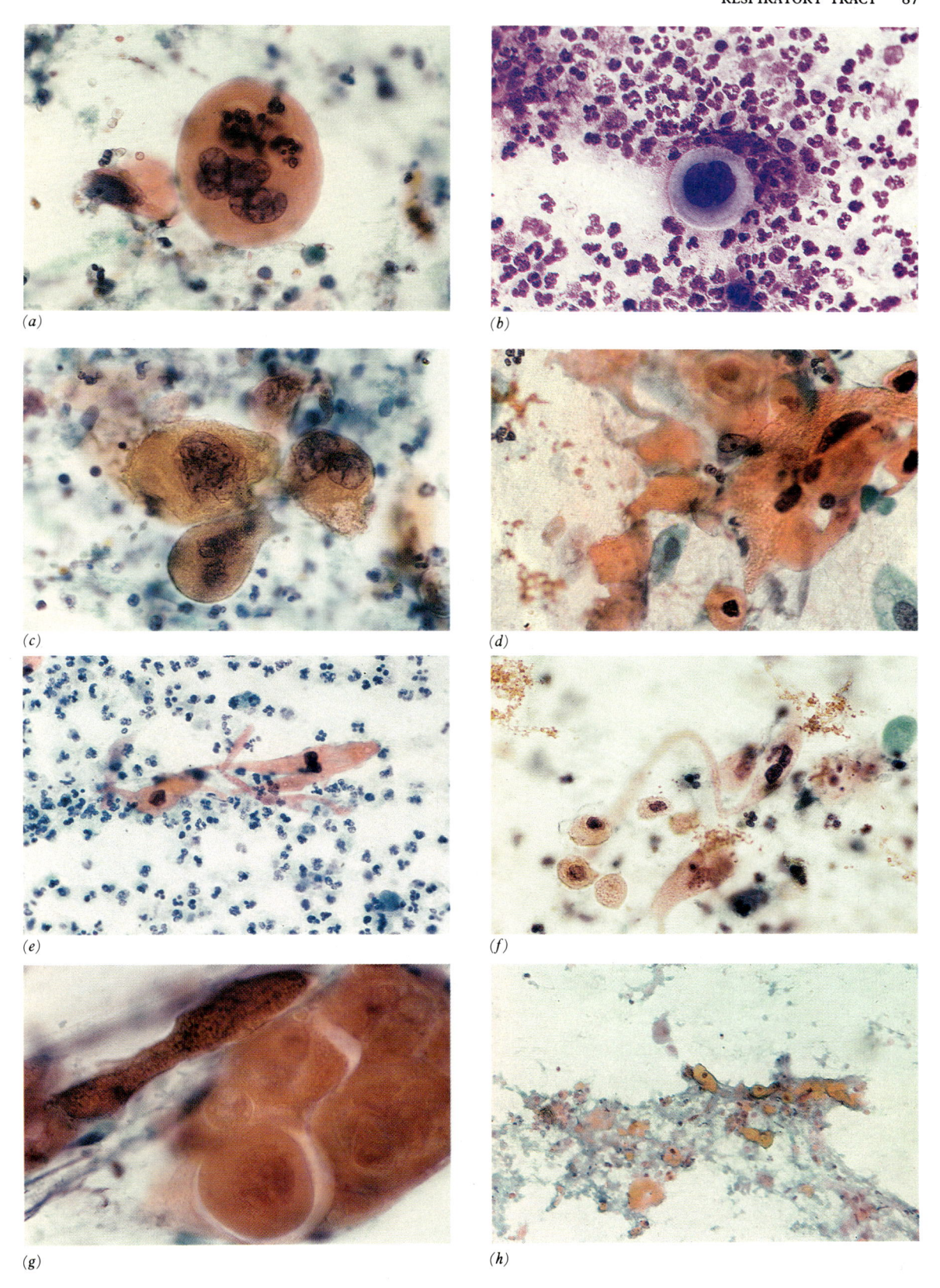

(a)

(b)

(c)

(d)

(e)

(f)

(g)

(h)

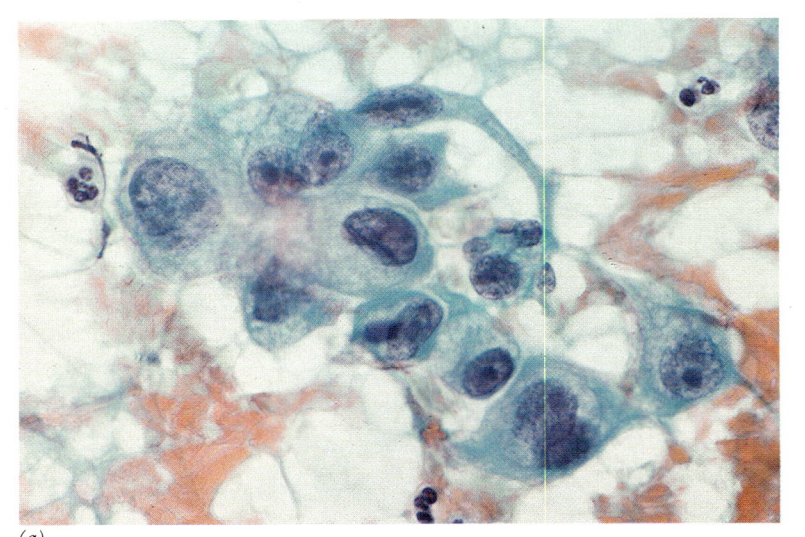

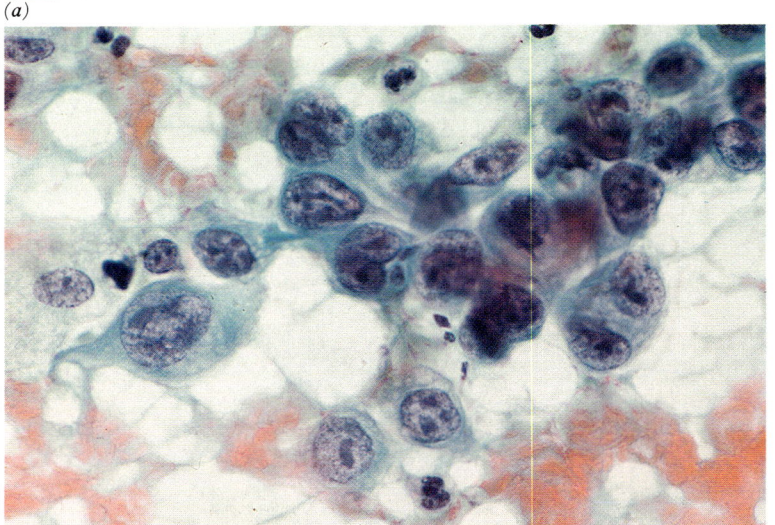

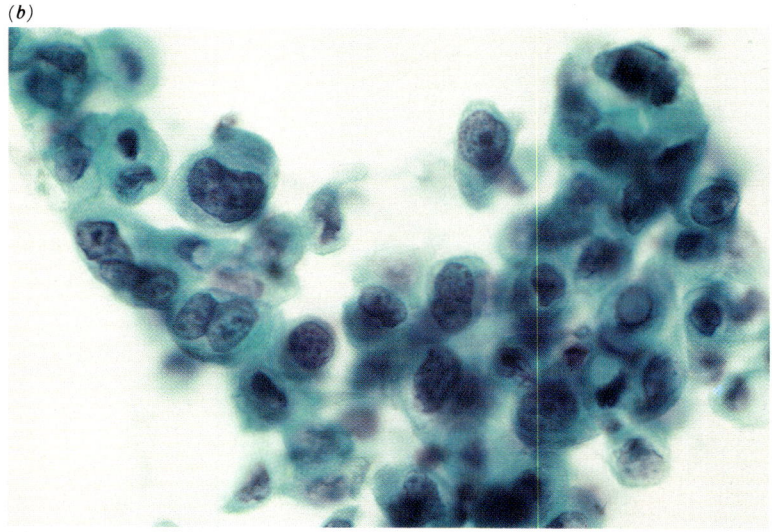

Fig. 3.48 Poorly differentiated squamous cell carcinoma

Papanicolaou ×720 (a) FNA; lung (b) same smear as (a) (c) sputum; another case (d) bronchial washings; another case (e) FNA; lung; another case (f) sputum; another case

Cells from the less differentiated squamous carcinomas cannot be graded or even typed with any consistency. Their cytoplasm is often delicate and translucent, and always cyanophilic. It may contain fine hydropic vacuoles.

The diagnosis of malignancy, based on nuclear abnormality, is seldom in doubt. The nuclei vary in size and staining intensity. A point to note is the relative hypochromasia of some of the aspirated nuclei (a), (e). The nuclear cytoplasmic ratio is high. Nucleoli, single or multiple, large and prominent (a), (b) or small and inconspicuous (d) are generally present.

Two features, when present, aid in the recognition of a squamous origin. The more important is the arrangement and inter-relationship of the cells. Unlike differentiated squamous cells, these remain cohesive and are recovered in small sheets which have ragged borders (a), (b), (c), (d), (e). Sharply angular projections of cytoplasm corresponding to intercellular bridges link the cells (a), (b). Similar angular extensions may be seen at the free edge of a cell (a), (b), (c).

The other indication of probable squamous origin, although less reliable, is the relative firmness of cytoplasmic texture of some of the cells in a cluster.

In the absence of such fine points, (e), discrimination between a poorly differentiated squamous carcinoma and a large cell carcinoma is not possible.

On occasion, poorly differentiated squamous cells may appear in clusters with smooth outlines; identification of the cell type is then even more difficult. The production of minute quantities of mucin does not, according to the World Health Organization, invalidate a diagnosis of squamous carcinoma. Degenerative cytoplasmic vacuoles coupled with smooth outlines (f) may result in an appearance rather more suggestive of adenocarcinoma.

(d)

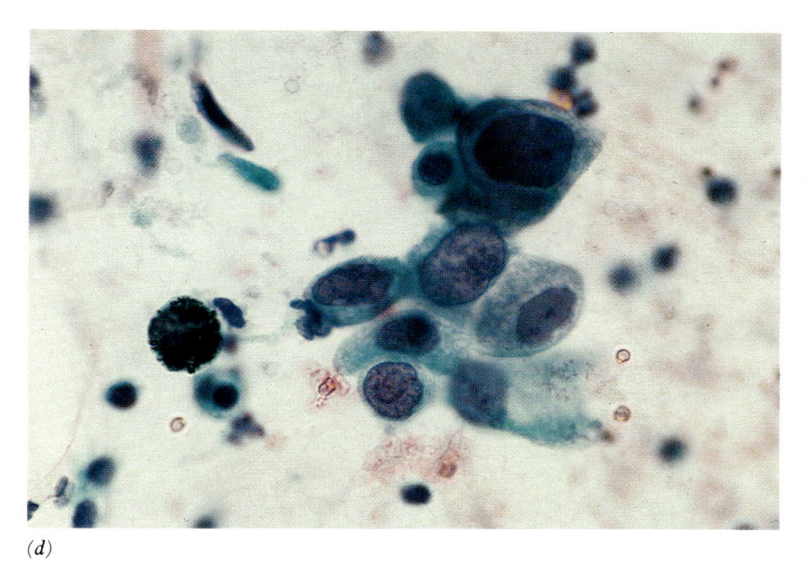

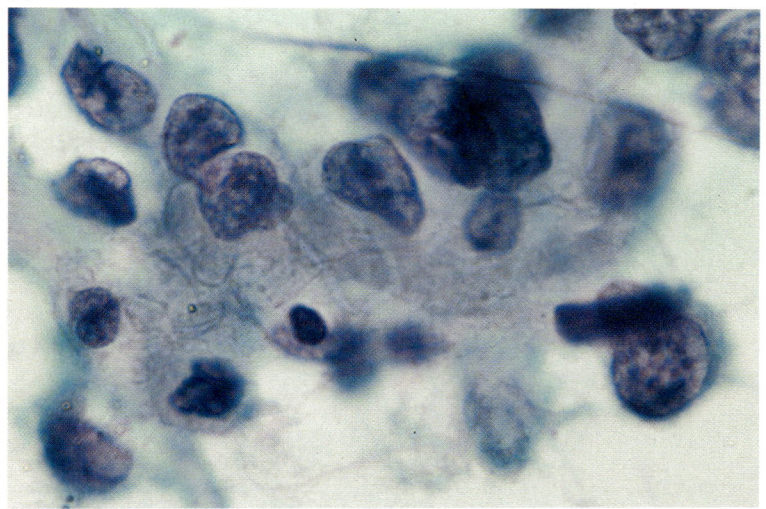

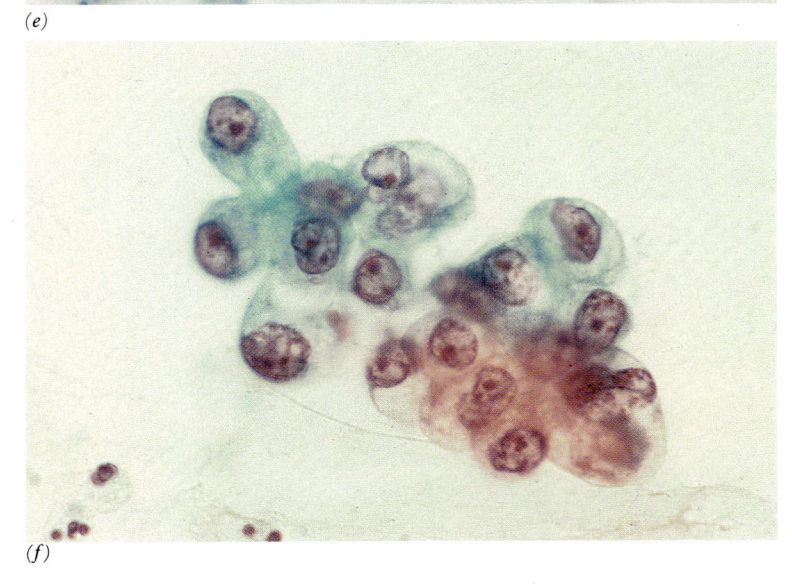

(e)

(f)

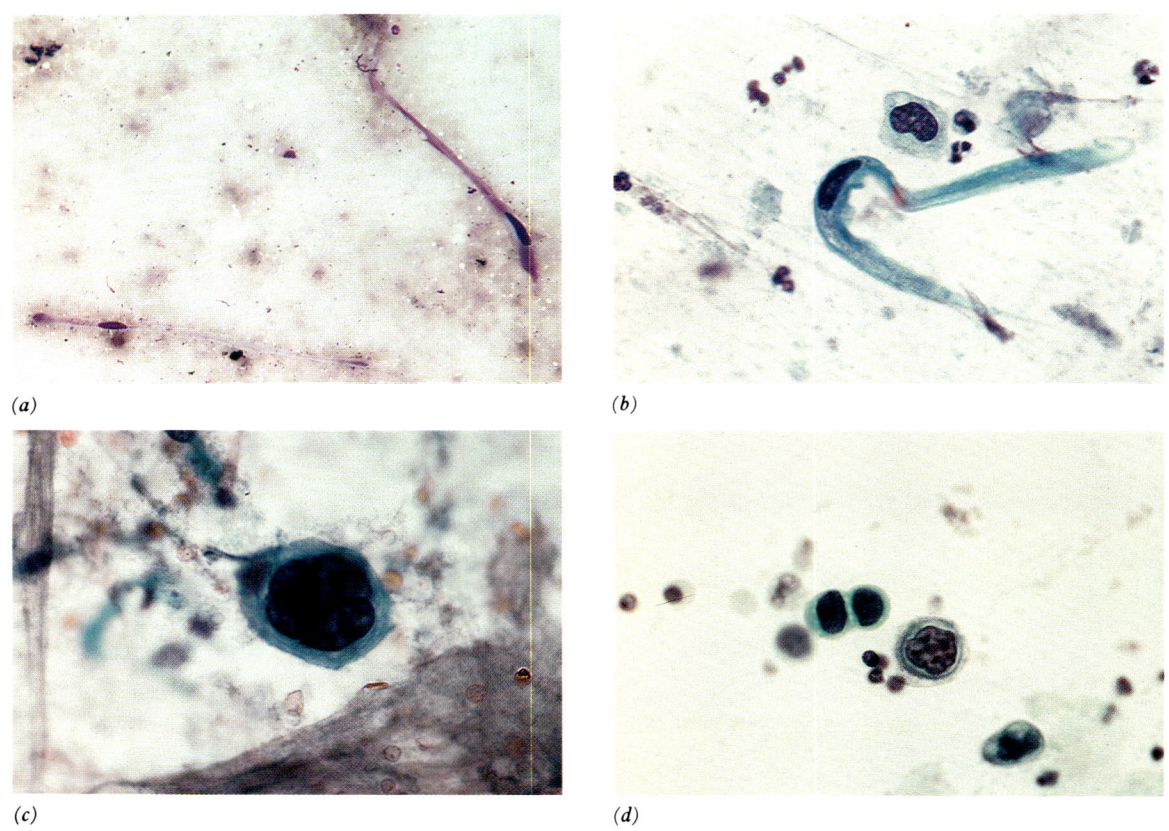

Fig. 3.49 Moderately differentiated squamous cell carcinoma

(a) MGG ×525: FNA; lung (b) Papanicolaou ×525: sputum; another case (c) Papanicolaou ×525: bronchial washings; another case (d) Papanicolaou ×525: sputum; another case

Two morphological features indicative of squamous differentiation may be recognized in a cell that is not yet keratinized. One is a coiled fibrillary apparatus, seen in the tail of some caudate cells, and known as the Herxheimer spiral (a), (b). The other is the presence, in a round cell, of one or more perinuclear lamellations (c), (d) which resemble the rings in a cross-section of a tree trunk. Both probably represent closely packed thick tonofilaments.

Squamous cells as they begin to differentiate tend to dissociate from their neighbours, and appear as single forms.

Small cell carcinoma

Small cell carcinoma (SCC) of the lung is a highly aggressive tumour which spreads rapidly, metastasizes early and most patients have disseminated disease when first seen. For this reason, surgical resection is contra-indicated and combined chemotherapy with or without radiotherapy is the treatment of choice. For the same reason, identification of the cell type and discrimination from other small-celled tumours is of particular importance.

In light microscopic preparations, the cells of SCC are said to resemble oat grains. Its earlier name of oat cell carcinoma, based on this resemblance, is still in current usage in many centres as a generic term, but is used by the World Health Organization to denote one of three sub-types:

1. *Small cell carcinoma, oat cell carcinoma*: a malignant tumour composed of uniform small cells, generally larger than lymphocytes, having sparse cytoplasm, dense nuclei and inconspicuous nuclei

2. *Small cell carcinoma, intermediate cell type*: a tumour of less regular appearance with fusiform, polygonal or round cells with more abundant cytoplasm. The nuclear characteristics are the same as in oat cell carcinoma. A large cell element may be present in some tumours

3. *Combined oat cell carcinoma*: a tumour with a definite component of oat cell carcinoma with squamous cell and/or adenocarcinoma.

The origin of small cell carcinoma is still a matter of debate. SCC and bronchial carcinoid were both considered to arise from the Feyrter or Kultschitsky (K) endocrine cell of the APUD (amine precursor uptake decarboxylation) system of cells which secrete peptide hormones. Ultrastructurally, APUD cells have membrane bound dense core granules similar to granules present in some nerve endings, and they were considered to derive from the neural crest. More recently, it has been postulated that all benign and malignant bronchial mucosal cells have a common endodermal stem cell origin. The stem cell undergoes progressive differentiation along several different pathways, one of which is endocrine, and may switch from one pathway to another under different stimuli. This would explain the similarity and the difference between SCC and bronchial carcinoid, the presence within SCC of large cell elements, combined tumours and the not infrequent emergence of a different malignant cell type in patients treated with chemotherapy protocols appropriate to SCC. Tumour-related endocrinopathies are not uncommonly associated with SCC which may secrete a variety of ectopic hormones, notably ACTH and ADH.

The cytoplasmic dense core granules of SCC are small in size, sparse in number or altogether absent. When seen, they are generally located near the cell membrane and are usually argentaffin with silver stains.

In cytological materials, the size and shape of the SCC cell, the amount of cytoplasm and nuclear characteristic appear to be affected more by the nature and preparation of the specimen than by the histological sub-type.

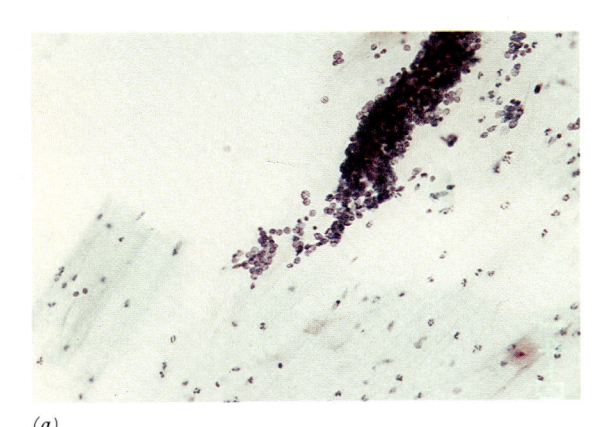

(a)

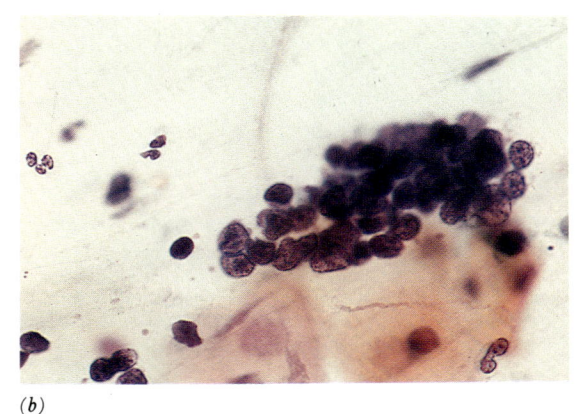

(b)

Fig. 3.50 Small cell carcinoma

Papanicolaou (a) ×133: sputum (b) ×525: sputum; another case

Sputum from a patient with SCC is often clear, or it may be flecked with blood. The tumour cells are seen aggregated in clumps or flat sheets, often against a clean background free of mucus and macrophages. The cluster often thins out at one or both ends, so that the cells appear in linear streaks (a). The individual cell appears to consist almost entirely of nucleus with virtually no cytoplasm (b).

92 DIAGNOSTIC CYTOPATHOLOGY

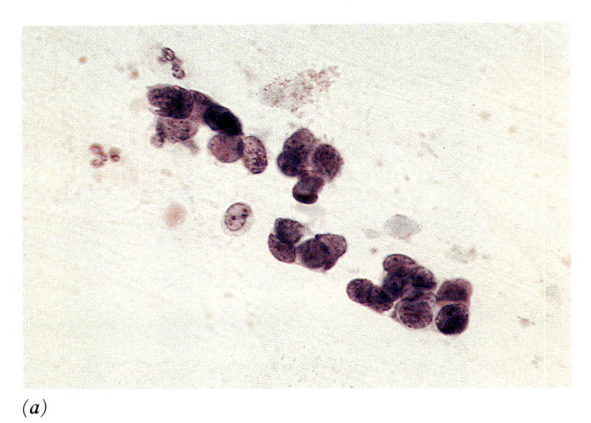

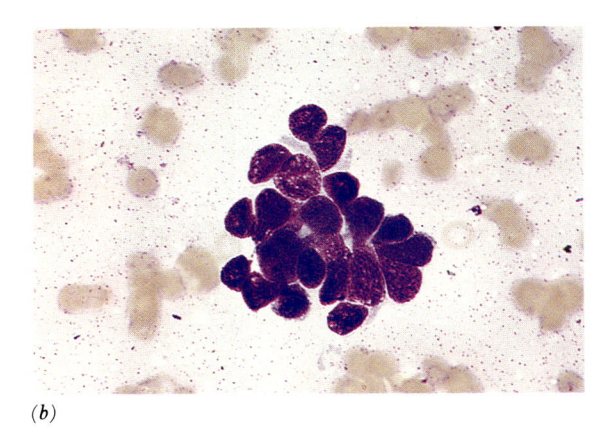

(a)   (b)

Fig. 3.51 Small cell carcinoma
(a) Papanicolaou ×525: sputum (b) MGG ×525: FNA; lung; another case

Compression of one or more sides of closely adjacent cells results in the characteristic moulding of oat cells. The space between two moulded nuclei is minimal, almost linear. However, it should be clearly seen – as overlapping nuclei or a wider space does not constitute the typical moulding of SCC. More often than not, one nucleus of a moulded pair is round while its neighbour has one semilunar margin (a). Nuclear moulding, considered to be virtually diagnostic of SCC, is almost always seen in bronchial secretions; it may be present in brush and aspiration smears (b), but is inconstant and often inconspicuous.

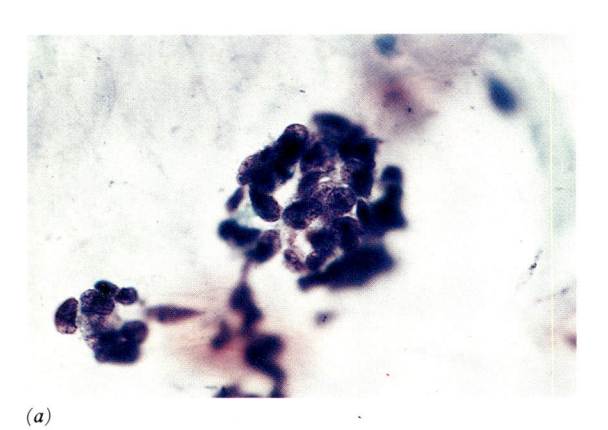

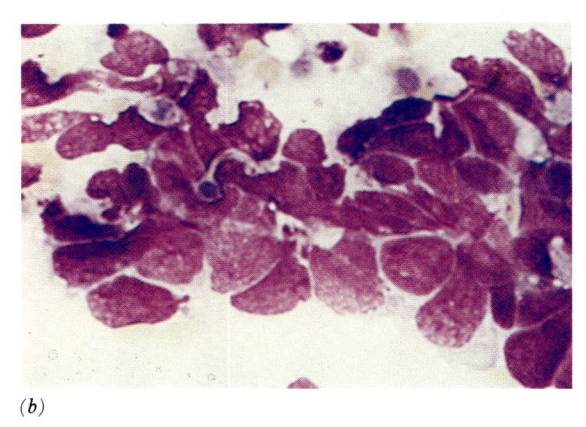

(a)   (b)

Fig. 3.52 Small cell carcinoma
(a) Papanicolaou ×525: sputum (b) MGG ×525: FNA; lung; another case

The cell or rather the nuclear shape is generally round or cuboidal. Elongated spindle cells or pear-shaped cells, rounded at one end and pointed at the other, are only occasionally seen in sputum (a) and bronchial washings, but are quite common in brush and aspiration smears. It is likely that this feature is exaggerated by the spreading of the smear, and is more marked in air-dried smears (b). The artefact is not restricted to the fusiform cell sub-type and is not diagnostic of small cell carcinoma of the intermediate cell variety.

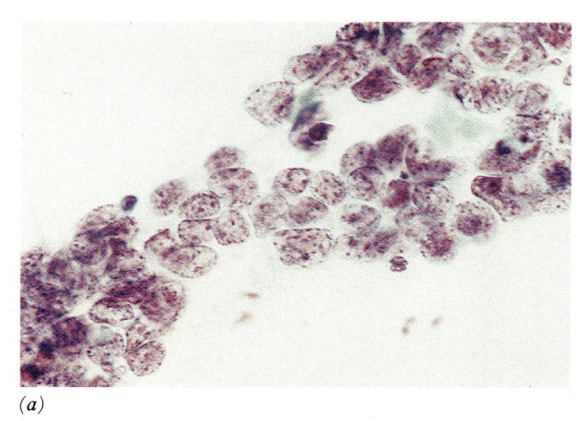

Fig. 3.53 Small cell carcinoma

Papanicolaou ×525 (a) sputum (b) bronchial brush; another case

The chromatin of the well preserved SCC cell is distinctive. It is invariably granular; the granules are very fine or slightly coarse, sharply defined and often spiculated. They are dispersed through the entire nucleus right to the margin.

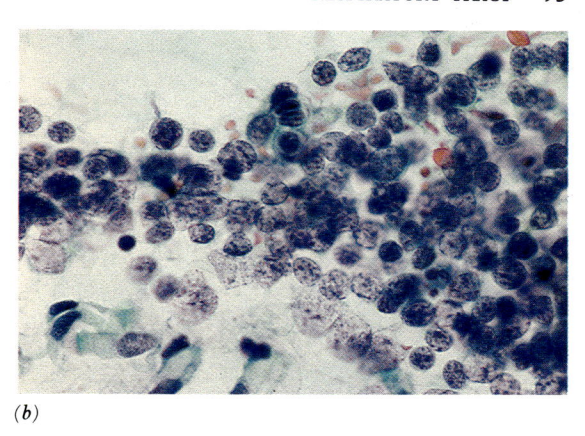

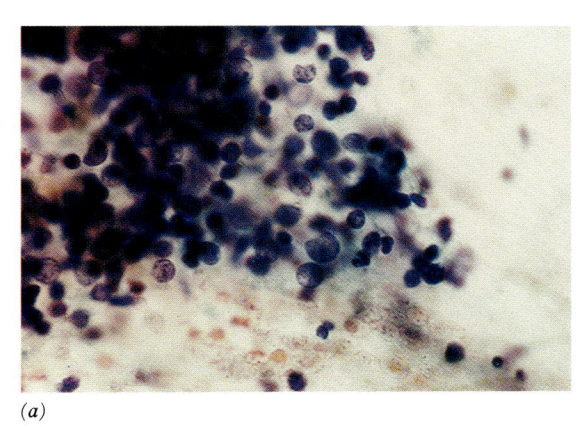

Fig. 3.54 Small cell carcinoma

Papanicolaou ×525: (a) bronchial washings; same case as Fig. 3.53b (b); bronchial brush; another case

Necrosis is common in SCC and the cells often show degenerative changes. These are more marked in cells which lie near the edge of the tumour and are shed spontaneously or in bronchial washings (a) (b). The degenerate nuclei are hyperchromic and tend to pyknosis. The cells appear even smaller and the difference in the size of the degenerate cells in washings (a) and the cells obtained from the same tumour by brushing (Fig. 3.53b) may be quite considerable. The distinctive salt and pepper chromatin is lost and only a few granules may remain against a homogenous violet background (b). As the nucleus retracts into a pyknotic mass, the cytoplasm becomes more evident (b).

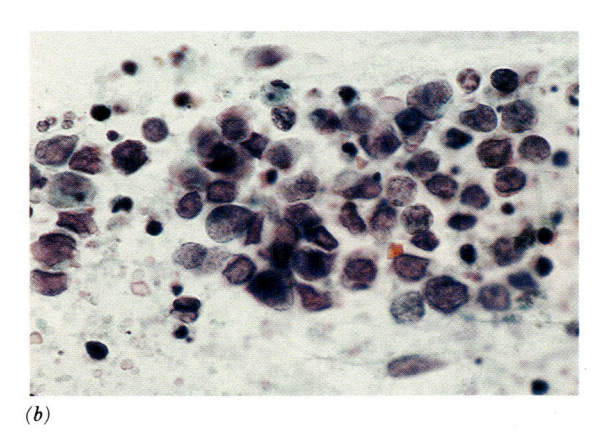

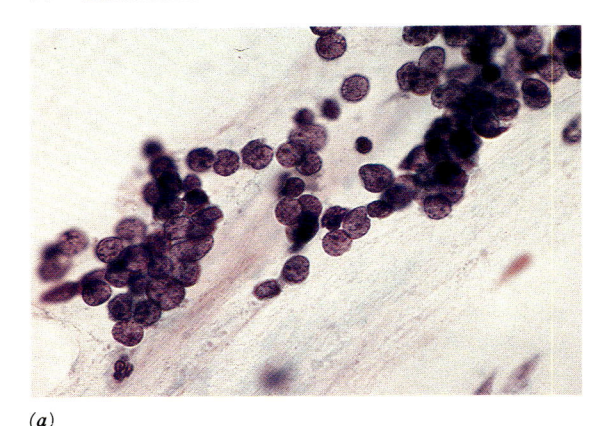

94 DIAGNOSTIC CYTOPATHOLOGY

(a)

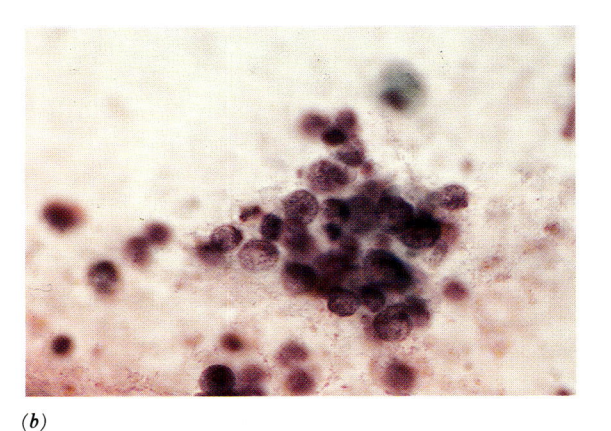

(b)

Fig. 3.55 Small cell carcinoma

Papanicolaou ×525 (a) sputum (b) bronchial brush; another case

Nucleoli which are inconspicuous in sections, may be seen in some of the better preserved SCC cells in almost all types of cytological specimens. Generally, the nucleolus is basophilic, small and single (a). Occasionally, it is eosinophilic, large and prominent. As a rule, only one or two cells in an aggregate have large nucleoli. The presence of prominent red nucleoli in all the cells in one cluster in a specimen with classical oat cells is suggestive of a small cell carcinoma with a large cell component.

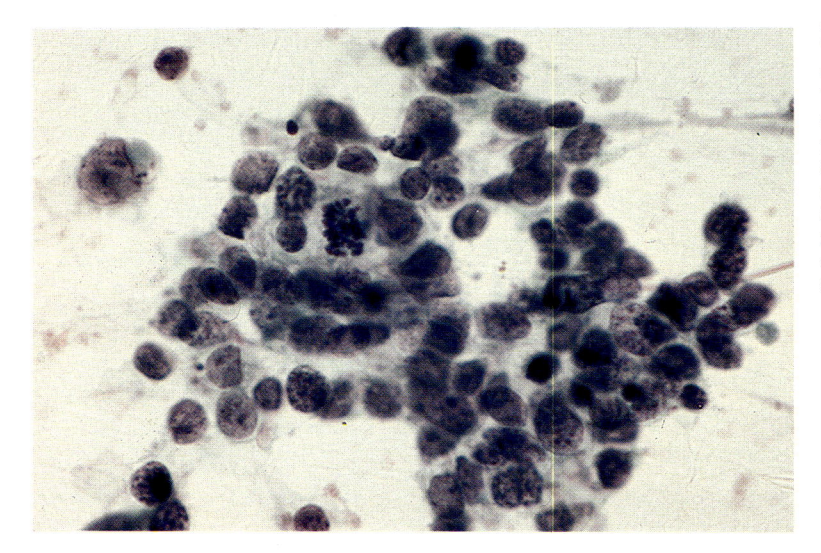

Fig. 3.56 Small cell carcinoma

Papanicolaou ×720: FNA; lung

The appearance in this micrograph is suggestive of the intermediate cell sub-type. The cells show some variation in size and more cytoplasm is evident. The nuclei have the stippled chromatin of SCC. Mitotic activity seen here, may be met with in oat cell carcinoma, but is often greater in the intermediate cell sub-type.

(a)   (b)

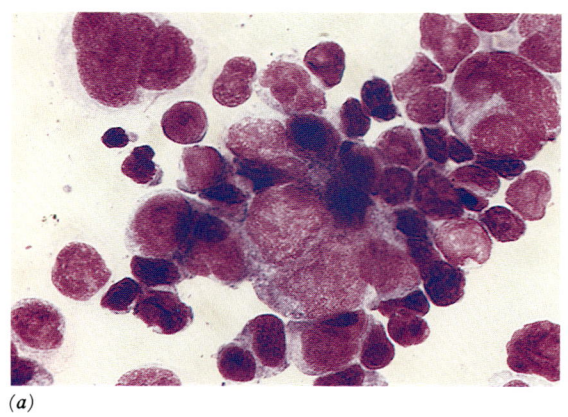

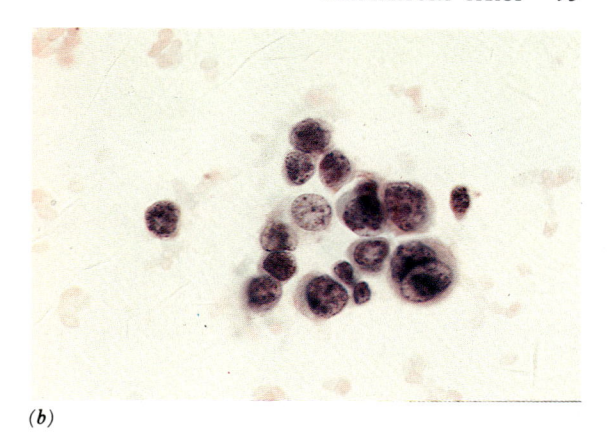

Fig. 3.57 Small cell carcinoma
(a) MGG ×525: FNA; lung (b) Papanicolaou ×525: same specimen; another smear

Some small cell carcinomas display considerable pleomorphism. A single tumour may be composed of small oat like cells, spindle shaped cells, small and large polygonal cells and a few multinucleated giant cells. The anisocytosis and anisonucleosis is enhanced by air drying (a). These tumours may be examples of small cell carcinoma with a large cell component. Note the cell within cell (b); this feature is frequently seen in all variants of SCC.

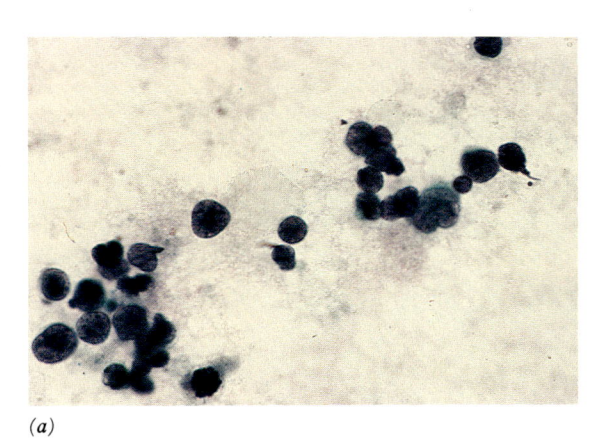

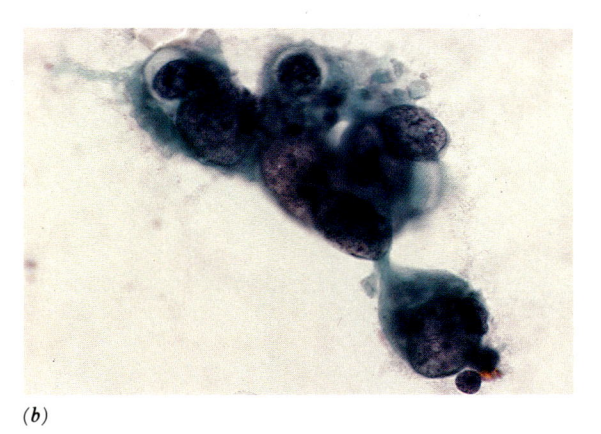

(a)   (b)

Fig. 3.58 Combined oat cell carcinoma
Papanicolaou ×525 (a) transbronchial FNA: small cells (b) same smear; another field; large cells

These micrographs are from a single smear made from a small transbronchial needle aspirate. Two types of cells were present. Micrograph (a) shows classical oat cells with nuclear moulding and virtually no cytoplasm and a couple of slightly larger cells. The cells in (b) are very much larger and more pleomorphic; they have substantial deeply cyanophilic cytoplasm and coarsely granular nuclei. The transbronchial biopsy contained a definite component of oat cell carcinoma with large malignant squamous cells which were connected with each other by obvious intercellular bridges.

96 DIAGNOSTIC CYTOPATHOLOGY

(a)

(b)

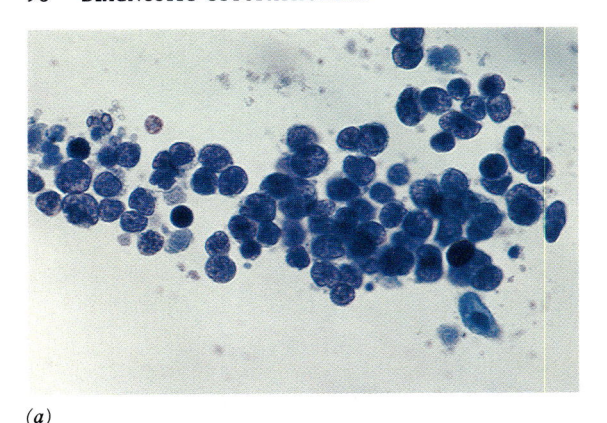

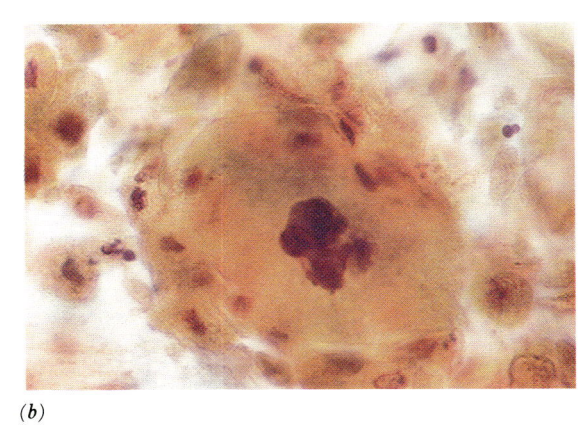

Fig. 3.59 Oat cell carcinoma and squamous cell carcinoma

Papanicolaou ×525 (a) sputum; oat cell carcinoma (b) same smear; another field; squamous cell carcinoma

Two distinct and pathognomonic cell types were present in a sputum sample. The majority of the cells were classical oat cells (a). In addition, the sputum contained several large keratinized malignant squamous cells (b). The patient, an elderly man with a long history of chronic bronchitis, had one radiological lung opacity. The question as to whether he had one mixed tumour or two separate primary bronchogenic carcinomas remained unanswered.

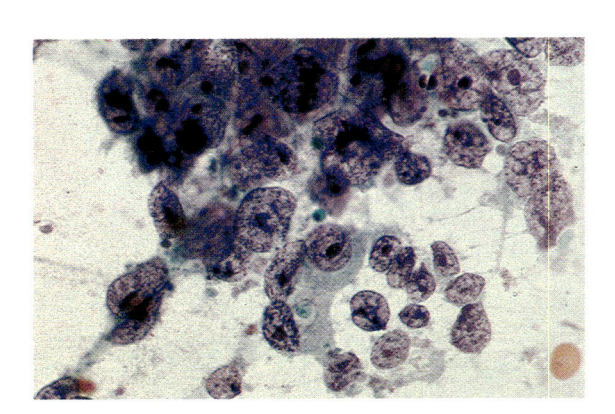

Fig. 3.60 Treated small cell carcinoma

Papanicolaou ×525: bronchial brush

Large undifferentiated malignant cells with prominent polymorphic nucleoli were recovered in a bronchial brush specimen from a patient who had shown partial response to chemotherapy administered for a histologically confirmed small cell carcinoma. Emergence of a refractory large cell element and even another malignant cell type after treatment for SCC has been well documented.

Bronchial carcinoid

Bronchial carcinoids are neoplasms of low grade malignancy. With few exceptions, they are centrally located and 90% are visible through a bronchoscope. They are generally circumscribed and present either as a fleshy endobronchial polyp or have a locally infiltrating 'ice-berg' pattern of growth. Both types develop in the bronchial sub-mucosa and are covered with epithelium which may be normal, but is more often metaplastic. The so-called atypical carcinoid is more anaplastic and may show a histological and clinical similarity to the highly malignant small cell carcinoma.

Pulmonary carcinoids resemble intestinal carcinoids. Their most important secretory product is serotonin (5 hydroxytryptamine) and they may be associated with the carcinoid syndrome. Their relationship to small cell carcinoma is not clear. Both tumours contain ultrastructural dense core secretory granules with an endocrine function. The granules of a carcinoid are larger, variable in size and shape, abundant and are distributed through the cytoplasm. The majority are argyrophilic, i.e. they require an external reducing agent to convert a silver solution to metallic silver. They may also be demonstrated by the alkaline diazo method; a few are argentaffin.

Cells from a pulmonary carcinoid are not exfoliated in bronchial secretions unless the covering mucosa is ulcerated. Brush smears taken after a biopsy forceps has disrupted the epithelium and transbronchial and percutaneous needle aspirations are more likely to yield diagnostic material.

RESPIRATORY TRACT 97

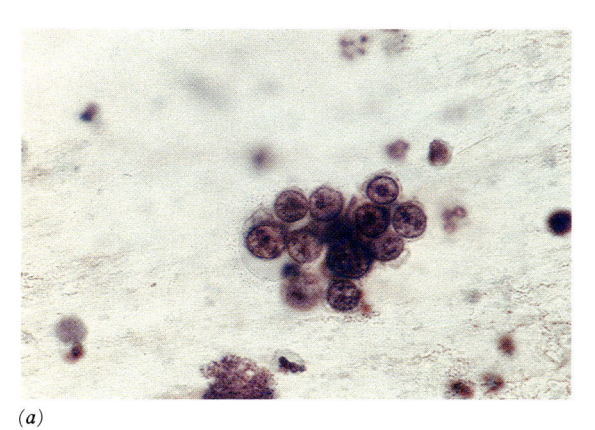

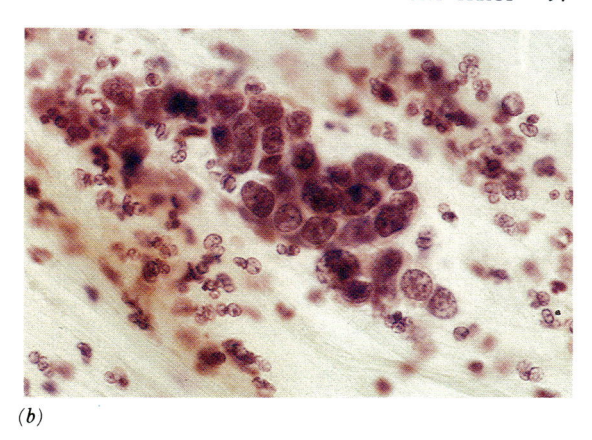

(a) (b)

Fig. 3.61 Carcinoid tumour
Papanicolaou ×525 (a) sputum (b) sputum; another specimen from the same case

The cells illustrated were present in the sputum of a patient with local recurrence several months after resection of a circumscribed carcinoid tumour. They were abundant and formed clusters. The cells in (a) are typical of carcinoid tumours. They are small and uniform and have a narrow rim of cytoplasm. The round nuclei contain prominent nucleoli. The nuclear borders are thick and moulding is not seen. The cells in another sample of sputum from the same patient are less regular, the nuclei have a 'salt and pepper' chromatin, there is a suggestion of nuclear moulding and nucleoli are not seen. Further surgery was performed on the patient and the recurrent tumour was seen to be more anaplastic and had infiltrated the adjacent lung parenchyma.

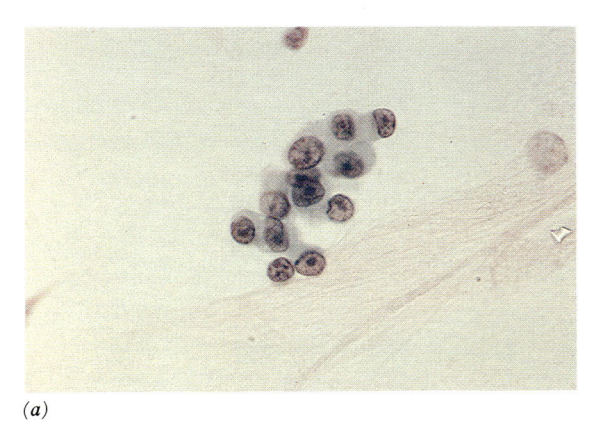

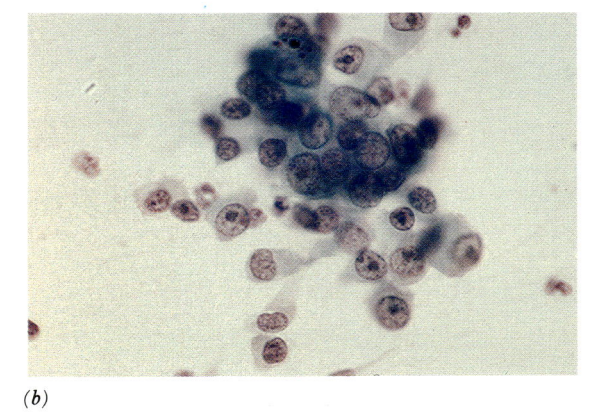

(a) (b)

Fig. 3.62 Carcinoid tumour
Papanicolaou ×525 (a) bronchial brush (b) same smear; another field

These micrographs show a bronchial carcinoid with some atypia. The cells in (a) appear somewhat larger than in the preceding example, but are uniform. The eccentrically situated nuclei show minimal variation in shape and size and contain conspicuous nucleoli. Compare the normochromasia and the near absence of a chromatin deposit on the nuclear margin of these viable tumour cells with the hyperchromasia and thick nuclear membrane of the degenerating exfoliated cells in Figure 3.61 (a). Another field in the same smear is seen in (b). The variation in the size of the cells and nuclear pleomorphism is greater.

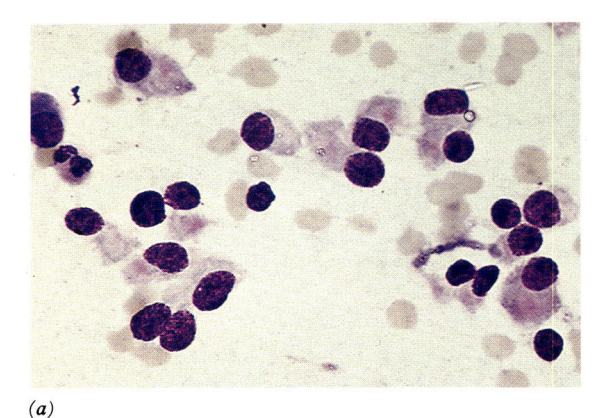

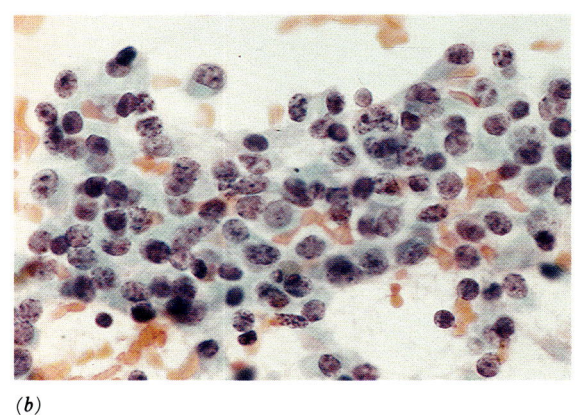

Fig. 3.63 Carcinoid tumour

(a) MGG ×525: FNA; lung (b) Papanicolaou ×525: same specimen; another smear

The case illustrated was not recognised as a carcinoid and the cells were considered to be lymphoplasmacytoid. Many of the round or oval nuclei are eccentric, a common feature of carcinoids in cytological smears. The nuclei have coarsely granular chromatin and the very occasional nucleolus present is small and inconspicuous.

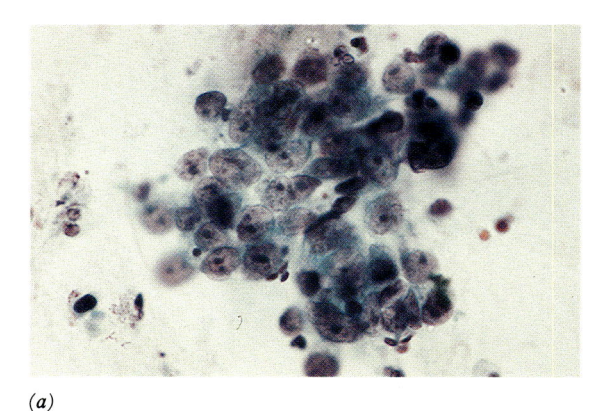

Fig. 3.64 Carcinoid tumour

Papanicolaou ×525 (a) sputum (b) FNA; lung; same case

This is an example of a pleomorphic, high malignant, atypical carcinoid which was diagnosed by aspiration and sputum cytology as a poorly differentiated adenocarcinoma. The correct diagnosis was established by histological and ultrastructural examination of the resected specimen. The patient developed widespread metastases and died of disseminated malignancy 14 months later.

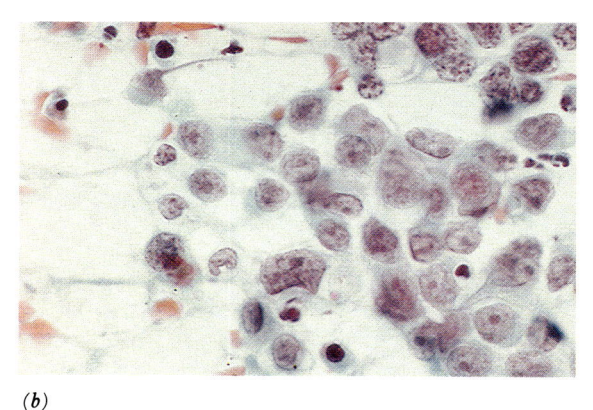

Adenocarcinoma (including broncho-alveolar carcinoma)

Adenocarcinoma is the least common of the three major primary lung carcinomas and one that occurs in non-smokers. An increasing incidence has been reported in recent years, and it is now considered to be provoked to some extent by cigarette smoking.

Approximately three-quarters originate in the smaller bronchi at the periphery of the lung fields. They have a special propensity for scar tissue and most of the scar cancers that arise in chronic interstitial fibrosis (honeycomb lung) or in areas of focal fibrosis that result from pneumoconiosis or treated tuberculosis are adenocarcinomas.

Three basic histological patterns of growth are seen. The acinar type shows a predominance of glandular structures, the papillary type consists of fronds of tumour with cells covering a fibrovascular stalk; the solid carcinoma lacks a distinctive pattern but has many mucous-secreting cells. A tumour may exhibit mainly one pattern and may be typed accordingly, or it may have a mixed pattern.

Broncho-alveolar carcinoma is a rare sub-type of adenocarcinoma and constitutes approximately 1% of all primary lung cancers. It may present as a single coin lesion or a mass in the vicinity of a pre-existing scar, as multi-centric nodules or exhibit a diffuse extensive intrapulmonary spread and lobar consolidation. Broncho-alveolar carcinoma may have a papillary pattern, but typically uses the walls of the alveoli as a scaffolding along which it grows. Some arise in the mucous or the Clara cells of the terminal bronchioles, others in the type 2 pneumocyte.

Two histological and clinical patterns are observed. In one, thin alveolar septa are lined by tall mucous-secreting cells and bronchorrhoea of 1–4 litres of clear fluid may be a major and troublesome symptom. In the other, the cells are cuboidal and peg-like and contain little or no mucin.

It has been claimed that the acinar and papillary sub-types of adenocarcinoma can be identified by cytology. In the author's view, a papillary tumour, whether benign or malignant, can be diagnosed with certainty, only when a fibrovascular stalk covered with malignant cells is seen. Such an appearance is seen in fine needle aspirations, but is exceedingly rare in other respiratory tract specimens. Similarly, cytological distinction between a localised broncho-alveolar carcinoma and the other adenocarcinomas is not consistent. The diffuse variety of broncho-alveolar carcinoma cannot be separated with certainty from primary large cell bronchogenic carcinoma or a metastatic gastrointestinal carcinoma that grows along the alveolar walls. In the absence of histological confirmation, a diagnosis of broncho-alveolar carcinoma can be suggested if cytological appearances are assessed in conjunction with radiological and clinical features.

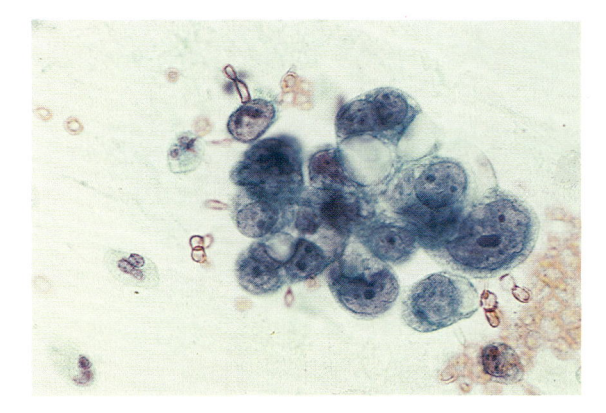

Fig. 3.65 Adenocarcinoma of lung
Papanicolaou ×525: sputum

This micrograph shows several typical features of an exfoliated cluster of well differentiated adenocarcinoma cells. An acinar space is seen in the right lower part. Several sharply circumscribed mucous vacuoles are present. There is a dipping down of the smooth outer margins to the points of junction between adjacent cells. This may be seen in cohesive benign glandular cells, but tends to be greatly enhanced in adenocarcinoma cells and gives a scalloped effect to the entire cluster (compare with Fig. 3.44). A wide variation is apparent in the size of the cells, the nuclei and the nucleoli and the nuclear cytoplasmic ratio.

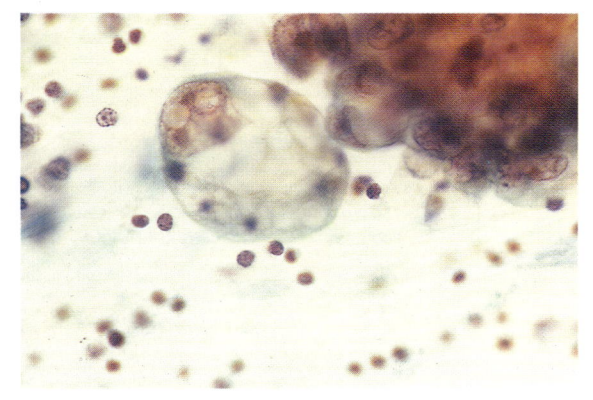

Fig. 3.66 Adenocarcinoma of lung
Papanicolaou ×525: sputum

The ballooned secretory cell in the centre of the field has a substantial depth of focus, the large nucleus being at a lower plane of focus than the overlying darkly outlined mucous vacuoles. The cells at the edge of the clump show all the stigmata of malignancy, i.e. disproportionate enlargement of the nucleus, anisonucleosis and a very high nuclear cytoplasmic ratio. One nucleus is depressed into a cup shape by a mucous globule. The small cells in the field are mature lymphocytes.

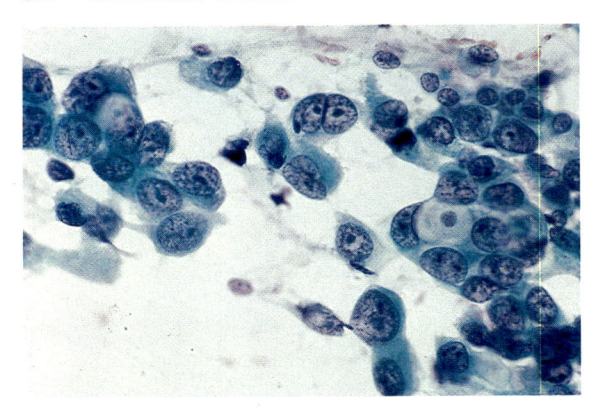

Fig. 3.67 Adenocarcinoma of lung

Papanicolaou ×525: bronchial brush

A two-dimensional spread of adenocarcinoma cells is the rule rather than the exception in brush smears. Distinction from a large cell carcinoma can be difficult and the presence of intracytoplasmic mucin may be the only clue to cell type. Unlike a hydropic vacuole, a mucous vacuole often indents the nucleus and may consist of a sharply demarcated clear area with a central dense body.

(a)

(b)

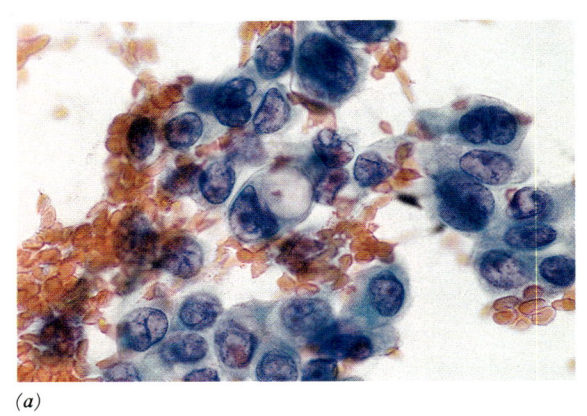

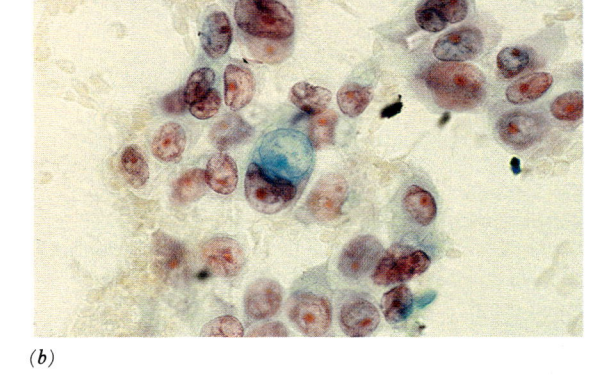

Fig. 3.68 Adenocarcinoma of lung

(a) Papanicolaou ×525: FNA; lung (b) Alcian blue ×525: same field

A similar problem is encountered in aspiration smears. The cells shown formed flat sheets, several contained intracytoplasmic vacuoles, some with a central condensation (a). The smear was decolourised in 1% HCL for 30 seconds, restained with 1.0% alcian blue and the presence of mucin was confirmed (b). For a correct interpretation of this procedure, the cells examined should be clear of free background mucin which is often present in a respiratory tract specimen, and the alcian blue positive secretory product should be clearly delineated within the limits of the cytoplasm.

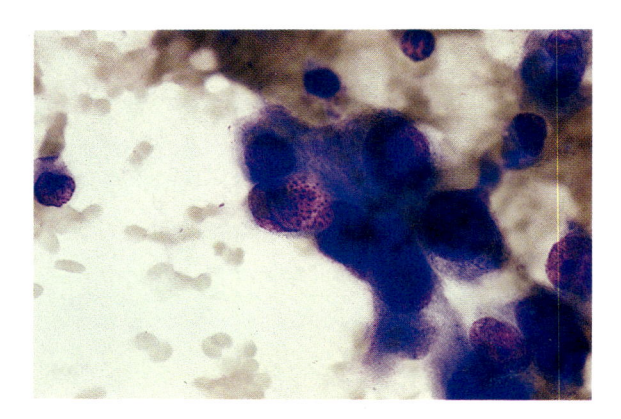

Fig. 3.69 Adenocarcinoma of lung

MGG ×525: same specimen as in Figure 3.68

A less common appearance of a mucous globule is seen in this micrograph. Instead of one large, central, dense condensation, there are several punctate inclusions against a clear or lavendar background. Note the hard edge of the vacuole and the indentation of the nucleus at its lower right.

(a)

(b)

(c)

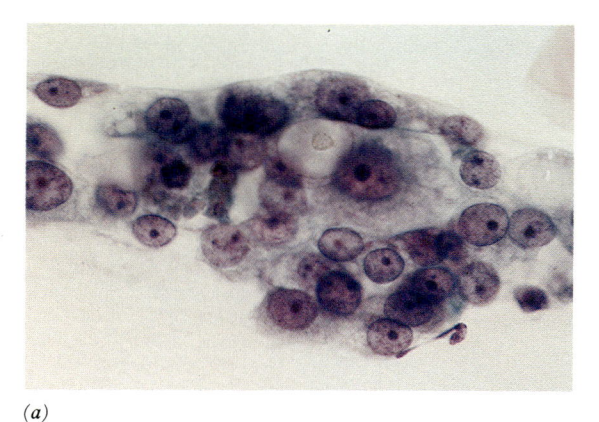

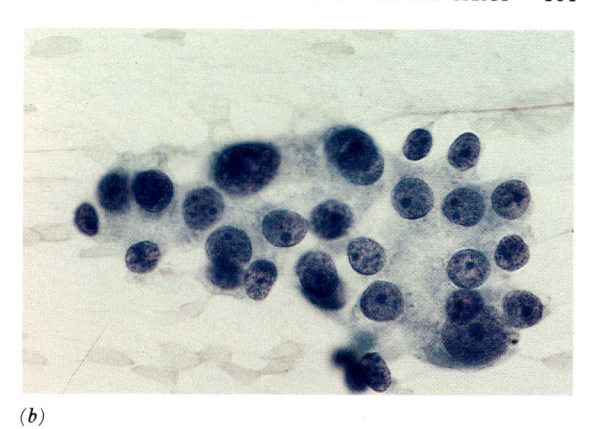

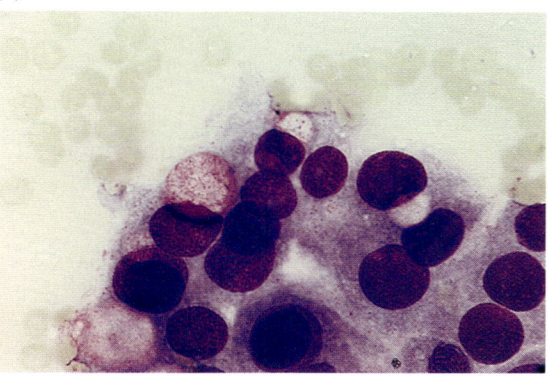

Fig. 3.70 Adenocarcinoma of lung

(a) Papanicolaou ×525: sputum (b) Papanicolaou ×525: FNA; lung; same case (c) MGG ×525: same specimen as (b) another smear

The large sheet of malignant epithelial cells with ill-defined intercellular borders and a haphazard distribution of nuclei shows an arrangement unusual in sputum (a). The thick nuclear membrane, the paucity of chromatin and the extreme hypochromasia of the main body of the nucleus are due to degenerative changes. Nucleoli are prominent against the pale nucleus. One mucous vacuole with a central condensation, resembling an erythrocyte is seen. The same basic morphological features, namely a fragile cytoplasm which appears almost syncytial, the random distribution of variable sized nuclei, differences in size and number of nucleoli, are seen in the lung aspirate (b). The chromatin pattern of the aspirated viable cells is significantly different. The chromatin is aggregated into granules, which vary in shape and size, some being exceedingly fine. Condensation of the chromatin on the nuclear membrane, an early indication of degeneration, is conspicuous by its absence. The relatively monomorphic malignant cells are identified as adenocarcinoma cells by the four finely stippled mucous vacuoles present in the Romanowsky-stained smear (c). The appearance seen in the sputum and the lung aspiration is suggestive of a poorly differentiated solid carcinoma with mucus secretion.

Fig. 3.71 Adenocarcinoma of lung

Papanicolaou ×525: FNA; lung

Much of the vacuolation in these flat, pleomorphic carcinoma cells is diffuse and taken in conjunction with the blurred cell outlines and loss of chromatin from several pale nuclei indicates advanced degeneration. Two of the better preserved cells contain well defined mucous vacuoles. Note that the edge of the vacuole in the right lower corner coincides with the periphery of the cell and mimics the terminal plate of a ciliated cell.

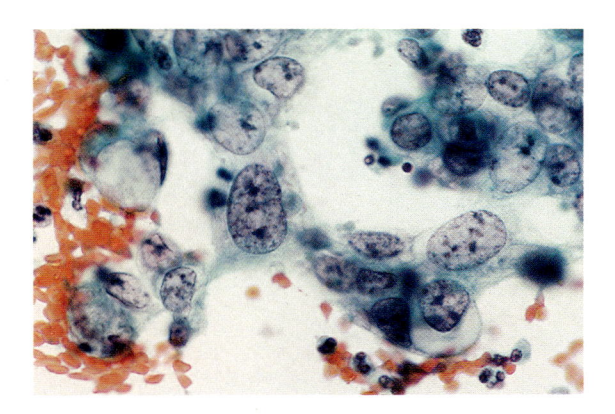

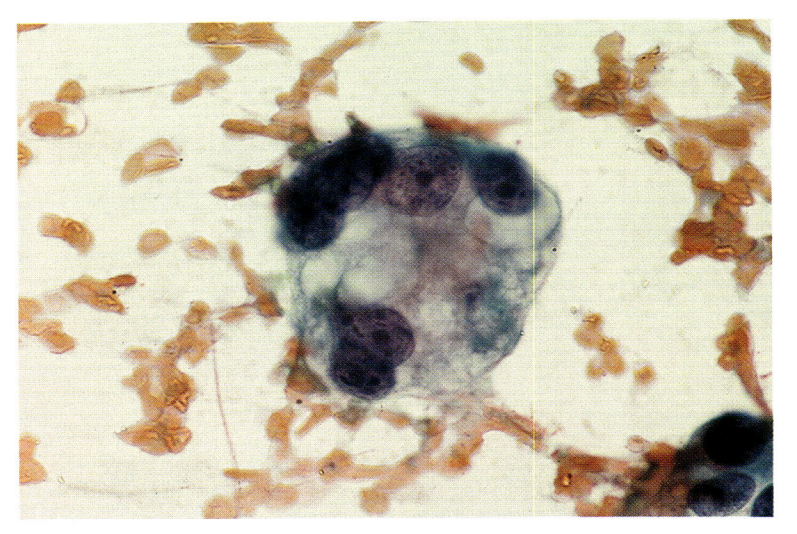

Fig. 3.72 Adenocarcinoma of lung

Papanicolaou ×720: FNA; lung

A similar impression of a terminal plate is created by the thickened eosinophilic right edge of this cluster of adenocarcinoma cells. Malignant cells do not form true physiological cilia but have been shown by electron microscopy to often have a covering of microvilli which are irregular in length and width. The firm edges of these obviously malignant cells represent the line of attachment of microvilli.

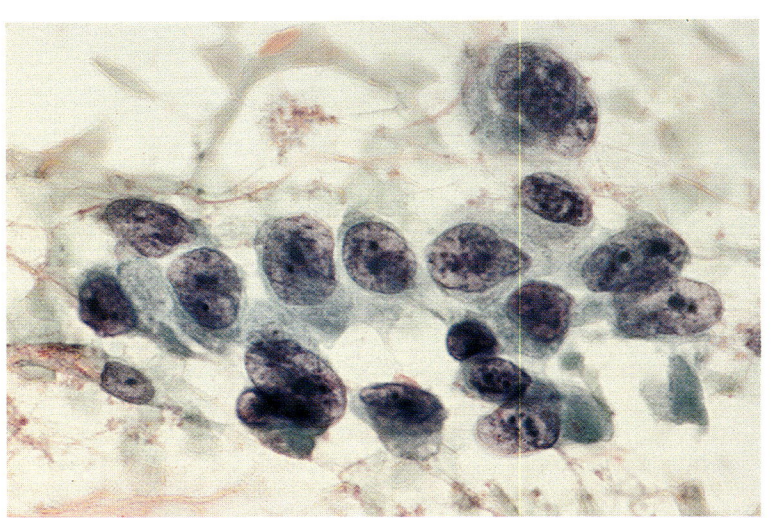

Fig. 3.73 Adenocarcinoma of lung

Papanicolaou ×720: Transbronchial FNA

In the absence of clear-cut mucous vacuoles, it is sometimes difficult to discriminate between a poorly differentiated adenocarcinoma, a non-keratinized squamous cell carcinoma or a large cell undifferentiated carcinoma. The problem is compounded in aspiration and brush smears by the absence of three-dimensional clumps. The cytological appearance in this case was suggestive of a large cell undifferentiated carcinoma; the correct diagnosis of adenocarcinoma was established by histological examination of a transbronchial biopsy.

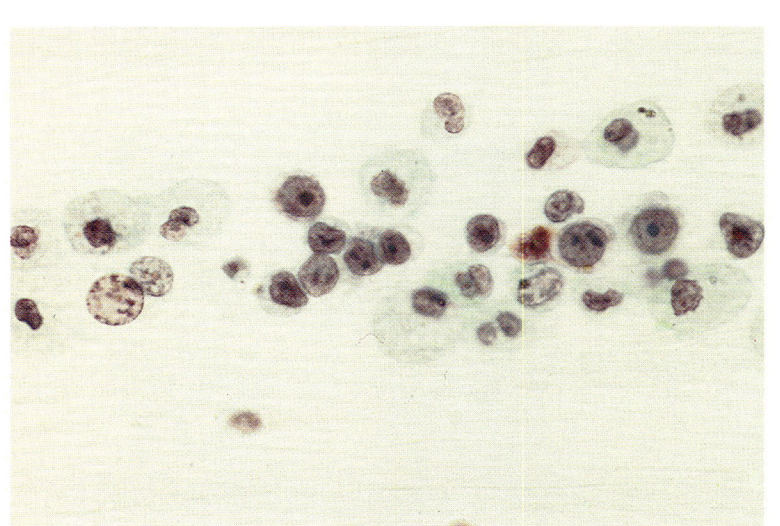

Fig. 3.74 Adenocarcinoma of lung

Papanicolaou ×720: sputum

Another area of cytological difficulty is distinction between an adenocarcinoma composed of small round or oval cells with one or two prominent nucleoli and a broncho-alveolar carcinoma composed of cuboidal cells. The latter sub-type was suggested in this case; autopsy findings showed a solid, very poorly differentiated adenocarcinoma with sparse intracellular mucin.

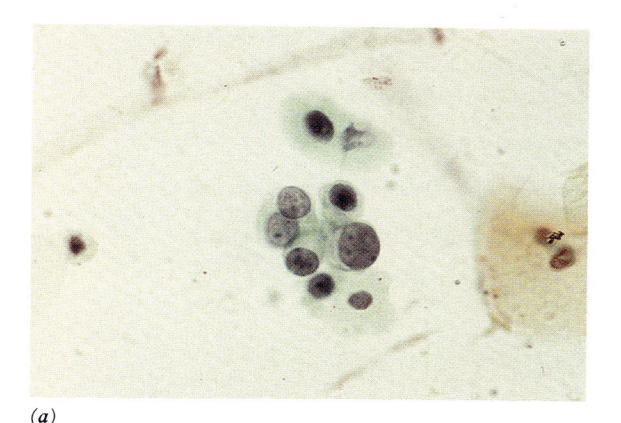

Fig. 3.75 Broncho-alveolar carcinoma

Papanicolaou ×525 (a) sputum (b) same smear; another field

Sputum is an eminently suitable medium for recovery of cells from a broncho-alveolar carcinoma. As a rule, large numbers of cells are exfoliated, mostly in clusters but single cells may be interspersed among macrophages. The cells of the variant illustrated are relatively small, round or ovoid. The nuclear cytoplasmic ratio is high but a certain amount of cytoplasm is quite clearly seen and nuclear moulding is never present. The nucleus may contain a few fine granules of chromatin against a homogenous background and have a surprisingly bland appearance. One to two nucleoli are generally present (a). Cells exfoliated from this type of tumour are often in an advanced stage of degeneration. The three larger nuclei in the cohesive clump of tumour cells appear to consist of violet nuclear sap without any chromatin granules, and with a single nucleolus. The other nuclei have retracted away from the cell border into structureless opaque masses (b).

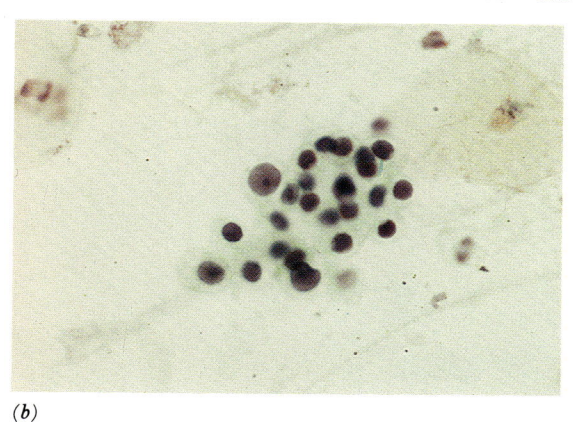

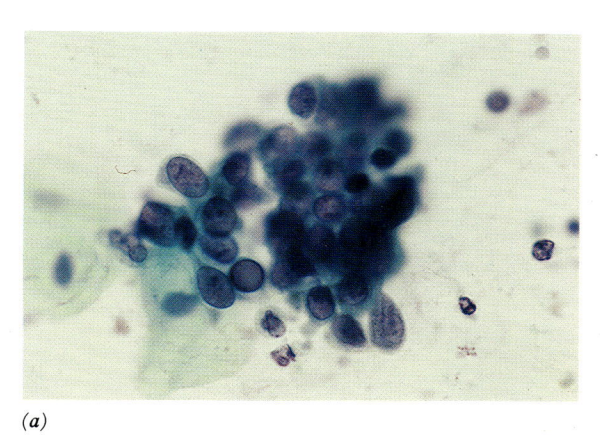

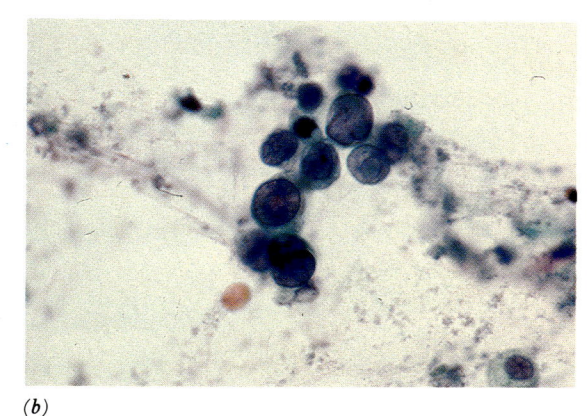

Fig. 3.76 Broncho-alveolar carcinoma

Papanicolaou ×525 (a) broncho-alveolar lavage (b) same smear; another field

Another type of specimen suitable for the identification of a broncho-alveolar carcinoma is lavage of the small bronchioles and the terminal air spaces. A very characteristic appearance is illustrated here. The cluster in (a) contains a large number of closely packed or overlapping cells. Intercellular borders are not clear and the outline of the tumour fragment is indistinct. Note again the relative paucity of chromatin granules, lack of clearing of the nuclear sap and scattered individual nuclear pyknosis. A moderate degree of anisocytosis and anisonucleosis can be appreciated when the cells are spread out (b). The two sharply defined vacuoles overlying two nuclei probably represent mucous globule.

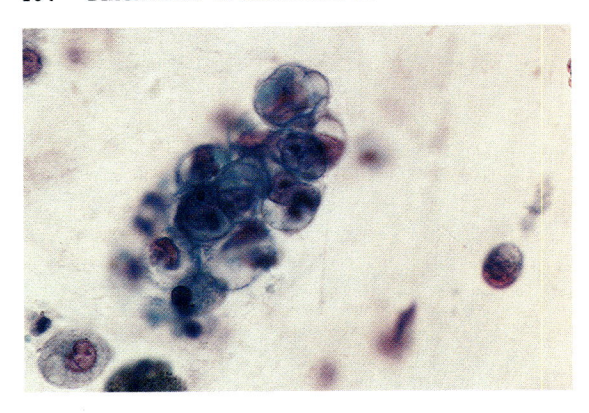

Fig. 3.77 Broncho-alveolar carcinoma
Papanicolaou ×525: sputum

In the more rapidly spreading variant of broncho-alveolar carcinoma, tall columnar cells with abundant cytoplasm line the alveolar spaces. In cytological smears of sputum, these cells become spherical, are quite large, have distinct intercellular borders and contain substantial amounts of mucin. Their nuclei have obvious malignant characteristics, and the nucleoli are larger and more prominent. The morphological features seen do not discriminate between a broncho-alveolar carcinoma and other types of adenocarcinomas.

Large cell carcinoma

Electron microscopy studies of large cell carcinoma of the lung have shown that very few are completely undifferentiated and that the majority have poorly developed features of squamous or glandular cells. These are not appreciated at light microscopy level and large cell carcinoma is classified as a distinct entity. Two variants are recognized. The clear cell carcinoma is similar to renal cell carcinoma. The giant cell carcinoma has a looser pattern of growth and contains many pleomorphic giant cells.

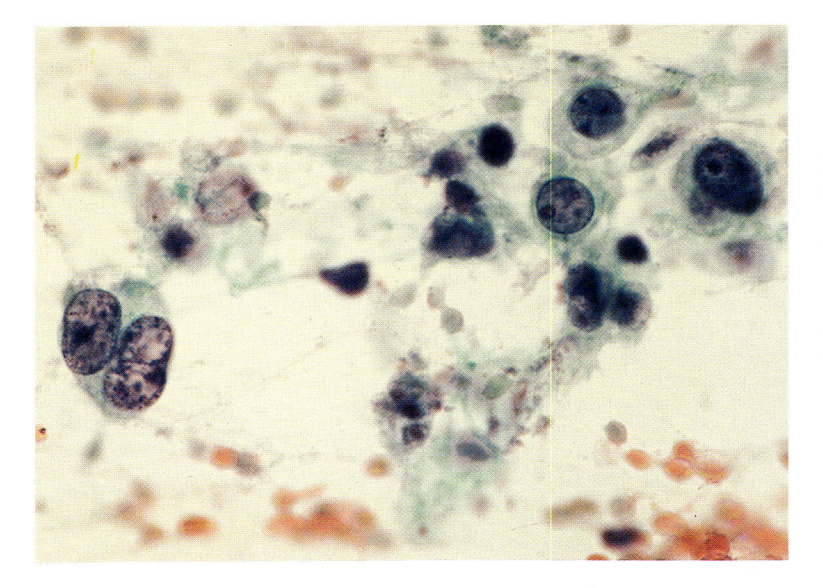

Fig. 3.78 Large cell carcinoma
Papanicolaou ×720: bronchial washings

The cells in this case with a cytological and histological diagnosis of large cell carcinoma are cyanophilic. They have abundant cytoplasm which is delicate but not clear and the cell outline is fairly sharp. The nuclei vary in size and in number from one to three. Two eosinophilic nucleoli are outlined by perinucleolar condensation of chromatin, the other nucleoli are basophilic. The loose cytoplasmic fragments, the scattered pyknotic and hypochromic nuclei are evidence of tumour necrosis.

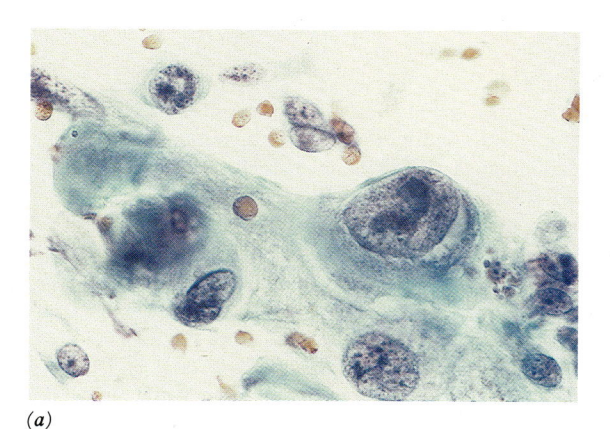

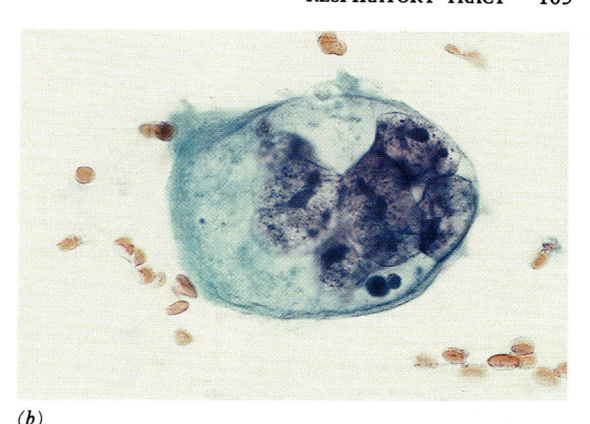

Fig. 3.79 Large cell carcinoma: giant cell carcinoma

Papanicolaou ×525 (a) bronchial brush (b) same smear; another field

An example of a pleomorphic large cell carcinoma is illustrated in the two micrographs. Discrete and cohesive cells are seen in (a). The single forms are fairly small. The intercellular borders of the attached cells are so poorly defined that the sheet appears to consist of a syncytium of cytoplasm. There is gross variation in the size of the nuclei. The plump fusiform nucleus opposite 11 o'clock has a sarcomatous appearance. A giant cell with bizarre pleomorphic nuclei and large irregular nucleoli is seen in (b).

Fig. 3.80 Large cell carcinoma: giant cell carcinoma

Papanicolaou ×720: bronchial brush

This micrograph shows another example of the giant cell variant. The specimen contained moderate-sized, mononuclear malignant cells which lacked definite cytological features of a squamous or glandular origin. Several giant cells with multiple large overlapping nuclei were present. Most of the nuclei contained prominent nucleoli which varied greatly in size and shape. Giant cells may be present in some poorly differentiated squamous cell carcinomas and adenocarcinomas, but do not usually have the appearance, as in this case, of giant sarcomatous cells.

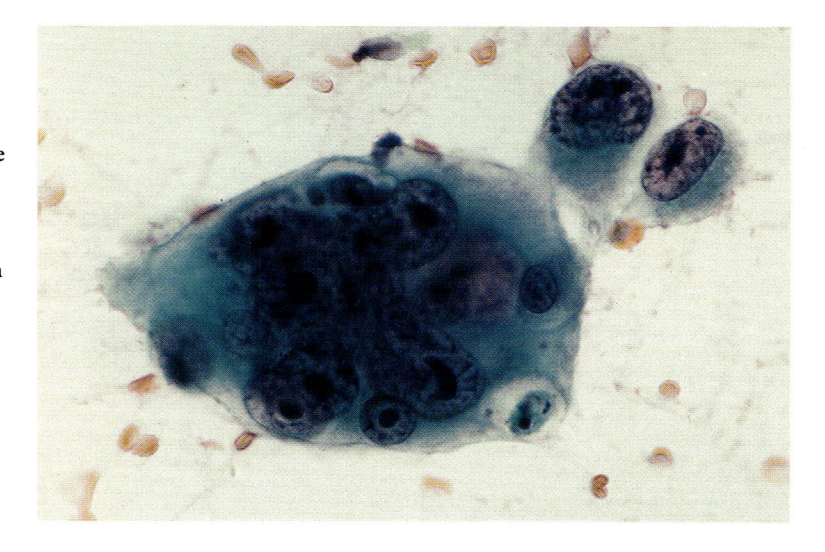

106 DIAGNOSTIC CYTOPATHOLOGY

METASTATIC CARCINOMA

The lungs have a vast capillary network through which the entire blood flow passes. They also possess an extensive network of lymphatics which have free anastomoses with the lymphatics of the upper abdomen. Cancer cells are easily carried to the lungs which are common sites of metastatic tumours. It has to be remembered, however, that the lung is itself a frequent primary site of the commonest malignancies, namely adenocarcinoma, squamous cell and anaplastic carcinoma. In addition, many other tumours which include extragonadal germ cell tumours, a variety of sarcomas and assorted epithelial and mesenchymal neoplasms, benign or of border-line malignancy, develop in the lung. The cytopathologist required to give an opinion on a lung lesion needs to bear this in mind. Cytomorphological appearances seen in respiratory tract specimens may be diagnostic or suggestive of any of the lesions that occur in the lung, and may even direct attention to a silent extrapulmonary primary. In common practice, however, a cytopathological diagnosis of a metastatic pulmonary deposit is not made in isolation, but is correlated with clinical and radiological assessment.

A few examples of metastatic tumours and the associated diagnostic problems are illustrated and discussed below.

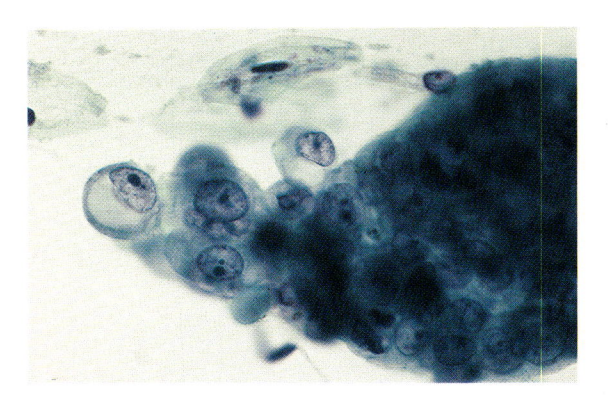

Fig. 3.81 Adenocarcinoma

Papanicolaou ×525: bronchial washings

Adenocarcinoma diagnosed in the bronchial washings of a man with a history of colon carcinoma was confirmed by bronchial biopsy histology. Primary adenocarcinoma of the lung more usually arises in peripheral bronchi or scars. Secondary carcinoma occasionally presents as single or multiple endobronchial tumours. In this case, neither cytology nor histology was able to determine whether the tumour was bronchogenic or metastatic.

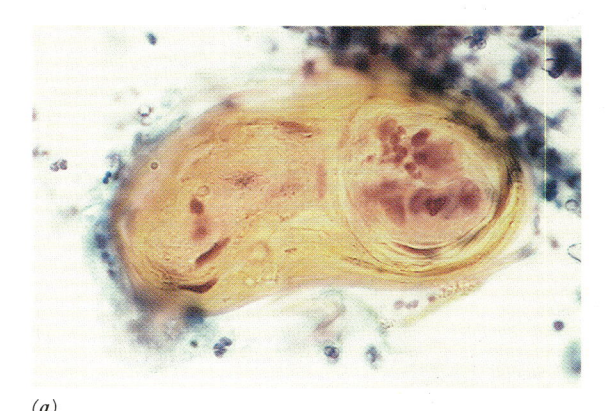

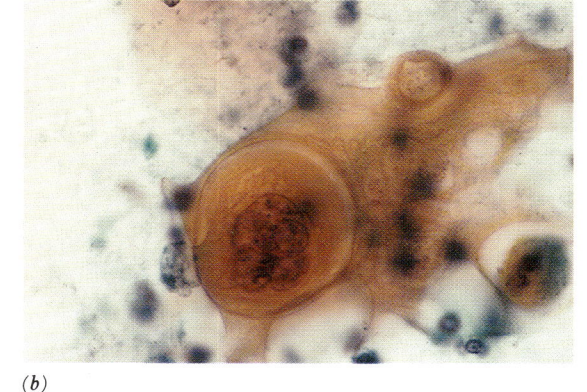

(a) (b)

Fig. 3.82 Squamous carcinoma of larynx

Papanicolaou ×525 (a) sputum: secondary (b) sputum: primary; another case

Squamous carcinoma of the larynx is usually well differentiated and epithelial pearl formation (a) is a notable feature. It may contain many refractile dyskeratotic cells, ghost nuclei and bizarre anucleate keratinized cells (b) indistinguishable from the cells of a keratinized bronchogenic carcinoma (see Fig. 3.47). The cells in (a) came from a patient who had multiple lung nodules, rheumatoid arthritis of long standing and a history of carcinoma of larynx treated by radiotherapy. The differential diagnosis which lay between rheumatoid lung and mestastatic disease was resolved by the presence of numerous unequivocal squamous carcinoma cells in the sputum (a). The cells in (b) were found in the sputum of a patient with clear lung fields and a tumour seen through a laryngoscope to be confined to one vocal cord.

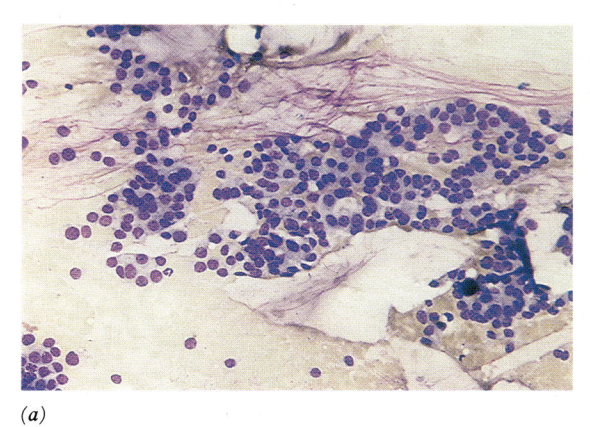

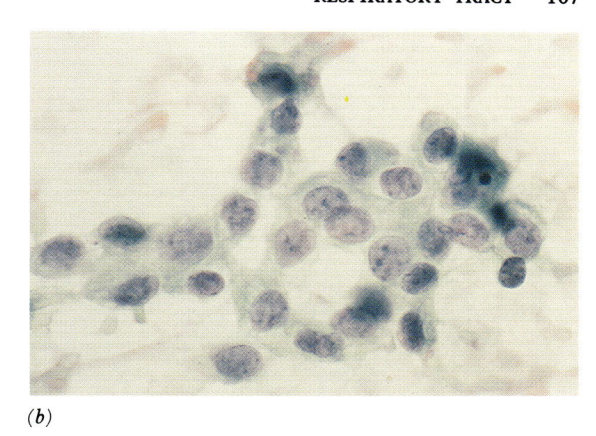

Fig. 3.83 Adenocarcinoma of breast
(a) MGG ×133: FNA; lung (b) Papanicolaou ×525: FNA; lung; another case

Carcinoma of the breast metastasizes readily to the pleural spaces. A deposit in the lung may develop from blood-borne tumour emboli direct from the primary site or via the pleural cavity. The tumour cells are often monomorphic, arranged in an acinar pattern and do not secrete much mucin but may contain an occasional intracellular mucin droplet. Both the patients, whose cells are shown, had undergone mastectomy for breast carcinoma; both had intrapulmonary masses with smooth contours. The chest X-ray appearances of these patients were highly suggestive of metastatic deposits and the cytological features were considered to be consistent.

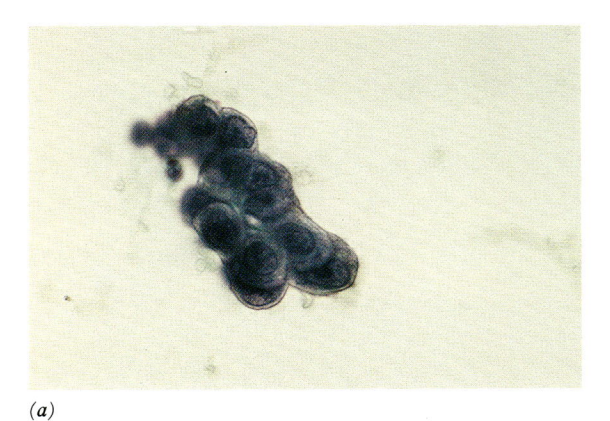

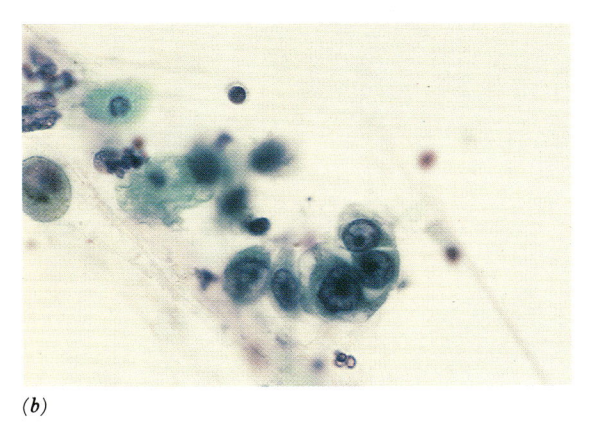

Fig. 3.84 Adenocarcinoma of colon
(a) Papanicolaou ×525 bronchial washings (b) FNA; abdominal mass; same case

The malignant cells in the bronchial washing are arranged in a row with a suggestion of palisading and with firm luminal borders (a) and were reported to be from a poorly differentiated adenocarcinoma. The patient underwent a lobectomy; the tissue diagnosis was poorly differentiated squamous cell carcinoma. Six weeks later, an abdominal mass was detected by ultrasound carried out as the patient had developed signs of intestinal obstruction. Needle aspiration of the mass yielded identical cells (b). The histology of the lobectomy specimen was reviewed, scattered mucin vacuoles demonstrated with alcian blue and the diagnosis revised to metastatic mucin-depleted colon carcinoma.

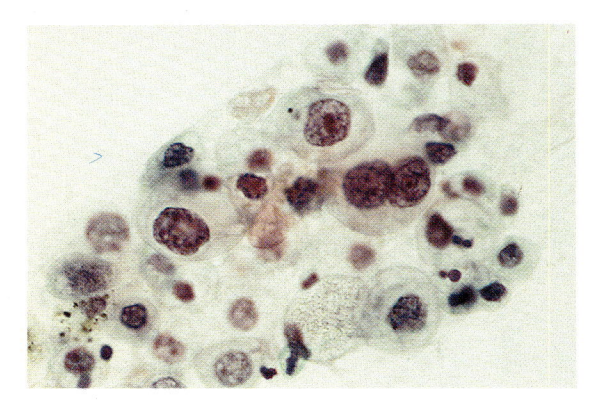

Fig. 3.85 Adenocarcinoma of pancreas
Papanicolaou ×525: sputum

The pancreas is probably the commonest source of a silent primary which spreads to the lung. An adenocarcinoma was diagnosed on sputum cytology, and broncho-alveolar carcinoma was suggested as the chest X-ray showed diffuse infiltration. Development of further symptoms in the patient led to the discovery of a pancreatic carcinoma.

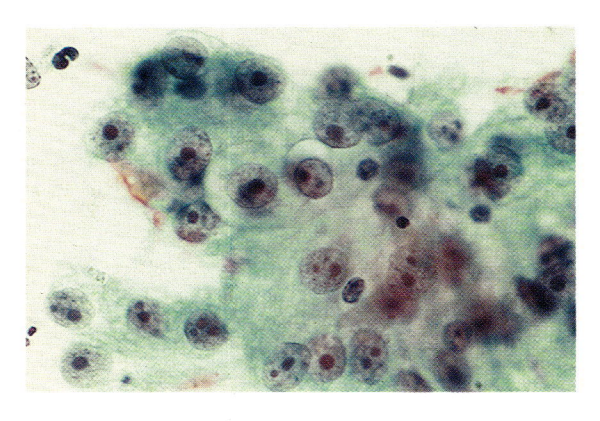

Fig. 3.86 Renal cell carcinoma
Papanicolaou ×525: sputum

Malignant renal cells have abundant cytoplasm, which may be granular but is more often clear. The nuclei may appear relatively bland, but contain prominent nucleoli. A diagnosis of metastatic renal cell carcinoma, rather than a primary clear cell carcinoma of lung, was consistent with the cannon ball appearance of the lung mass in a patient with a proven carcinoma of the kidney.

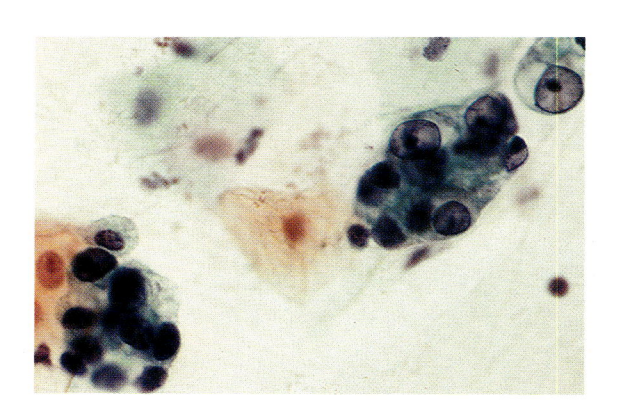

Fig. 3.87 Mesonephroid carcinoma of ovary
Papanicolaou ×525: sputum

The sputum of a woman with a history of a mesonephroid carcinoma of ovary contained several adenocarcinoma clusters. The cells in some clusters were small and virtually filled with deeply staining nuclei without obvious nucleoli. Other clumps were composed of significantly larger cells with substantial clear cytoplasm, paler vesicular nuclei and large conspicuous nucleoli. The appearance was considered to be diagnostic of a metastatic mesonephroid tumour.

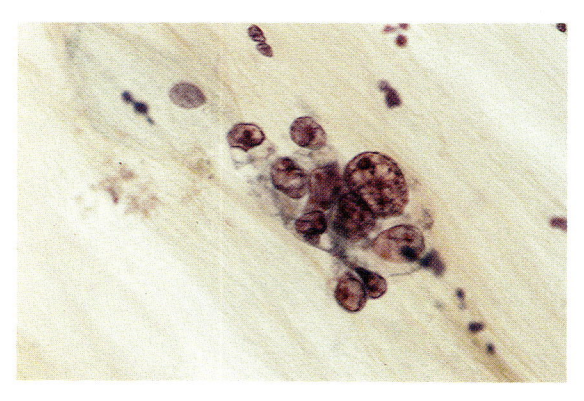

Fig. 3.88 Adenocarcinoma of endometrium
Papanicolaou ×525: sputum

This micrograph illustrates an example of an adenocarcinoma which cannot be distinguished from a primary lung adenocarcinoma. The diagnosis of metastatic disease in this patient was based on the radiological appearances of the multiple lung shadows in a patient with a history of endometrial carcinoma. The cytological findings lent support to the diagnosis but are not specific.

LYMPHOPROLIFERATIVE DISORDERS

Fig. 3.89 Hodgkin's disease

(a) Papanicolaou ×720: FNA; lung (b) MGG ×720: Same specimen; another smear (c) Papanicolaou ×720: same smear as (a)

The exact cell of origin of Hodgkin's disease, a lymphoproliferative disorder, is uncertain. The lymphocytes that accompany the neoplastic cells are benign and reactive. The diagnostic cell is the Reed-Sternberg (R-S) cell. In its classical form the R-S cell is binucleate (a), (b) or appears multinucleated (c) in light microscopy preparations, although ultrastructural studies have shown a single polylobated nucleus in some instances. Each nucleus contains a prominent macronucleolus linked by fine strands of chromatin to the condensed chromatin on the nuclear margin. The cytoplasm is darkly-staining and may be amphophilic. The mononuclear form, referred to as the Hodgkin's cell (a), (b) is non-specific as it occurs in other lymphoproliferative malignancies. The treatment and prognosis of Hodgkin's disease is different from lymphocytic lymphomas and a diagnosis of Hodgkin's lymphoma should not be made in the absence of the R-S cell. Primary Hodgkin's lymphoma of the lung is rare, but secondary involvement of pulmonary tissue is common. The fine needle aspiration illustrated was obtained from a new shadow which appeared in the lung of a patient with established extrapulmonary Hodgkin's disease.

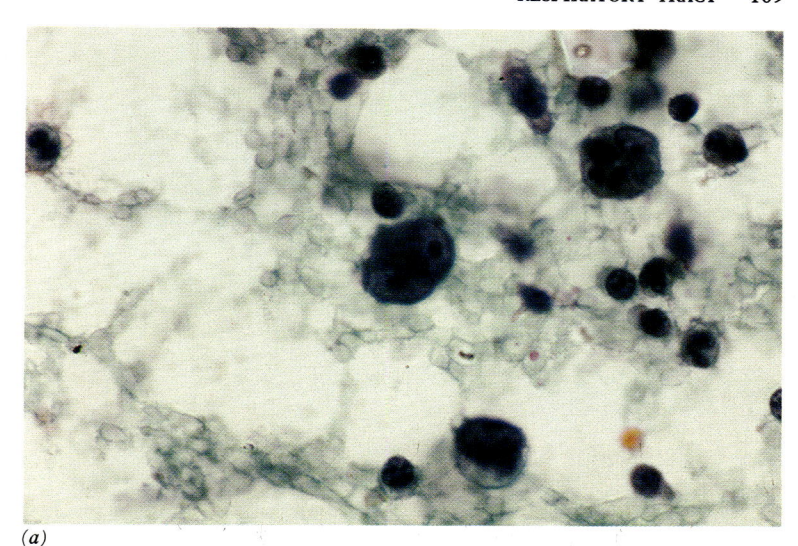

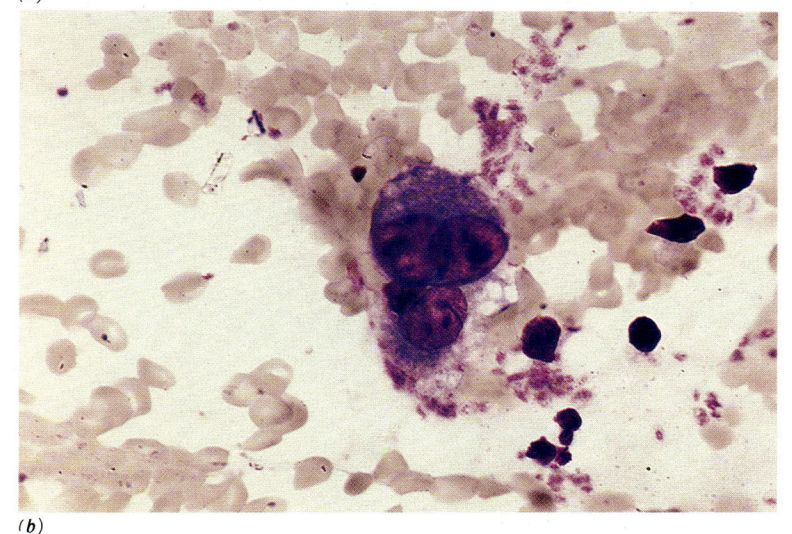

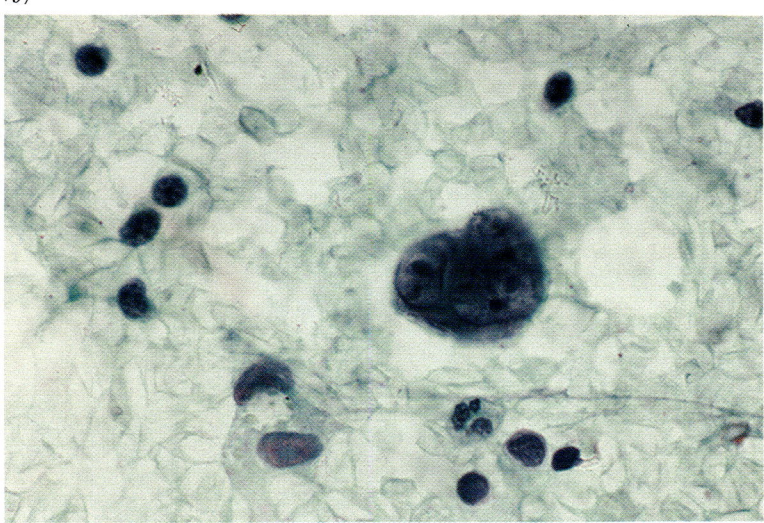

110 DIAGNOSTIC CYTOPATHOLOGY

(a)

(b)

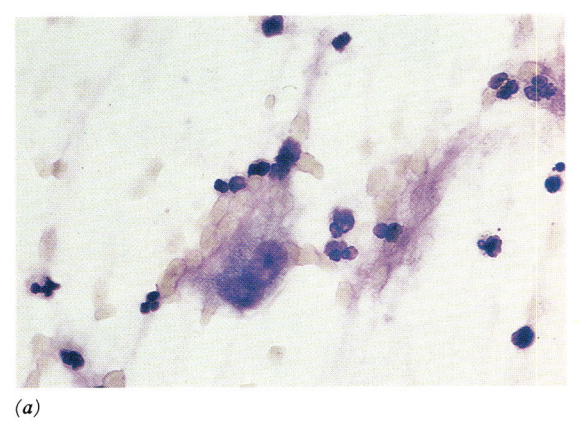

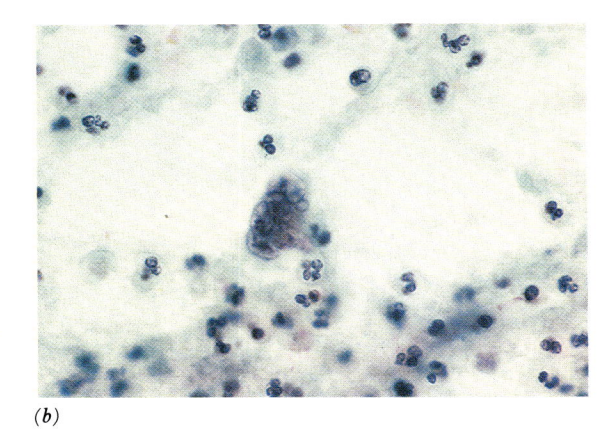

Fig. 3.90 Hodgkin's disease
(a) MGG ×525: FNA; lung (b) Papanicolaou ×525: same specimen; another smear

The binucleate (a) and polylobated (b) R-S cells illustrated are two of a dozen tumour cells identified in pus aspirated from a lung abscess in a 19-year-old male with a history of Hodgkin's lymphoma. Culture of the abscess fluid yielded a growth of *S. pneumoniae*, an infection to which patients with this disease are particularly prone. The shadow diminished in size on antibiotic therapy but did not resolve completely and enlarged again shortly after. The flimsiness of the cytoplasm and the somewhat ragged appearance of the neoplastic cells is due to necrotic changes in a purulent specimen.

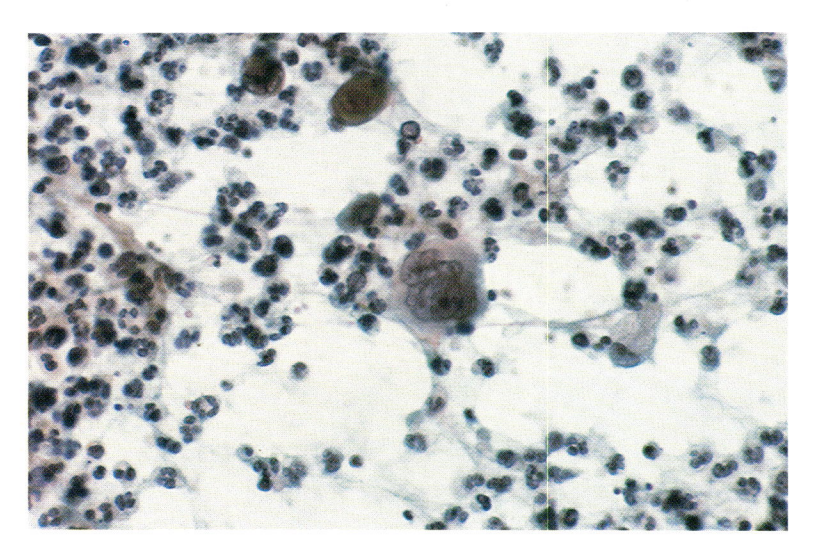

Fig. 3.91 Hodgkin's disease
Papanicolaou ×458: FNA; lung

The characteristic cell of nodular sclerosing Hodgkin's is a variant of the R-S cell, known as the lacunar cell. This type of cell has abundant pale cytoplasm, a polylobated nucleus and a smaller nucleolus than the classical R-S cell. The name derives from the tendency of the cell to shrink away from the surrounding structures in formalin-fixed tissues to lie within a clear lacuna. This appearance is not seen in alcohol-fixed cytological preparations and the cell is difficult to distinguish from other bizarre malignant cells of lymphoid origin. The diagnosis of primary nodular sclerosing Hodgkin's of the lung was established by open biopsy histology.

Fig. 3.92 Non-Hodgkin's lymphoma

Papanicolaou (a) ×183: sputum
(b) ×720: same field

Precise classification of non-Hodgkin's lymphoma is established by combined immunocytochemical and morphological analyses of the malignant lymphoid cells. In the absence of the former, a reliable, if limited diagnosis, is often possible in cytological material and an opinion may be given on the grade of the tumour. Small-celled lymphomas are generally of low grade malignancy; larger neoplastic cells with nucleoli indicate a high grade lymphoma. A shower of tumour cells (a) covered the smears made from the sputum of a woman with a bronchial biopsy diagnosis of small cell carcinoma. High power examination (b) shows discrete neoplastic cells with narrow rims of cytoplasm surrounding large nuclei. The majority of the nuclei are round, a few show the indentation or cleft seen in cells of lymph follicle centre origin. The nucleoli vary in size and number and are seen in all the cells in the field (b). A cytodiagnosis of a high grade centroblastic lymphoma was confirmed by repeat biopsy histology.

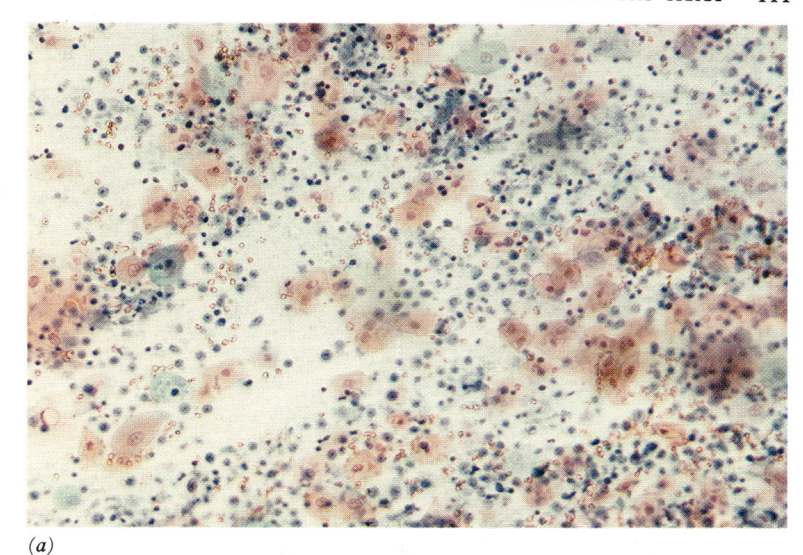

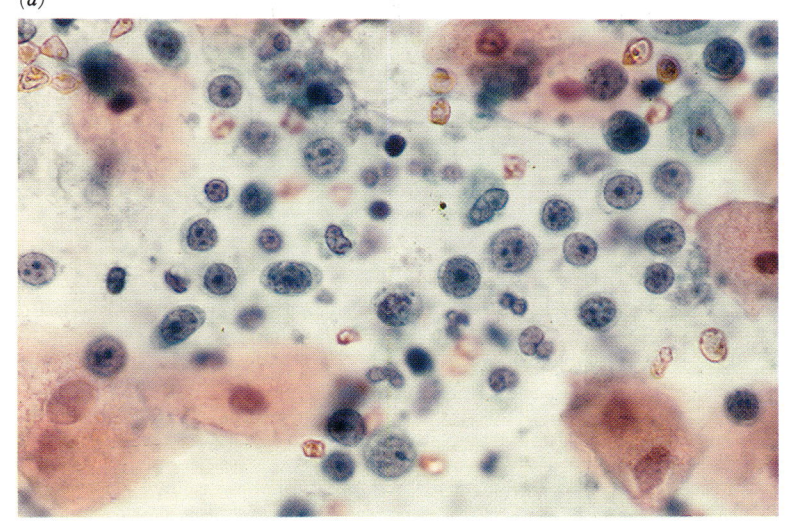

(a)

(b)

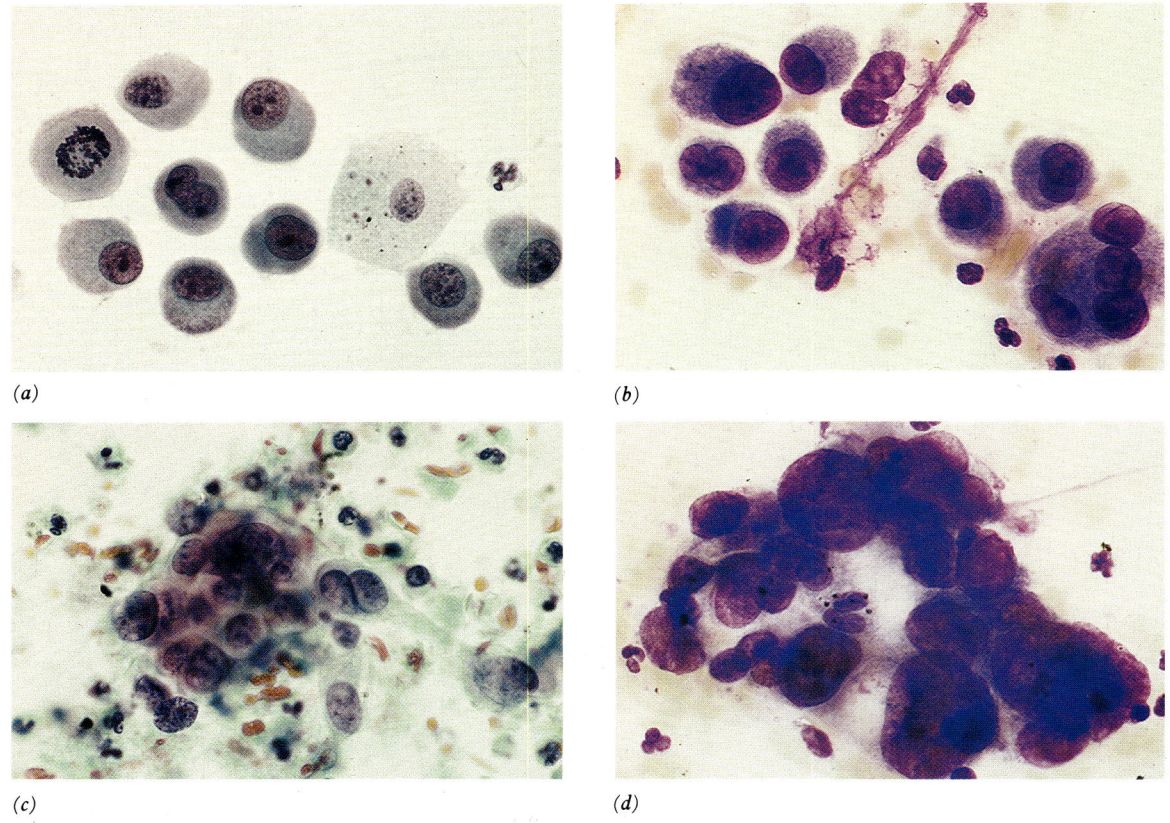

Fig. 3.93 Multiple myeloma and primary bronchogenic carcinoma

(a) *Papanicolaou ×525: FNA; lung; myeloma cells* (b) *MGG ×525: same specimen; another smear; myeloma cells* (c) *Papanicolaou ×525: same smear as (a); carcinoma cells* (d) *MGG ×525: same smear as (b); carcinoma cells*

Two malignancies in the same organ are exceedingly rare, but not unknown. A diagnosis of double pathology should be based on clear cut evidence especially in cancers which can be extremely pleomorphic. The lung aspirate of an elderly patient contained two separate populations of malignant cells, myeloma and carcinoma cells.

Myeloma is a lymphoreticular neoplasm of plasma cells, develops from a single clone and produces large quantities of a monoclonal antibody. It may form a solitary lesion (plasmacytoma) or present as multiple osteolytic foci or a diffuse infiltrate of marrow, lung and other organs. Light chains of the antibody may be excreted in the urine (Bence-Jones protein). The tumour cells may be differentiated plasma cells or they may be immature and pleomorphic.

The cells in (a) and (b) are large and discrete, the cytoplasm is basophilic and the nuclei are eccentric in position. A cell in mitosis is seen in (a). Two binucleate forms and one large multinucleated cell are shown in (b). A kidney-shaped nucleus is seen in (a) and in (b). The prominent nucleoli indicate immaturity of the malignant plasma cells. The patient had dysproteinaemia and Bence-Jones proteinurea.

Sheets of cohesive pleomorphic carcinoma cells with high nuclear-cytoplasmic ratios, granular chromatin and inconspicuous nucleoli were identified in the same smear (c), (d).

In the terminal illness, the patient developed a pleural effusion which yielded mucin positive adenocarcinoma cells, and heart failure induced by increasing viscosity of blood caused by a rapid rise in circulating myeloma proteins.

4. Serous effusions

The body cavities, the right and left pleural, the pericardial and the peritoneal have a common origin from the coelom. Each lies within a double-layered serous membrane derived from the embryonal mesenchyme. The inner layer of the membrane invests the organs within the cavity and is known as the visceral layer; reflected back over the internal wall of the body cavity, it becomes the outer parietal layer.

The three thoracic cavities containing the two lungs and the heart are self-contained. In the female the peritoneal cavity communicates with the genital tract through the fimbrial ends of the Fallopian tubes; in the male, it consists of an additional small sac applied to the abdominal parietes. A potential space separates the closely apposed parietal and visceral layers of the pleura and pericardium; the distance between the outer layer of the peritoneum, which has a complex anatomical structure, and the serosal covering of the abdominal organs is greater.

The serous membrane is made up of loose connective tissue carrying capillaries, lymphatics and nerves, and is covered on its free surface by a simple pavement epithelium which is lubricated by a small quantity of serous fluid. The fluid between the two layers of the pleura is the result of the net hydrostatic oncotic pressure of the capillaries of the parietal pleura which favours flow of a relatively protein-free fluid from these capillaries into the pleural space and its reabsorbtion by the venous capillaries of the visceral pleura (80–90%) and the pleural lymphatics (10–20%). It is likely that a similar mechanism operates in the pericardium and peritoneum. Disturbances of the mechanism that normally maintains this dynamic flow may result in accumulation of excess fluid, i.e. a serous effusion. Free fluid in the peritoneal cavity is referred to as ascites (Gr. *askos*, belly).

Two types of effusions are recognized, transudates and exudates.

A transudate results when hydrostatic pressure is increased and oncotic pressure is reduced, as in congestive cardiac failure, cirrhosis, peritoneal dialysis, hypoproteinaemia of malnutrition or hypoalbuminaemia of the nephrotic syndrome. The fluid is generally straw coloured and clear, occasionally opalescent, has a protein count of < 3 g/dl, a specific gravity of 1015 or less and contains relatively few cells. Some long standing transudates in heart failure and cirrhosis may be very cellular.

An exudate is formed when capillary permeability is increased, lymphatic flow is decreased, or both mechanisms operate. Malignant involvement of the serous membrane, which may, additionally, disrupt the capillary endothelium, is a common cause of an exudate. Other aetiologies include inflammatory disease due to infective agents, bacterial, viral, parasitic or fungal, connective tissue disease such as rheumatoid disease and lupus, pulmonary infarct, drug sensitivity and vasculitides such as Wegeners granulomatosis. The protein content of an exudate usually exceeds 3 gm/dl, the specific gravity is greater than 1015 and the cell count is generally high.

Differences in the specific gravity and protein content are fairly useful in determining whether an effusion is a transudate or an exudate, but are unreliable in approximately 10% of cases.

METHODS OF PREPARATION

Most serous effusions will clot on standing, particularly exudates which have a high protein content and are rich in fibrin. The clot may be large and jelly-like in consistency or form one or more firm, thin strands. A considerable proportion of the cells are likely to become enmeshed in the clot. To prevent clot formation, an effusion should be placed immediately in a sterile container with an anticoagulant. Satisfactory anticoagulants for 20 ml of fluid are EDTA (ethylene diamine tetra-acetic acid dipotassium salt) 20 mg; heparin, 2 mg or 200 units; 3.8% sodium citrate, 2 ml. Oxalate and liquoid are unsuitable as they distort cell morphology.

In the laboratory, the volume, colour and consistency should be noted. It is desirable but not essential to estimate the specific gravity and total protein content. A differential cell count is useful in a sterile, benign effusion. The usual methods of preparation are as follows:

1. The fluid is centrifuged in a conical tube at 600 g or approximately 1500 rpm for 5–10 minutes. The supernatant is discarded and smears made from the virtually fluid free sediment, rapidly wet-fixed in 95% ethanol, for Papanicolaou and H & E staining, air-dried and fixed in methanol for a Romanowsky stain. Spare wet-fixed and air-dried smears are kept in reserve for any special staining procedures that may be required. Some cytologists

recommend re-suspension of the cell button in normal saline, and a second spin to wash the cells free of protein before spreading the smear.

2. Cytocentrifugation.
3. Concentration of cells on membrane filters.
4. Preparation of cell blocks for histology.

A heavily blood-stained fluid can be treated with 1% acetic acid to lyse the cells. A preferable method is to make smears from the buffy coat of nucleated cells that separates out between the supernatant and the erythrocyte layer. If necessary, Wintrobe tubes may be used to obtain several buffy coats of reasonable depth.

A clot in the fluid can be used to make a succession of dabs on one or more grease-free slides until all the fluid has been squeezed out. The last two or three imprint smears from the practically dry clot are usually satisfactory. Alternatively, it can be processed for histological sections.

BENIGN CONDITIONS

Mesothelial cells

The pavement lining of a serous membrane is formed by a single row of cuboidal mesothelial cells which are the only cells of epithelial origin native to a serous effusion. Other benign epithelial cells may, in rare instances, enter an effusion through a fistula or be accidentally introduced during a surgical procedure. A metastatic tumour is the most likely source of non-mesothelial epithelial cells. Almost all effusions, benign or malignant, also contain blood derived cells.

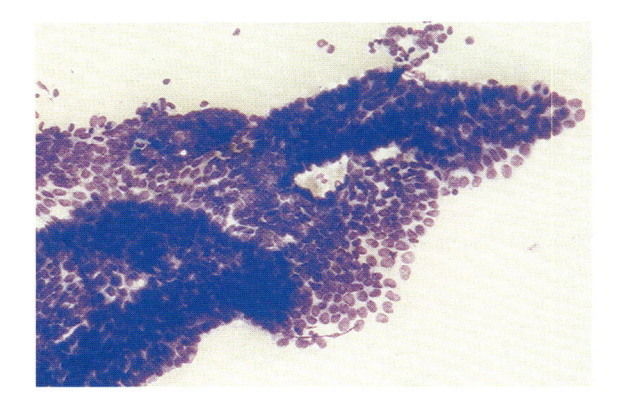

Fig. 4.1 Mesothelial cells
MGG ×133: fluid from the Pouch of Douglas

It is virtually impossible to obtain fluid from a normal pleural or pericardial space. A small quantity of free peritoneal fluid is often present in the Pouch of Douglas from which normal mesothelial cells may be recovered. These are often single or they may appear in a sheet of uniform cells with round or oval nuclei.

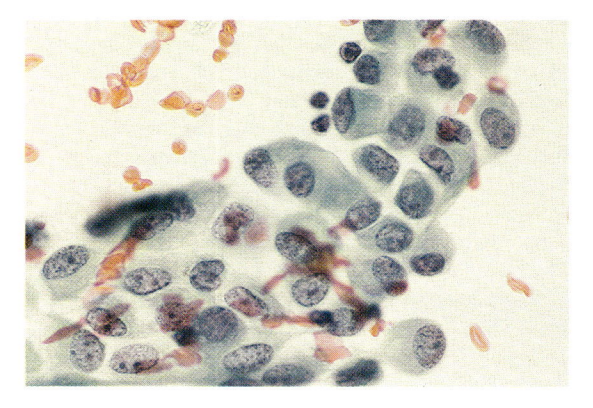

Fig. 4.2 Mesothelial cells
Papanicolaou ×525: peritoneal washing

Sheets of normal mesothelial cells may be dislodged by mechanical means which include washing the serous cavity with sterile normal saline. The cells are cuboidal in shape and have a translucent cytoplasm which sometimes contains small vacuoles. The nuclei are regular in size, finely reticulated and may have one to three small nucleoli. Normal mesothelial cells have been shown by electron microscopy to have microvillous brush borders.

SEROUS EFFUSIONS 115

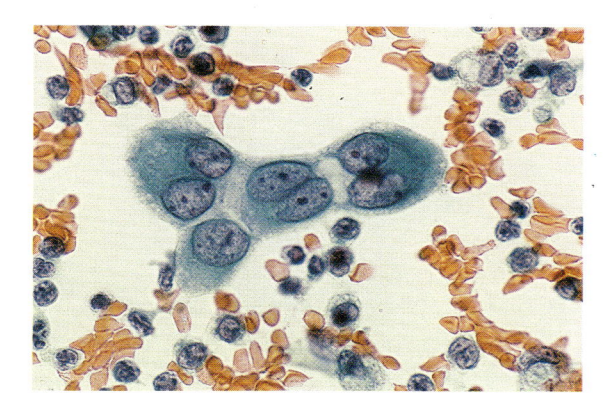

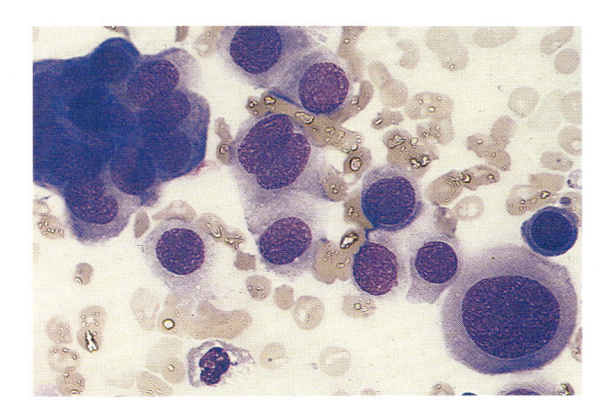

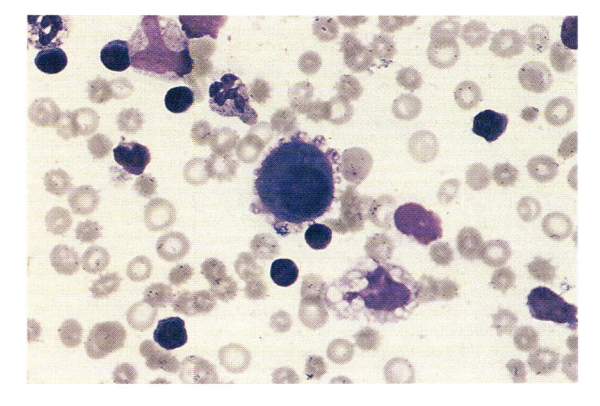

Fig. 4.3 Active mesothelial cells

Papanicolaou ×525: pleural fluid; case of congestive cardiac failure

In a pathological collection of fluid, mesothelial cells display morphological changes which suggest that they have been shed from a hyperplastic mesothelium; these cells have many of the characteristics of proliferative cells and are referred to as active or reactive forms. The cells are larger than their normal counterparts. An increase in the amount of RNA is reflected in greater basophilia of the cytoplasm. This may be uniform in colour or two-toned with a darker and a paler zone. In some cells, the zone of pallor is perinuclear while in others it is peripheral. Another indication of increased RNA is seen in nucleoli. These are more prominent, may be increased in number and size, and show variations of size and shape.

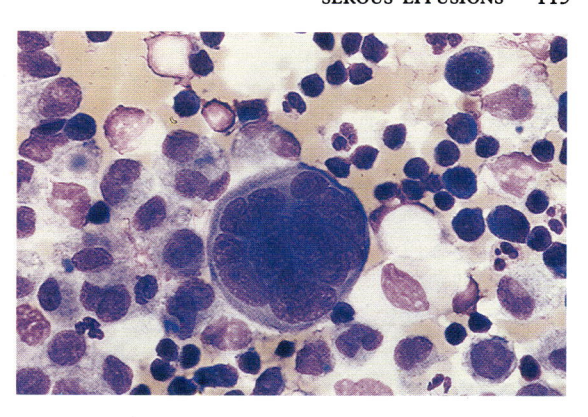

Fig. 4.4 Multinucleated mesothelial cells

MGG ×525: pleural fluid; case of left ventricular failure

The nucleus of the active mesothelial cell shows a proportionate increase in size and the nuclear cytoplasmic ratio is relatively constant. The majority of cells have one nucleus but two or three nuclei are not uncommon (Figs. 4.3 and 4.5). Large multinucleated forms packed with 20 or more nuclei can occur; these show minor variations in size but have a comparable chromatin pattern.

Fig. 4.5 Active mesothelial cells

MGG ×525: ascitic fluid; case of active chronic hepatitis

Variations in the size of the active forms within one specimen can be quite considerable. While a fair proportion of the cells are uniform, the odd cell may be disconcertingly large. A comparison of its nuclear and cytoplasmic characteristics with intermediate forms which progressively bridge the differences between it and a typical mesothelial cell is useful in identifying the cell.

Fig. 4.6 Active mesothelial cell

MGG ×525: pleural fluid; a treated case of lymphosarcoma

The brush border of the active mesothelial cell is more easily appreciated in a light microscopy preparation. Its appearance can vary according to the state of the cell, method of preparation and the staining procedure. It may consist of several distinct hairs of variable length or a shaggy 'beard' on one side or round the perimeter of the cell, as an indistinct halo, as a finely striated border (Fig. 4.3) or as, in this micrograph, a coronet of uneven knob like projections.

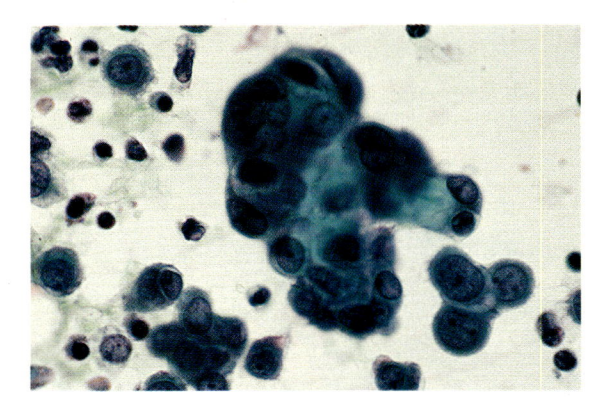

Fig. 4.7 Active mesothelial cells

Papanicolaou ×525: pleural fluid; case of active chronic hepatitis

Mesothelial cells often adhere to each other in small collections. Larger clumps can occur and these are a notorious source of diagnostic difficulty, leading even to false positive reports of malignancy. Shed into a fluid medium, the clump becomes rounded with some depth of focus. The fine vacuoles present in a normal mesothelial cell may be enhanced in size and number. An overall impression of a glandular structure may be created.

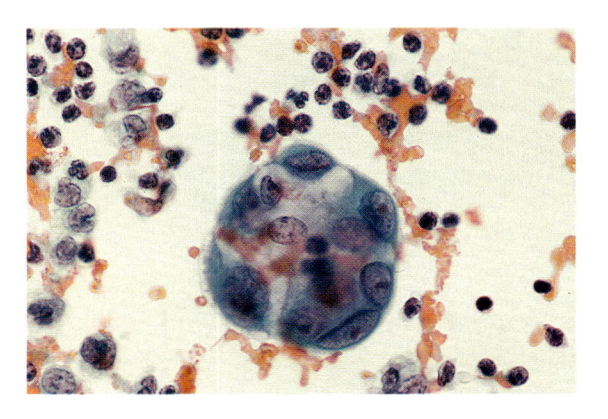

Fig. 4.8 Active mesothelial cells

Papanicolaou ×525: pleural fluid; case of congestive cardiac failure

The normal slit-like intercellular space may be widened between cells with well developed microvilli into what is referred to as a 'window'. This is generally crossed by several hair-like bridges, (presumably microvilli) connecting the neighbouring cells (see also Figs. 4.7 and 4.9).

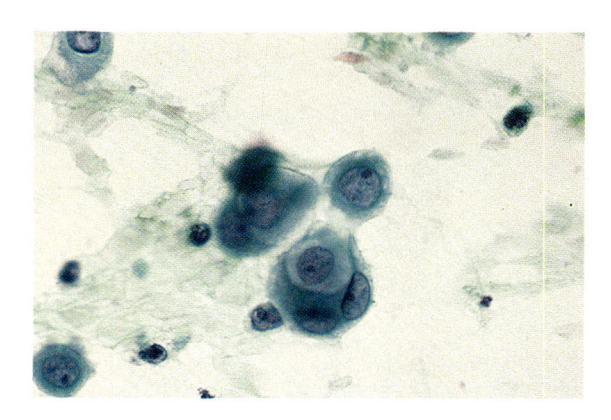

Fig. 4.9 Reactive mesothelial cells

Papanicolaou ×525: post-operative pleural effusion

Yet another situation in which a misleading appearance is encountered is the post-operative collection of fluid. The irritation of the mesothelium during the surgical procedure provokes reactive changes. The fluid is generally rich in cells which are basophilic, have conspicuous nucleoli, and which form pseudoglandular structures. Note the sharp edges that mark the line of attachment of microvilli. The specimen illustrated came from a man who, 2 days earlier, had undergone a diagnostic thoracotomy for a nodule which proved benign.

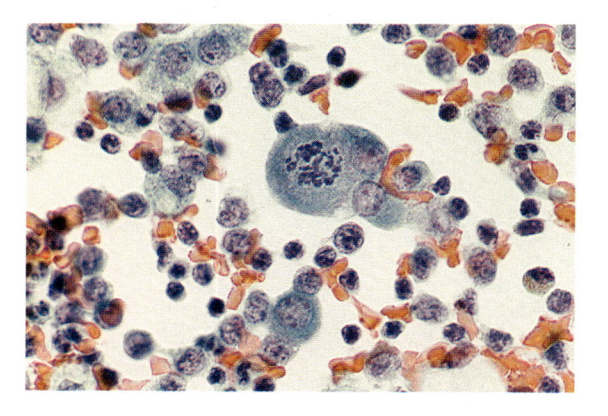

Fig. 4.10 Mesothelial cell in early metaphase

Papanicolaou ×525: same case as in Figure 4.3

A sterile serous effusion can serve as a suitable cell culture medium; cells in it will continue to live and grow for some time and, on occasion, divide. A mitotic figure in an effusion, should never be assumed, in the absence of diagnostic cancer cells, to indicate malignancy unless the diagnosis is supported by cytogenetic studies. The mitotic cell illustrated is adherent to two typical benign mesothelial cells and is itself of mesothelial origin.

Fig. 4.11 Degenerate mesothelial cells

MGG ×720: same case as in Figures 4.3 and 4.10

While some mesothelial cells continue to proliferate in an effusion, others undergo degenerative changes. The degenerate forms are a shade larger than their viable fellows. Their foamy cytoplasm is distended with multiple hydropic and fatty vacuoles. The nucleus is usually eccentric, paler in colour and has a smudged chromatin. One or two nucleoli are generally visible. Foamy mesothelial cells may contain particulate matter and this has been attributed to phagocytic properties.

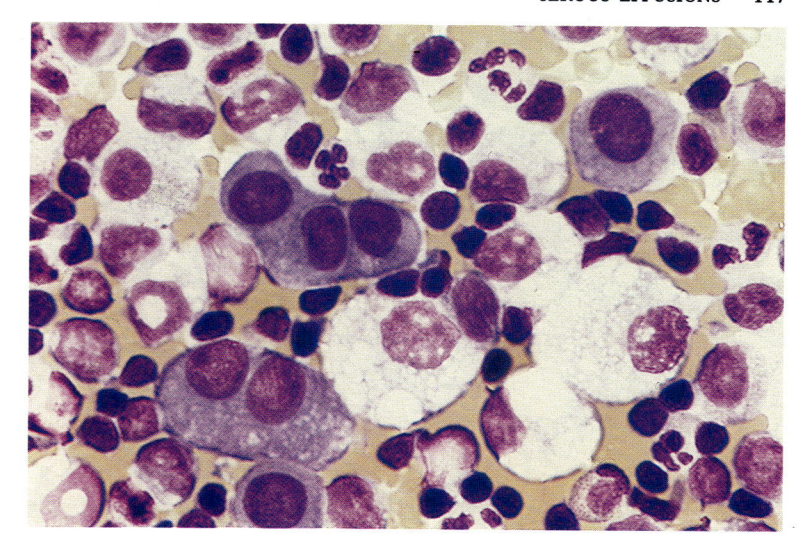

Fig. 4.12 Degenerate mesothelial cells: signet-ring forms

MGG: ×720: ascitic fluid; case of chronic hepatitis B and cirrhosis

In an extreme degree of degenerative vacuolization of the cytoplasm, the nucleus is compressed against the edge of the cell which acquires a signet-ring form. This type of cell occurs in any type of effusion, but is more plentiful and more often seen in ascites due to primary liver disease. A misdiagnosis of metastatic signet-ring carcinoma is avoided by careful assessment of the chromatin pattern.

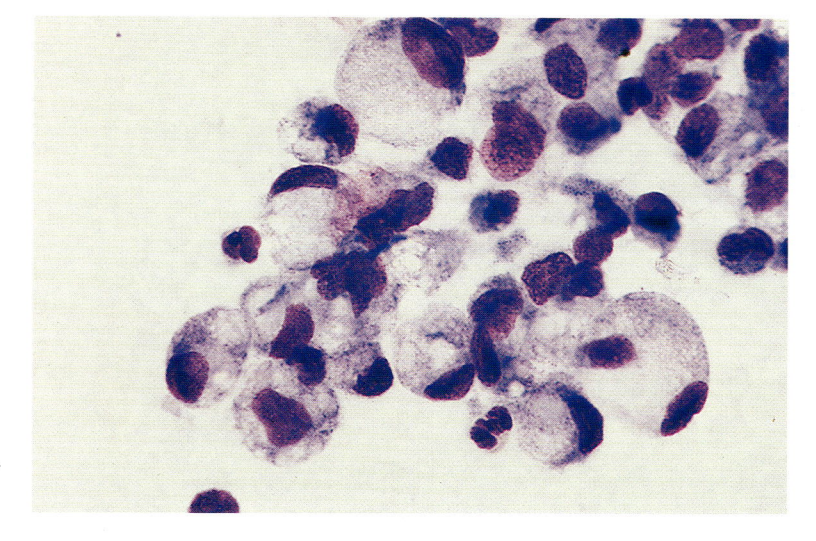

Marrow-derived cells

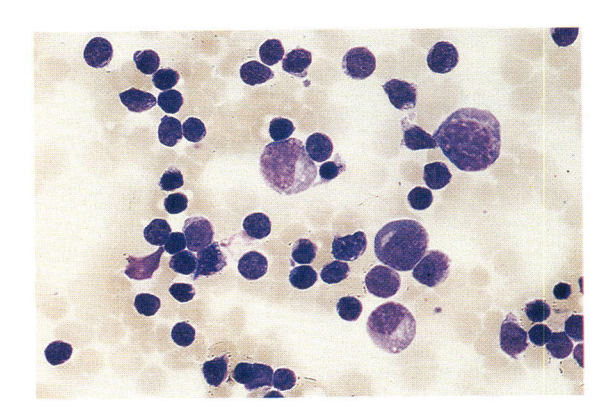

Fig. 4.13 Lymphocytes: lymphoplasmacytoid cells

MGG ×525: pleural fluid; case of squamous cell carcinoma of lung

The one cell which is present in every serous effusion is the lymphocyte and it often constitutes the largest single group of a mixed cell population. A tuberculous effusion may consist almost entirely of lymphocytes; most are small and mature, but some prolymphocytes and a few lymphoblasts are generally present; mesothelial cells are conspicuous by their near total absence. In some cases of lung carcinoma, a pleural effusion contains a preponderance of lymphoid cells including plasma and plasmacytoid cells; the latter have the nuclear characteristics of fully mature or slightly immature lymphocytes and the cytoplasmic features of plasma cells.

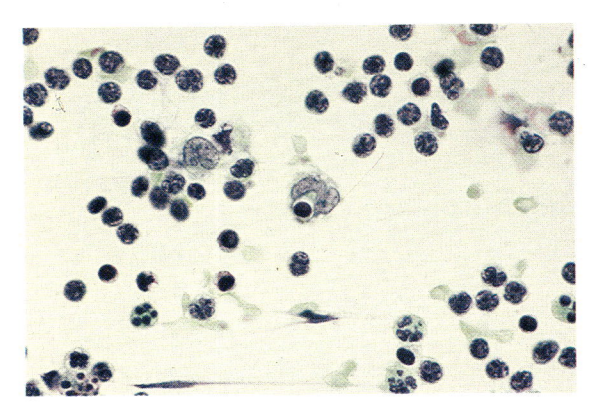

Fig. 4.14 Macrophages: neutrophils: lymphocytes

Papanicolaou ×525: pleural fluid

The true macrophage, a wandering scavenger, is derived from the bone marrow monocyte which it closely resembles. It is smaller than the mesothelial cell and has a pale grey deeply indented nucleus. It phagocytoses debris and other smaller cells; in this case, a lymphocyte. Macrophages are present in fluids in variable numbers, together with neutrophils, lymphocytes and occasionally eosinophils and basophils

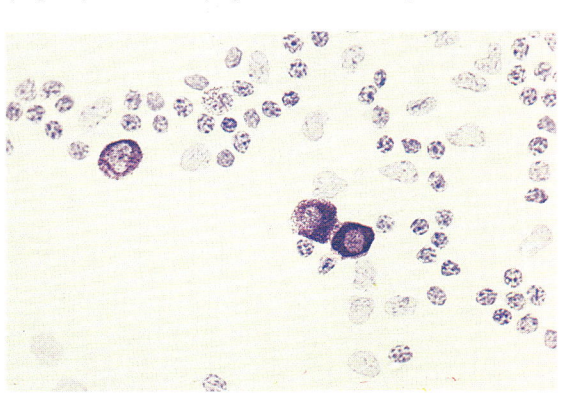

(a) 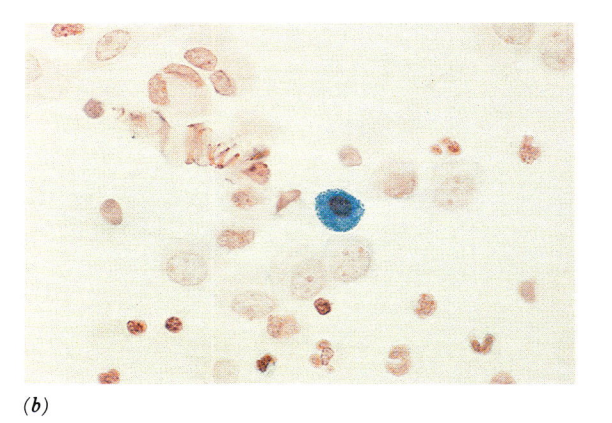 (b)

Fig. 4.15 Mast cells

(a) Toluidine blue ×333: pleural fluid (b) Alcian blue ×525: pleural fluid

Mast cells, derived from the primitive haemohistioblast via the histioblast, resemble basophil leucocytes but are much larger. They are found in bone marrow and loose connective tissue especially near blood vessels and may find their way into effusions in very small numbers. Mast cells contain numerous metachromatic granules, probably heparin, which stain bright purple with toluidine blue (a). They also react with alcian blue (b) to give the same blue colour as acid mucin. Mast cells are concerned with the release of histamine and heparin, but their full function is not known, and their significance in effusions remains unexplained.

Fig. 4.16 Eosinophils
Hansel's stain ×720: pleural fluid

A small number of eosinophils may be met with in an effusion obtained at the first tap and have no significance. Repeated taps result in the introduction of minute quantities of air and this provokes an increase in the number of eosinophils. Significant pleural eosinophilia is much more common than peritoneal eosinophilia and is associated with parasitic infestations or hypersensitivity states. The fluid illustrated came from a young male with a history of bronchial asthma: eosinophils constituted 80% of the cell population.

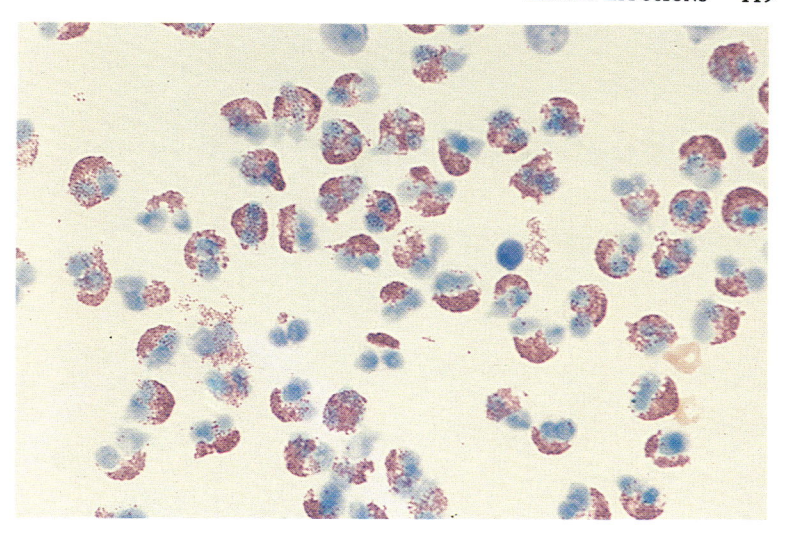

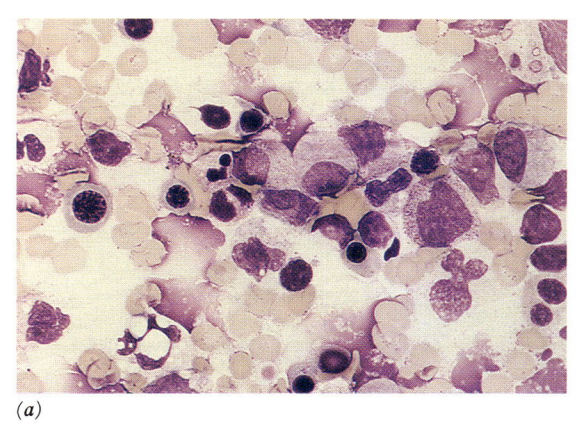

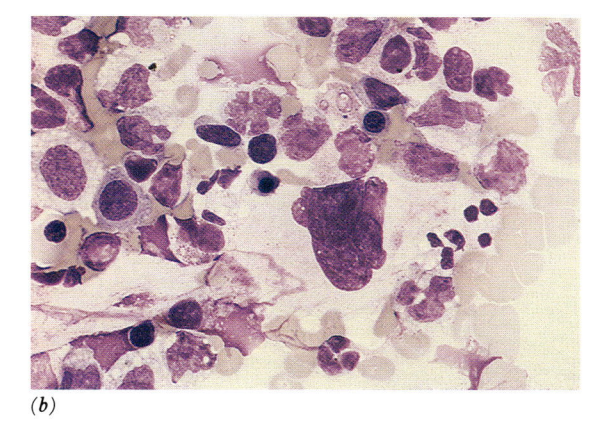

(a)   (b)

Fig. 4.17 Myeloid metaplasia
MGG ×525: ascitic fluid (a) normoblasts; myelocyte (b) megakaryocyte nucleus

A very occasional early neutrophil granulocyte may be present in some effusions, but they and immature blood cells in appreciable numbers are more likely to be present in effusions associated with leucoerythroblastic anaemia. The case illustrated is of a male patient with chronic myelofibrosis, hepatosplenomegaly and ascites.

Extramedullary haematopoiesis is an integral part of chronic myelofibrosis. The ascitic fluid (a) contained large numbers of normoblasts in different stages of maturation, a fair number of finely granular myelocytes (a) and one free convoluted megakaryocyte nucleus (b).

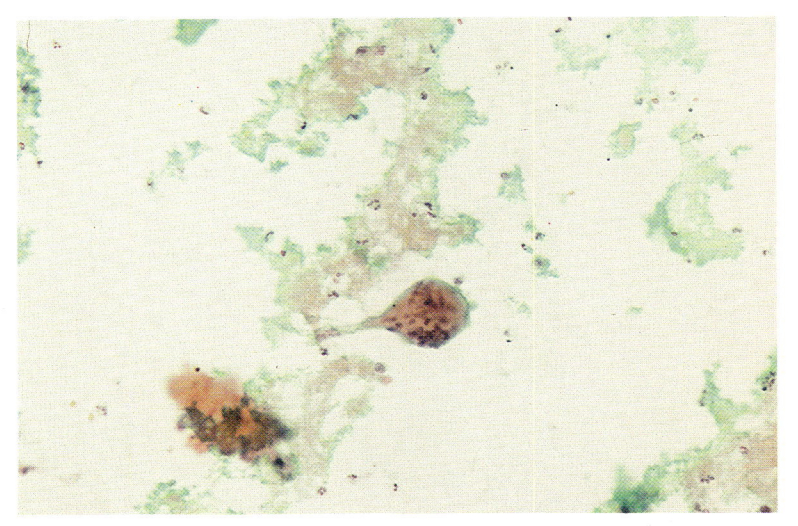

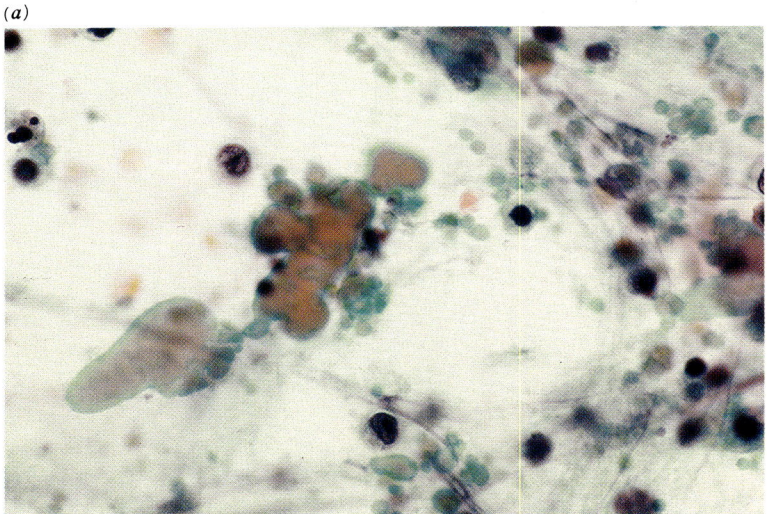

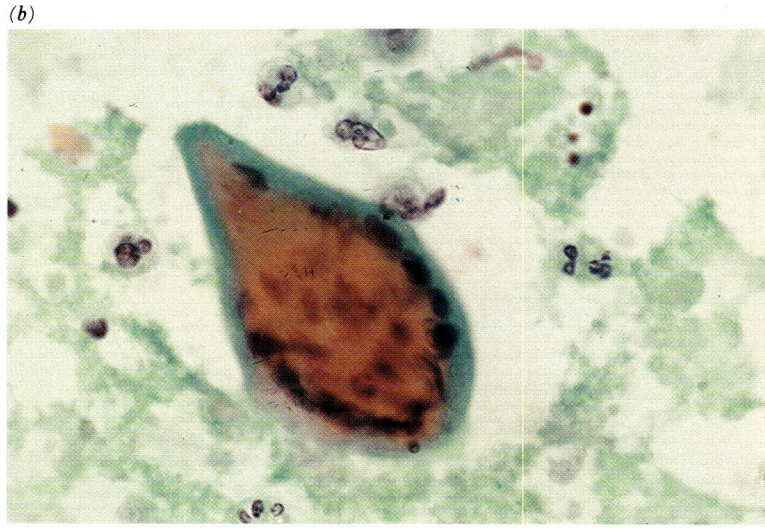

Inflammatory disease

Fig. 4.18 Rheumatoid effusion

Papanicolaou (a) ×183: pleural fluid (b) ×720; another case (c) ×720: pleural fluid; same case as (a) (d) ×720: pleural fluid; same case as (a) and (c) (e) ×720: pleural fluid; another case (f) ×720: pleural fluid; same case as (e)

The pulmonary manifestations of rheumatoid disease, a systemic disorder of probable immunological aetiology, include lung nodules and pleuritis, both of which may precede the onset of joint symptoms. The rheumatoid nodule is formed by an initial proliferation of mesenchymal cells, followed by a fibrinoid change in the collagen, which is loosened into simpler products consisting of mucopolysaccharides and glycoproteins; these form the core of the necrobiotic nodule. The cheesy centre is surrounded by a palisade of histiocytic spindle cells and occasional giant cells. This layer is in turn surrounded by fibroblasts, lymphocytes and plasma cells. The rheumatoid lesions of the pleura may be nodular or linear, and may be associated with a serous effusion.

A rheumatoid effusion is an exudate with a low glucose content (1.65 mmol/l, 30 mg%) and high lactic dehydrogenase values. It is usually small and unilateral and may be persistent or recurrent. The cytological appearance may be non-specific, the fluid being predominantly lymphocytic or with an excess of plasma cells or it may resemble pus.

A rheumatoid nodule occasionally calcifies, and calcium may be seen in the serous fluid. Cholesterol crystals may be formed in an unabsorbed effusion. Often enough, the several components of a rheumatoid nodule are released into the fluid to produce a virtually pathognomonic picture.

A typical rheumatoid effusion contains amorphous debris, epithelioid macrophages and leucocytes. The debris is usually abundant and dominates the picture. Its colour is variable in a Papanicolaou-stained smear. It may be basophilic (a), (c) or eosinophilic (d) and may coalesce into large irregular masses which are orange with green edges (b). Consisting as it does of mucopolysaccharides and glycoproteins, it is positive with alcian blue and PAS after digestion with diastase (see Fig. 12.9(c) and (d)).

The epithelioid cells are variable in number, size and shape. The tailed tadpole (a) or fish-shaped (c) epithelioid cell is distinctive to a rheumatoid effusion. It may be small and mono-nuclear, but usually has more than one nucleus and is often large and multinucleated. Its staining reaction may be similar to that of the orange and green aggregates of debris (a), (c). Elongated forms are seldom numerous; generally a greater number of round multinucleated giant forms (d), (e), (f) occur. These often contain several well circumscribed vacuoles (d), (e). Fragments of tissue consisting of spindle shaped fibroblasts intermingled with small and large multinucleated epithelioid cells (f) may be shed into the effusion.

The leucocytic infiltrate varies from case to case. In some cases, the majority of leucocytes are polymorphonuclear neutrophils. Most of these show a shift to the right and have four or five lobed nuclei (a), (c) which disintegrate into small pyknotic fragments of chromatin (a), (c). In other cases, degenerating lymphocytes are more abundant (b), (e).

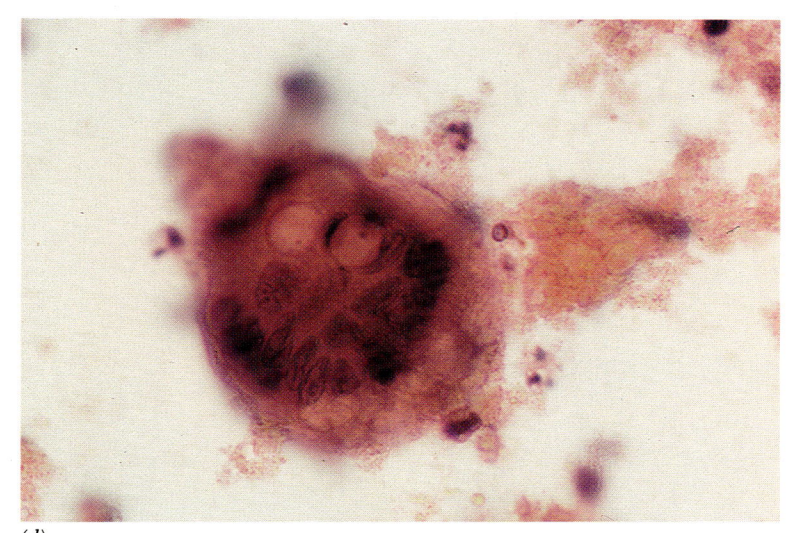

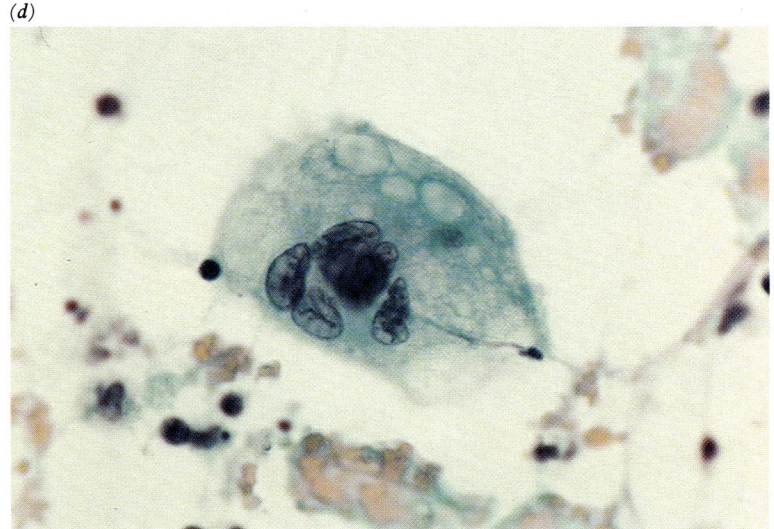

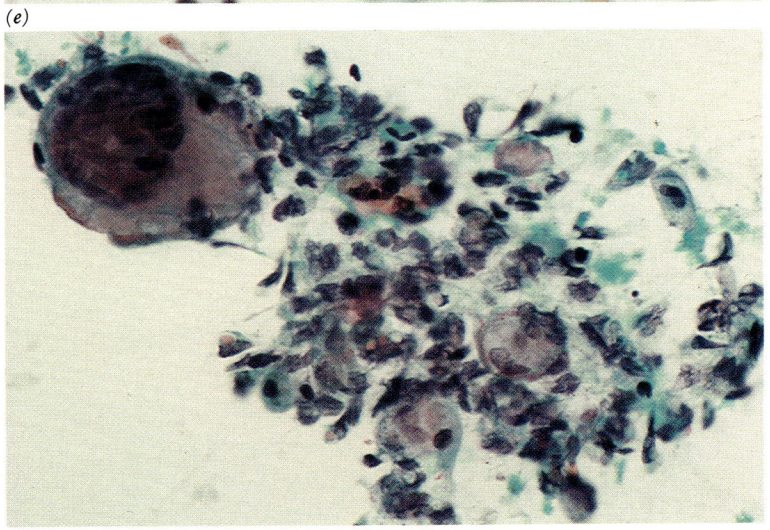

(d)

(e)

(f)

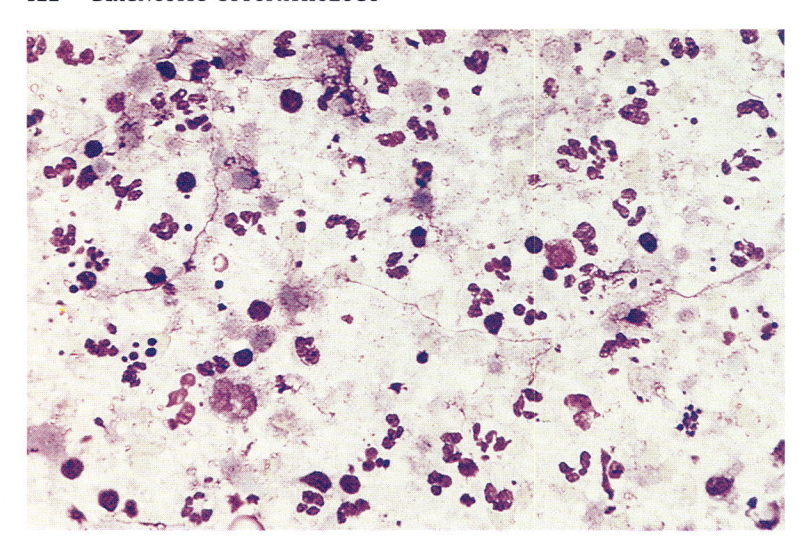

Fig. 4.19 Tuberculous empyema

MGG ×183: pleural fluid

A tuberculous effusion, as described earlier, is characterized by a preponderance of lymphocytes; neutrophils are few in number. With the onset of tuberculous empyema, this ratio is reversed. Degenerate neutrophils showing pyknotic degeneration and frank pus cells dominate the picture. A few macrophages and lymphocytes usually persist.

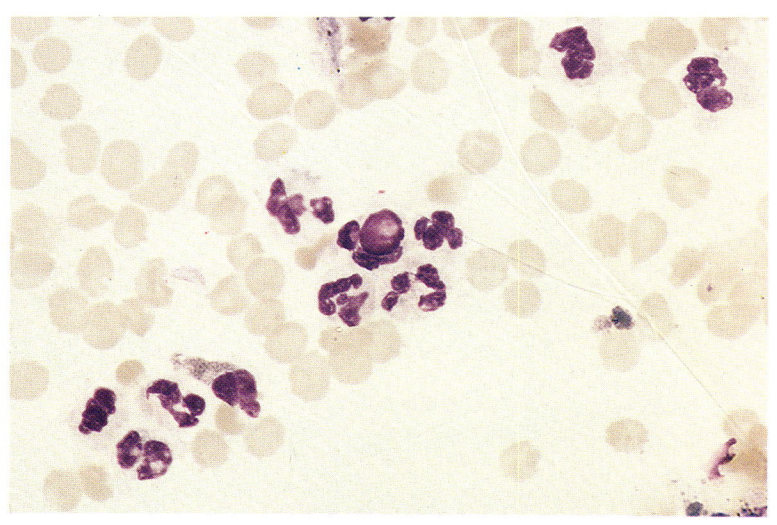

Fig. 4.20 LE cell

MGG ×720: pleural fluid

An lupus erythematosis (LE) cell is a neutrophil with ingested lysed nuclear material. The cytoplasmic inclusion is large, opaque and structureless. It fills the neutrophil and pushes its nucleus to the periphery. The LE phenomenon develops in drawn peripheral blood which has been allowed to stand. It has been reported in serous effusions but is exceedingly rare. The diagnosis of systemic lupus erythematosis was suggested by the finding of several LE cells in this ascitic fluid which was a few hours old when received in the laboratory (compare with the macrophage with an ingested lymphocyte in Fig. 4.14).

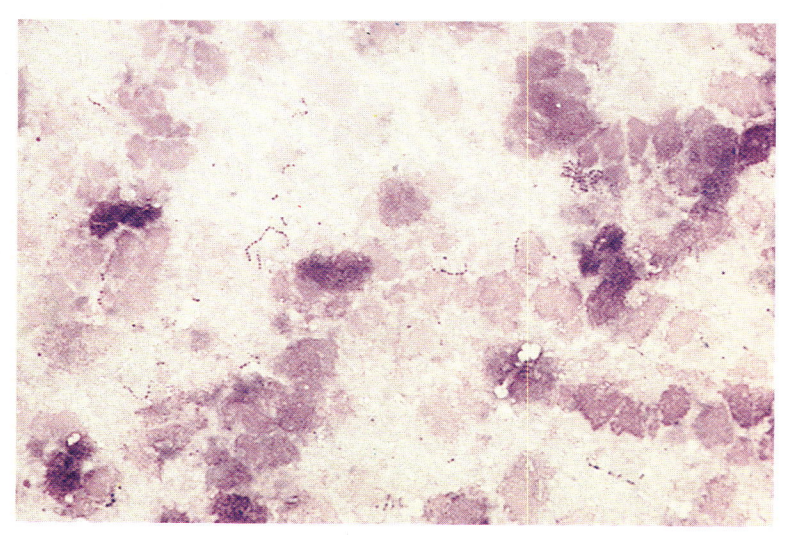

Fig. 4.21 Streptococcal empyema

MGG ×720: pleural fluid

Entry of pyogenic organisms into a serous effusion effects a dramatic change in its appearance and cellular composition. The fluid becomes turbid and may be quite thick. Mesothelial cells quickly disappear. The predominant cell is the pus cell; this is an extremely degenerate neutrophil which has an indistinct cell border and a pale, blurred, virtually amorphous nucleus. It disintegrates easily and the background of a smear of an empyema is covered with cellular and proteinous debris. The pathogenic organism may not always be evident. This empyema was due to a haemolytic streptococcus. Short chains of cocci are seen in this field.

METASTATIC TUMOURS

Carcinoma

The commonest cause of a malignant effusion is metastatic adenocarcinoma. This is as might be expected since the majority of human cancers are adenocarcinomas of one sort or another. In cytological smears as in small histological biopsies, there are a few appearances of individual cells, cell formations or distinctive secretory products which can pinpoint the primary. The increasing availability of monoclonal antibodies and application of immunocytochemical methods has extended the scope for a more precise definition of the nature and likely source of a metastatic deposit. In most cases, the primary, whether currently present or in the past, is known and the cytopathologist's immediate concern is to determine whether the effusion does or does not contain malignant cells. This is no idle exercise as an effusion in a cancer patient may be a transudate due to external pressure on blood or lymphatic channels, or hypoproteinaemia of cancer associated malnutrition or the effusion may be an exudate due to concomitant inflammatory disease.

Identification of tumour cells is usually obvious in 70–80% of malignant effusions and in a substantial proportion of cases, is practically a 'spot diagnosis'. Cancer cells are often larger than mesothelial cells and generally display greater pleomorphism. The individual malignant nucleus, except in small-celled tumours, is again usually larger than the nucleus of a mesothelial cell and occupies a disproportionately greater area of the cell. Nucleoli, which are almost always present in mesothelial cells, are not of great significance unless they are exceptionally large. Some cancer cells have macronucleoli and in such cases, the nucleolar-nuclear ratio is valuable in the assessment of malignancy. Biochemical characteristics such as mucin secretion are of considerable diagnostic value if interpreted with care. Both benign hyperplastic and malignant mesothelial cells may synthesize hyaluronic acid which reacts positively with acid mucin stains such as alcian blue; hyaluronic acid is digested by the enzyme hyaluronidase, but not diastase. Mast cells have alcian blue-positive granules (see Fig. 4.15b).

A useful exercise in a diagnostically difficult case is to compare the morphological features of the suspected malignant cells with typical mesothelial and similar cells. If intermediate forms can be traced, it is safer to assume that all the cells are of mesothelial origin. If, on the other hand, two distinct cell populations are clearly identifiable, it is reasonable to consider that one is native to the serous cavity and the other alien, i.e. metastatic.

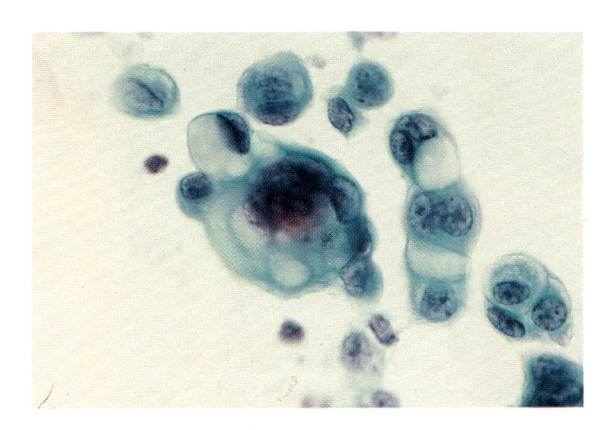

Fig. 4.22 Adenocarcinoma of lung
Papanicolaou ×525: pleural fluid

This micrograph illustrates malignant cells which are identifiable as adenocarcinoma cells, but are non-contributory as to the source of the primary. The tumour cells are larger than the degenerate histiocytoid mesothelial cells in size, the number of nuclei per cell and the nuclear cytoplasmic ratio. Nucleoli are not remarkable. The cell type is recognized by the presence of clearly bordered mucous vacuoles within some of the tumour cells. The two small cells are lymphocytes.

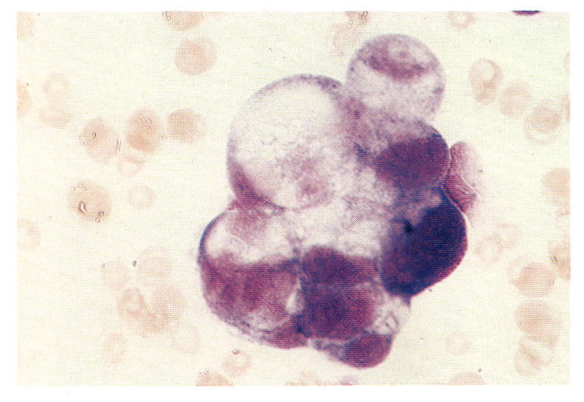

Fig. 4.23 Adenocarcinoma of lung
MGG ×525: pericardial fluid

A typical example of an adenocarcinoma cluster is shown. The large cells are aggregated into a three-dimensional cluster with a smooth, scalloped outline. Some cells have virtually no cytoplasm, others are distended with mucin, have peripheral nuclei and have assumed signet ring forms.

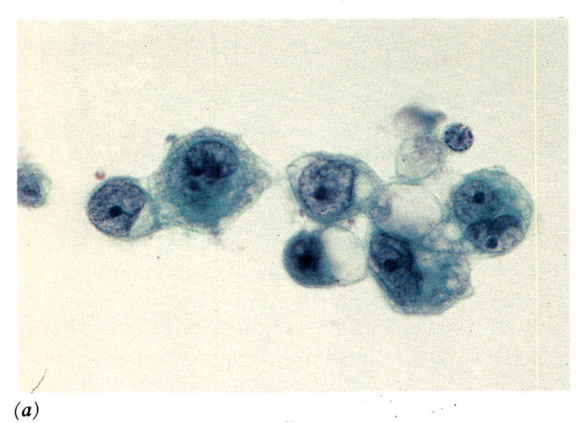

Fig. 4.24 Adenocarcinoma of lung

Papanicolaou ×525: (a) pleural fluid (b) pericardial fluid

In another example of a mucin-secreting adenocarcinoma of lung, the nuclei are large and variable in size. The cytoplasm is foamy (a). A few intracytoplasmic vacuoles are circumscribed and have the appearance of mucus droplets; most are hazy and are probably hydropic (a). The cells in the pericardial fluid are better preserved, and have a different appearance. The cell margins are well defined and the cytoplasm is deeply basophilic. One cell in the centre contains a cobweb of fine vacuoles which may be secretory or may have contained lipid. A few macrophages and leucocytes and many red blood cells are seen in the background.

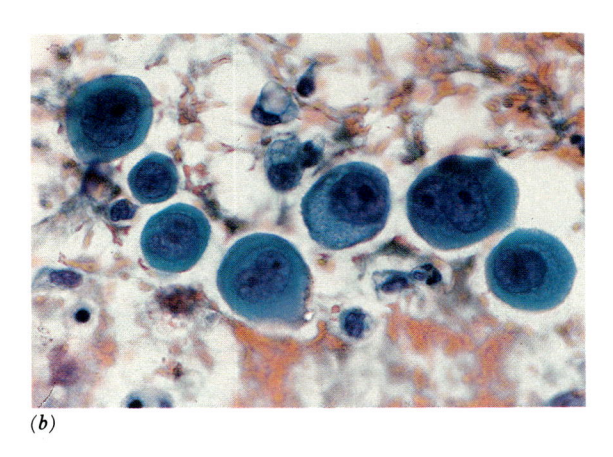

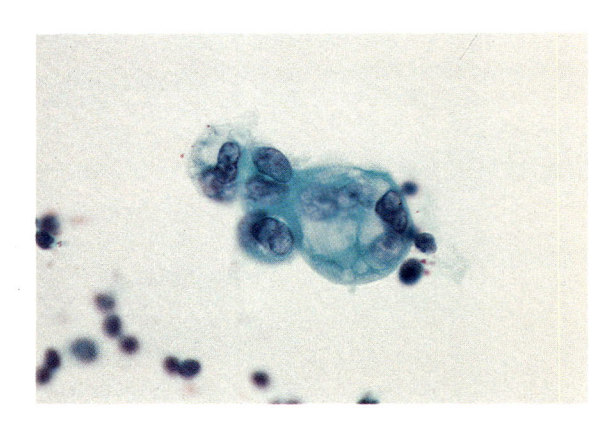

Fig. 4.25 Adenocarcinoma of pancreas

Papanicolaou ×525: ascitic fluid

A group of adenocarcinoma cells from a mucus secreting carcinoma of pancreas are illustrated. The nuclei are extremely hypochromic and have crenated outlines; both features indicate degenerative changes. The variation in cell size and the arrangement of the cells which contain mucin vacuoles is similar to that seen in Figure 4.23.

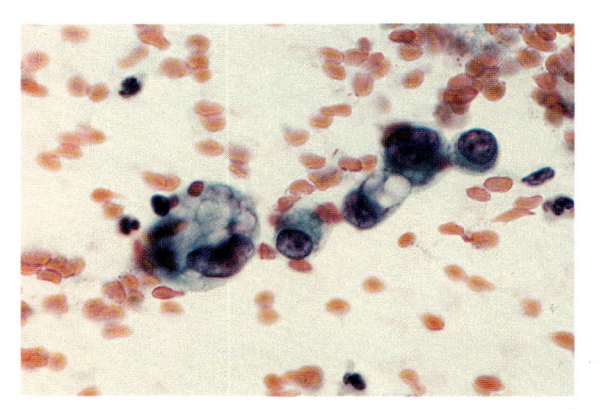

Fig. 4.26 Adenocarcinoma of breast

Papanicolaou ×525: pleural fluid

Breast carcinoma is one of the commonest cause of a metastatic malignant effusion. The cells from this case show all the stigmata of malignancy and two cells have vacuolated cytoplasm. They fulfil the cytological criteria of adenocarcinoma cells, but their appearance is not specific to any one organ.

Fig. 4.27 Mucinous cystadenocarcinoma of ovary

Papanicolaou ×720: ascitic fluid

This is another example of an adenocarcinoma which is immediately recognizable as such but is uninformative as to the source of the primary. The ballooning of the cells at the right upper border of the sheet appears to be of a hydropic nature; the sharply bordered vacuole at the lower border is a mucous vacuole. Note that while all the nuclei are hypochromic, several contain finely stippled chromatin and are not degenerate. One mitotic figure is seen in the centre of the field.

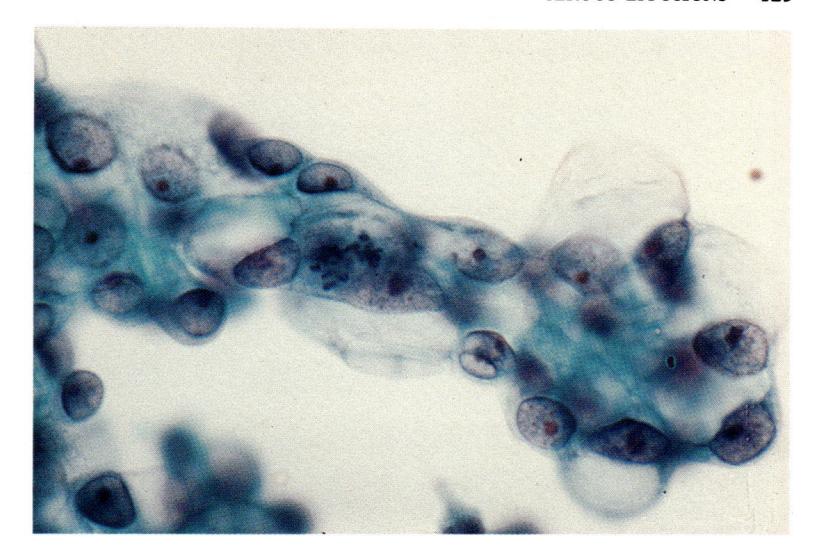

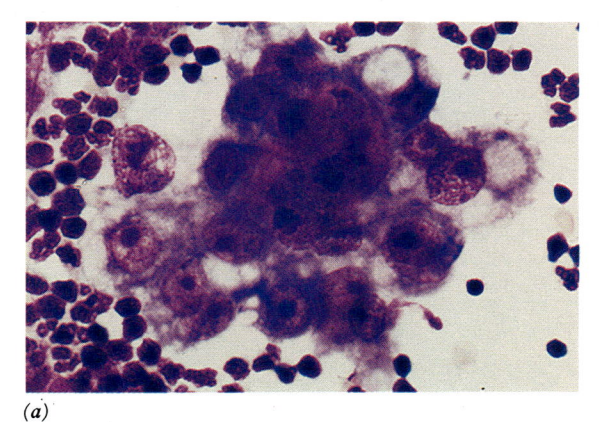

(a)   (b)

Fig. 4.28 Mesonephroid carcinoma of ovary

MGG ×525 (a) pleural fluid (b) same smear; another field

The pleural fluid of a woman with a history of mesonephroid carcinoma of ovary contained large adenocarcinoma cells and a few multinucleated carcinoma cells. The feature of note in the obviously malignant cells in (a) is the size of the nucleoli. These are larger than any nucleoli likely to occur in mesothelial cells. Despite the large size of each nucleus, the nucleolar-nuclear ratio in these epithelial cells is abnormal enough to be diagnostic of malignancy. Compare the giant multinucleated malignant cell (b) with the multinucleated mesothelial cell in Figure 4.4; note the difference between the granular chromatin of the malignant nuclei and the evenly reticulated chromatin of the mesothelial cell nuclei. The nucleoli are similar in both cells.

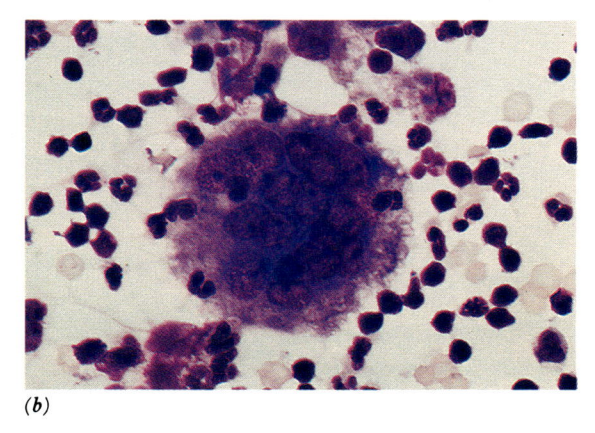

The peg-like cells which constitute the second cell type in a mesonephroma (see Fig. 3.87) were not evident in this case. The diagnosis of metastatic ovarian carcinoma was based therefore not on the cellular appearance but on clinical assessment. An ovarian tumour may be associated with a pleural effusion in the initial absence of ascites. In the syndrome first described by Meig and named after him, the ovarian tumour was a fibroma and the pleural effusion was benign. The condition in which a malignant ovarian tumour metastasizes to the pleural cavity is sometimes referred to as pseudo Meig's syndrome.

126　DIAGNOSTIC CYTOPATHOLOGY

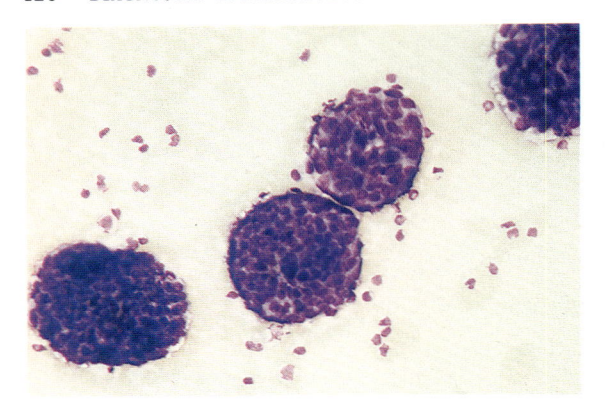

Fig. 4.29 Adenocarcinoma of breast
MGG ×133: pleural fluid

One of the few appearances seen in an effusion which is virtually diagnostic of the causative primary is produced by the type of breast carcinoma that used to be referred to as spheroidal cell carcinoma. The individual tumour cell has less cytoplasm than a mesothelial cell, a similar sized nucleus and a greater nuclear cytoplasmic ratio. Single forms are sparse and the typical picture is produced by numerous clusters of hundreds of tightly packed monomorphic cells. The size and shape of the clusters can vary, but the majority are large and spherical.

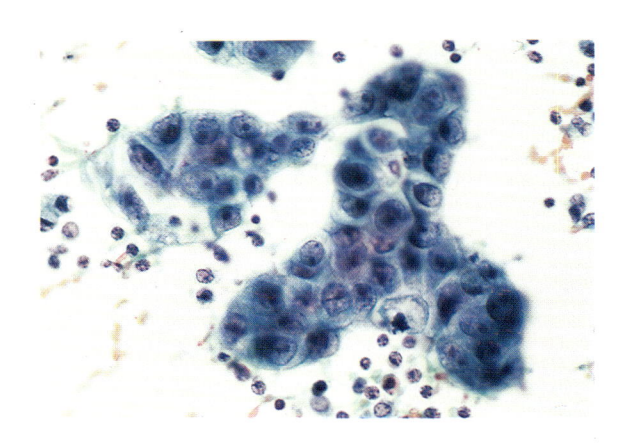

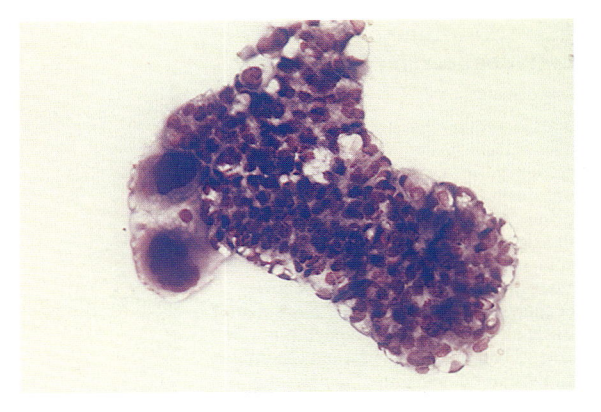

Fig. 4.30 Papillary cystadenocarcinoma of ovary
MGG ×133: ascitic fluid

It is by no means uncommon for a papillary carcinoma of ovary to shed fragments of tissue into an effusion, which acquires a granular turbidity. Microscopically, the fine granules which may be visible to the naked eye, are seen as cell aggregates which may be large enough to cover and extend beyond a low power field. These aggregates differ from the clumps of breast carcinoma cells illustrated in the preceding micrograph in several respects. Individual cells have more cytoplasm which is visible at the edge of the cluster and which results in greater separation of the nuclei. Some cells are finely vacuolated. Fairly often, substantially larger cells with one or several nuclei are seen in juxtaposition to the smaller cells and there may be some clumps composed predominantly of larger cells. The presence of smaller cells and significantly larger cells in an effusion from a female patient is most often seen in cases of ovarian carcinoma. The appearance is therefore suggestive of an ovarian primary but is not diagnostic as other tumours including the occasional breast carcinoma show a similar pattern (see Fig. 2.29).

Fig. 4.31 Papillary adenocarcinoma of gall bladder
Papanicolaou ×333: ascitic fluid

A papillary tumour, by definition, forms frond-like projections each of which has a slender fibrous stalk covered with layers of tumour cells. A true papilla with a central fibro-vascular core may be recovered in a needle aspiration but is seldom exfoliated. A papillary tumour may however, be identified in some cases by a cellular presentation which suggests that the cells have been shed from the tip of an outgrowth with a free surface. The cells appear in aggregates which may branch to form finger-like processes. The luminal border has an orderly configuration, the surface cells are palisaded and the distal nuclear borders are roughly equidistant from the free edge of the cell aggregate. A papillary carcinoma in this respect shows a cell arrangement which is usually more characteristic of benign glandular cells.

SEROUS EFFUSIONS 127

Fig. 4.32 Papillary adenocarcinoma of pancreas
MGG ×183: ascitic fluid
Not all papillary tumours show the appearance described above. The arrangement of the cells in this effusion from a histologically demonstrated papillary carcinoma of the pancreas is quite non-specific.

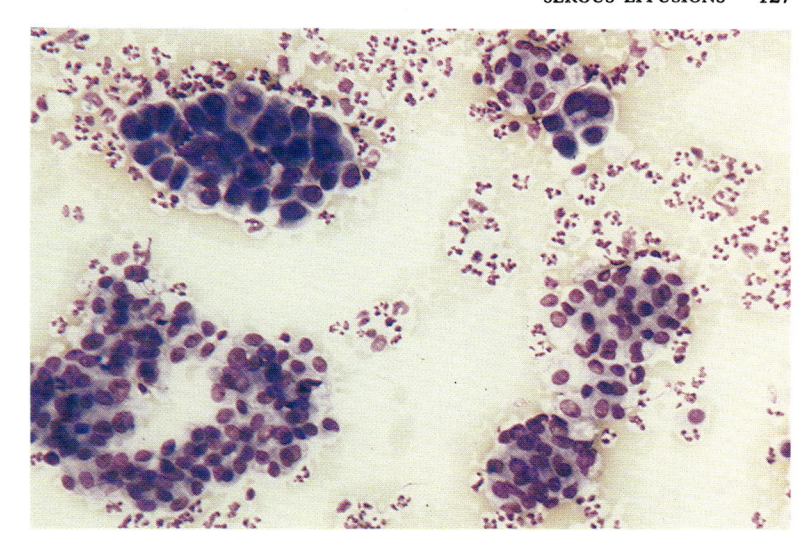

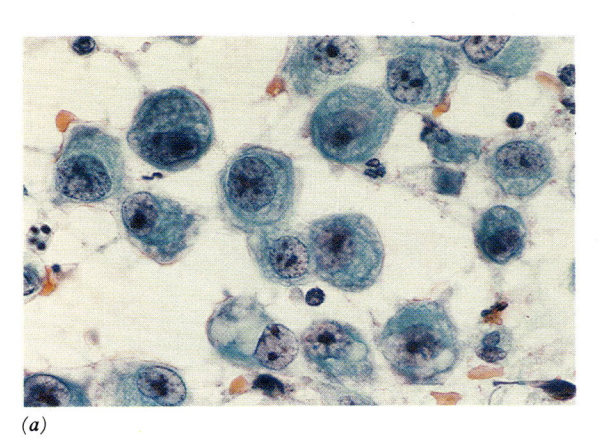

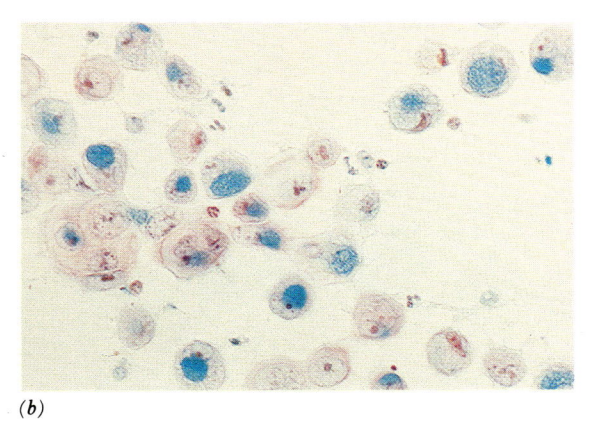

(a)   (b)

Fig. 4.33 Adenocarcinoma of stomach
(a) Papanicolaou ×525: ascitic fluid (b) Alcian blue ×333: same specimen; another smear

Biochemical activity of adenocarcinoma cells may be easily ascertained by the use of special stains. The metastatic stomach carcinoma cells in this micrograph have abundant foamy cytoplasm with the appearance of a large-meshed sieve.

Numerous mucin droplets are demonstrated with alcian blue; some form compact rounded masses, others are more diffusely stained.

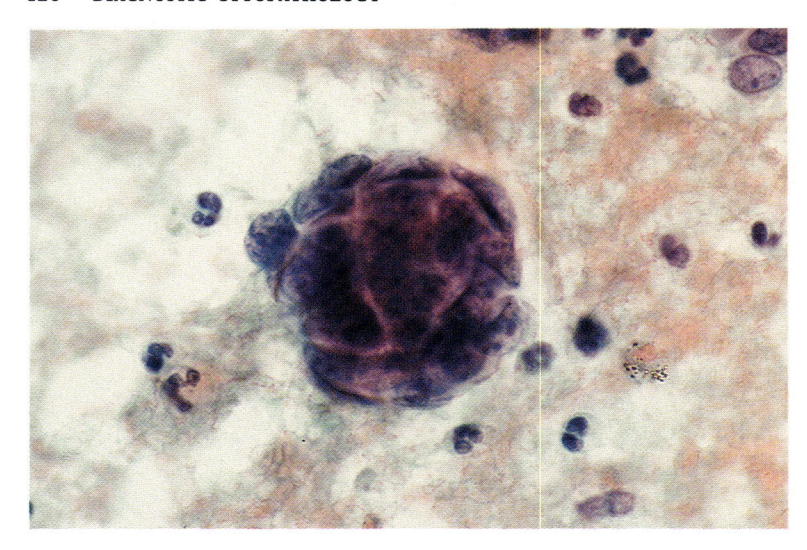

Fig. 4.34 Adenocarcinoma of colon

Papanicolaou ×720: ascitic fluid

In a very poorly differentiated adenocarcinoma, loss of distinguishing morphological features may be accompanied by loss of function. This micrograph illustrates an example of a poorly differentiated, mucin-depleted carcinoma of colon. The cells are packed together in a tight cluster. The spherical arrangement is suggestive of glandular origin but the scant cytoplasm lacks any morphological or functional feature that may identify the cell type. The malignant nature of the cells is indicated by the nuclei which practically fill the cells, are variable in size and have disorganized chromatin patterns.

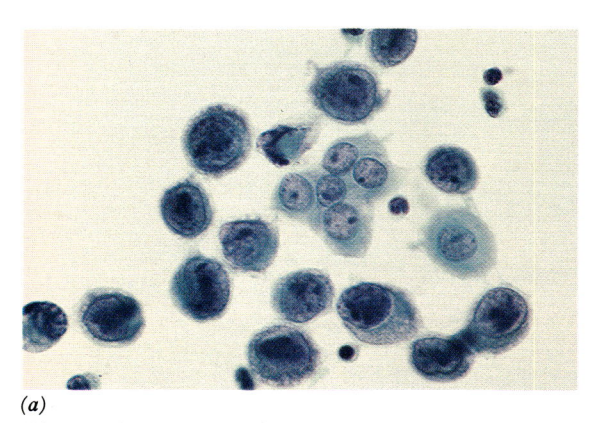

(a)

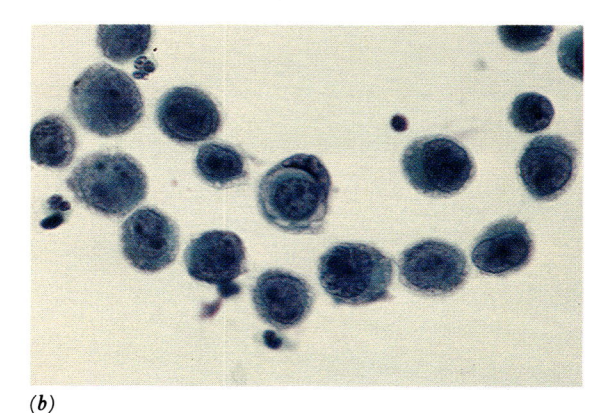

(b)

Fig. 4.35 Adenocarcinoma of stomach

Papanicolaou ×525: (a) ascitic fluid (b) same smear; another field

Reduced cohesiveness is one of the more notable characteristics of malignant cells. In some cases, this is so marked that the malignant effusion contains mainly dissociated cells. The carcinoma cells need to be distinguished from mesothelial cells and from high grade lymphoma cells.

Micrograph (a) shows malignant cells from a carcinoma of stomach, one discrete mesothelial cell (opposite 3 o'clock) and a group of five cohesive mesothelial cells in the centre of the field. The two cell types are roughly the same size. The significant differences between the malignant and benign cells are seen in the nuclei. The malignant nuclei are larger, variable and have hyperchromatic chromatin clumps which are irregular in size and distribution. The cell-within-a-cell formation (b), referred to as a bird's eye appearance, may be seen in a variety of tumours and in some benign cells.

SEROUS EFFUSIONS 129

(a)

(b)

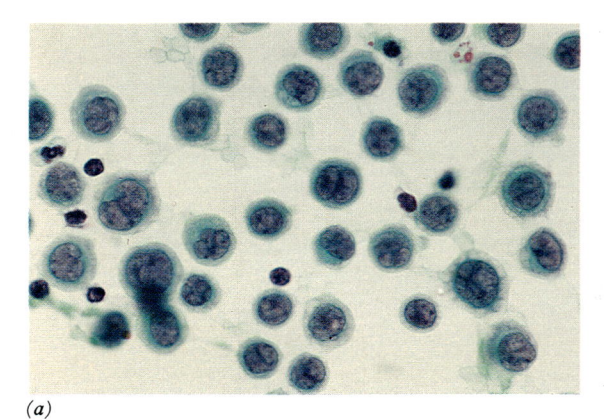

Fig. 4.36 Adenocarcinoma of breast

(a) Papanicolaou ×525: pleural fluid (b) MGG ×525: same specimen; another smear (c) Diastase PAS ×525: same specimen; another smear

The breast is one of several sources of dissociated metastatic carcinoma cells. The free cells often contain intracytoplasmic mucin vacuoles. The cells in this pleural effusion are discrete and moderately monomorphic. There is, however, variation in the morphology and the number of nuclei (a). Large diffuse mucous vacuoles are seen indenting or overlying a few nuclei in the Romanowsky-stained smear (b). The vacuoles are positive with PAS after diastase digestion (c). Note the variation in the mucin globules. The top two have dense central zones, the lower two are diffusely stained.

(c)

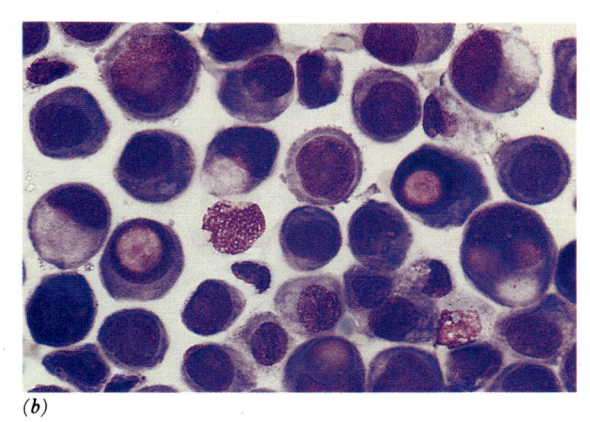

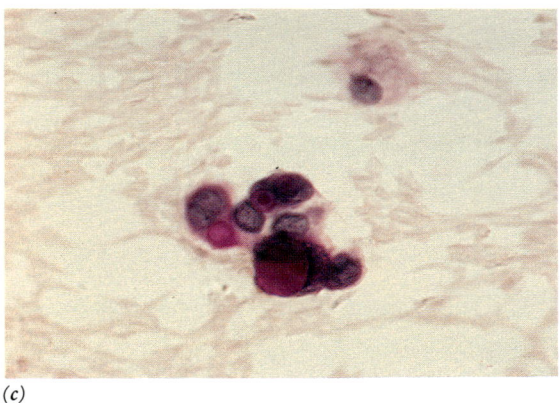

Fig. 4.37 Serous cystadenocarcinoma of ovary

Papanicolaou ×525: ascitic fluid

Another source of cells which either float free or form loose connections is a serous cystadenocarcinoma of the ovary. The cells with this type of presentation closely resemble mesothelial cells in size, shape and staining reaction. All epithelial tumours of the ovary are considered to arise from its serosal covering. Recognition of malignancy may be difficult on occasion; as a rule, the nuclei of the tumour cells are larger and more pleomorphic and the nuclear cytoplasmic ratio is fairly high. Two additional features which are sometimes met with in a malignant effusion due to a serous cystadenocarcinoma of ovarian origin are seen in this micrograph. A few cells contain mucin vacuoles. A serous tumour of ovary can be heterogenous and may contain foci of mucous differentiation. The other feature to note is the anomalous eosinophilia of some tumour cells. This is occasionally seen in degenerating cells, benign or malignant and does not indicate squamous differentiation.

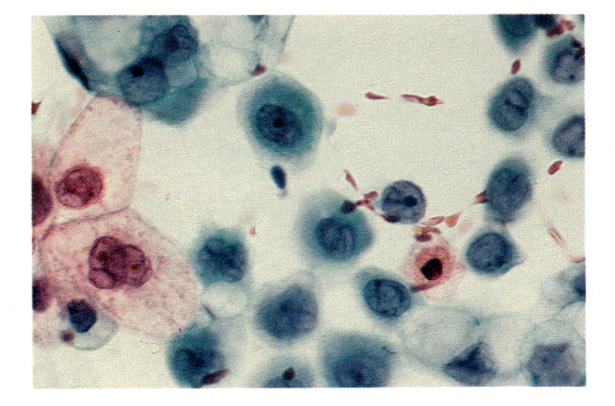

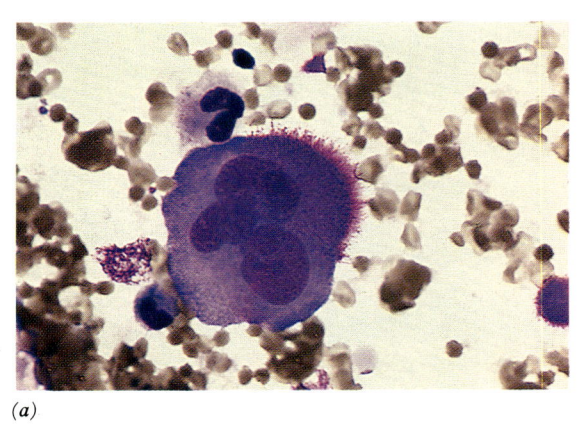

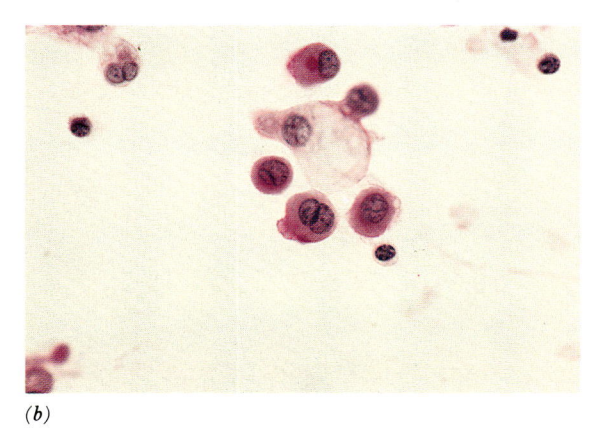

Fig. 4.38 Serous cystadenocarcinoma

(a) MGG ×525: ascitic fluid (b) PAS ×525: ascitic fluid; another case

Free floating tumour cells may occasionally have a covering of microvilli. These are generally uneven in length and considerably longer than the microvilli of benign mesothelial cells. The hair-like pseudo-cilia are usually present at one pole of the cell, but may entirely cover the cell. They may be seen in breast or gastric carcinomas, but are most frequently encountered in serous tumours of the ovary. They are difficult to see in Papanicolaou stained smears, but are clearly visible in Romanowsky stained smears (a). They react positively with the PAS reagent (b).

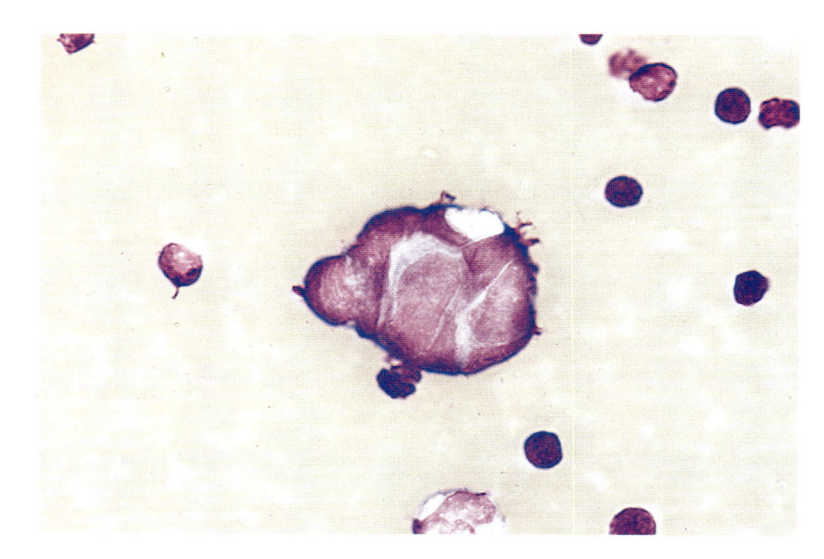

Fig. 4.39 Small cell carcinoma (SCC) of lung

MGG ×720: pleural fluid

The air-dried Romanowsky method of preparation is of particular value in the identification of small cell carcinoma of lung metastatic to an effusion. The cells form a flat monolayer. The nuclei have a homogenous almost smudged appearance and stain a uniform shade of purple appreciably paler than the accompanying lymphocytes. Adjacent nuclei are separated by a linear cleft which, unlike that in alcohol-fixed smear, is seldom crescentic in shape.

(a)

(b)

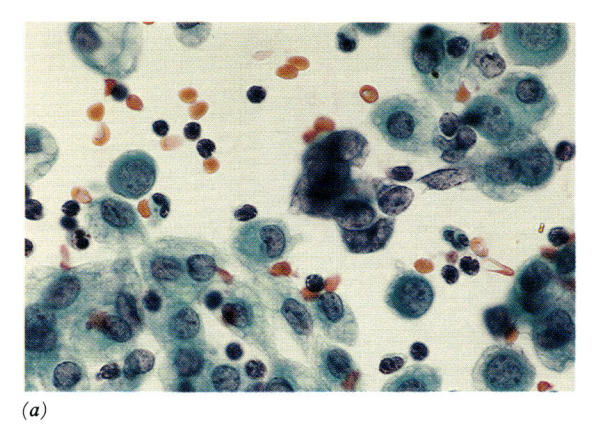

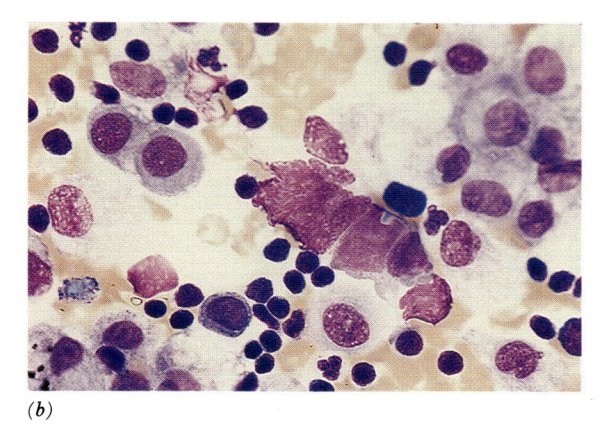

Fig. 4.40 Small cell carcinoma of lung

(a) Papanicolaou ×525: pleural fluid (b) MGG ×525: same specimen; another smear

Correct typing of SCC cells and distinction from a poorly differentiated adenocarcinoma may be difficult in a wet-fixed smear (a). Oat cells are said to be a little larger than lymphocytes. The comparison is based on appearances seen in sections. In an effusion, the individual oat cell appears substantially larger and approximates more closely to the mesothelial cell in size. The crescentic line of separation between moulded nuclei may be wider, the cytoplasm more abundant and lacy than in bronchial secretions.

The same cells appear even larger when air dried (b). Compare the central quadrilateral oat cell with the mesothelial cells in the field. The nucleus of the oat cell is 2–3 times the size of the mesothelial cell and 8–10 times the size of a lymphocyte.

(a)

(b)

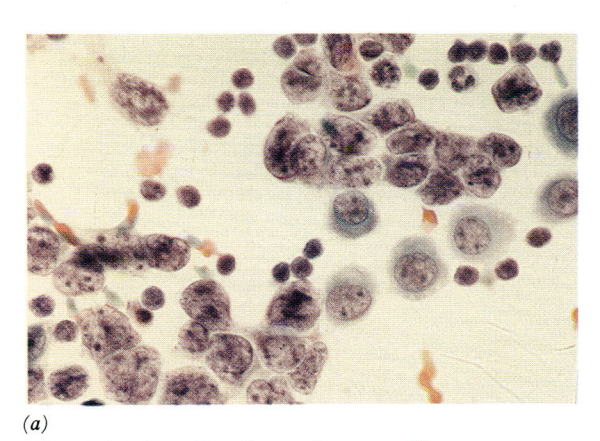

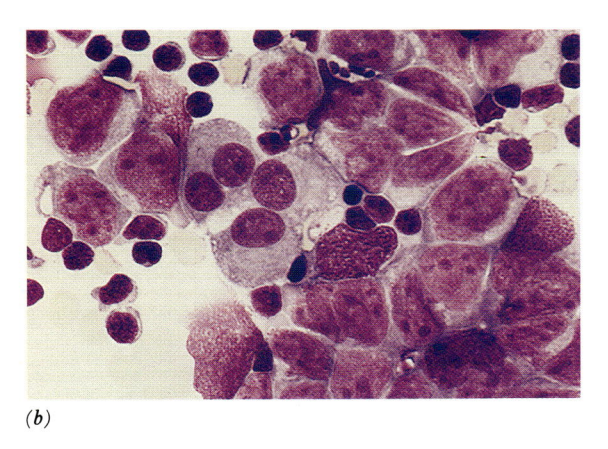

Fig. 4.41 Small cell carcinoma of lung

(a) Papanicolaou ×525: pleural fluid (b) MGG ×525: same specimen; another smear

The relatively greater size of the metastatic SCC cell in a fluid is even more evident when the tumour is composed of cells at the larger end of the spectrum. In this example (a), the neoplastic cells are moderately pleomorphic and several are larger than mesothelial cells. The nuclear moulding seen here is not usually remarkable in a Papanicolaou-stained fluid.

This specimen was unusual in as much as it contained a great number of carcinoma cells in large aggregates and was partially air dried.

The features seen in the alcohol fixed smear are greatly enhanced by air drying (b). Note the multiple conspicuous nucleoli and the large size of the malignant nuclei.

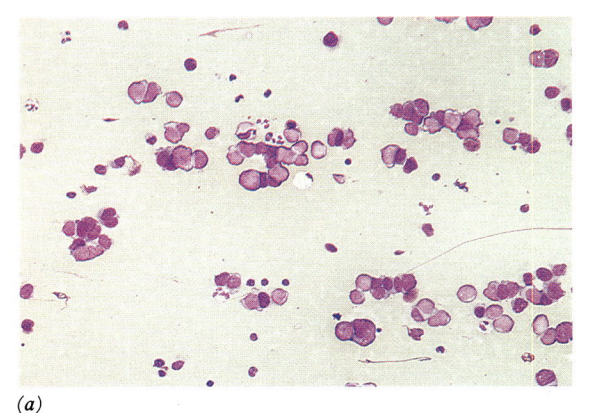

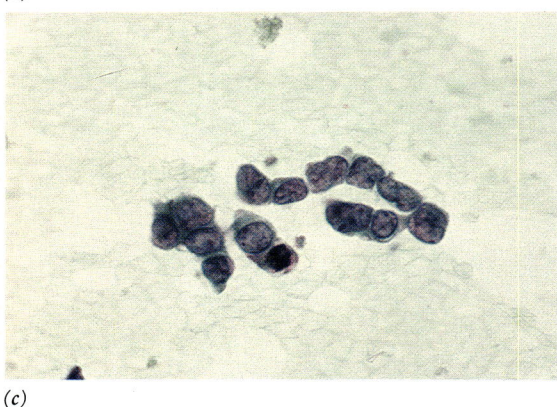

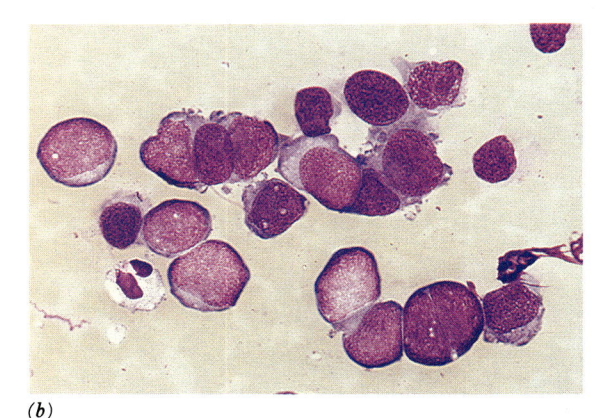

Fig. 4.42 Large cell carcinoma of lung

(a) MGG ×133 (b) MGG ×525: same field (c) Papanicolaou ×525; same specimen; another smear

The cells in micrograph (a) from a histologically proven large cell carcinoma appear, at first glance, to have features characteristic of SCC in an air-dried preparation. They are arranged in monolayers and separated by linear clefts.
A closer look reveals details which are not characteristic of SCC cells in a fluid stained by MGG (b). One is the anisochromasia of the nuclei; in SCC the nuclear staining is generally monochrome. The second is the shape of the cell. Excepting one triangular cell, the others are round or oval; in a cohesive sheet of SCC, the inner cells tend to a roughly rectangular shape. The third discrepant feature is the granular or stranded chromatin; in SCC cells, the chromatin is homogenous or ground glass.

The Papanicolaou smear is much more helpful in this case (c). The relatively abundant cyanophilic cytoplasm and the scanty stippled or coarsely granular chromatin are not characteristic of SCC.

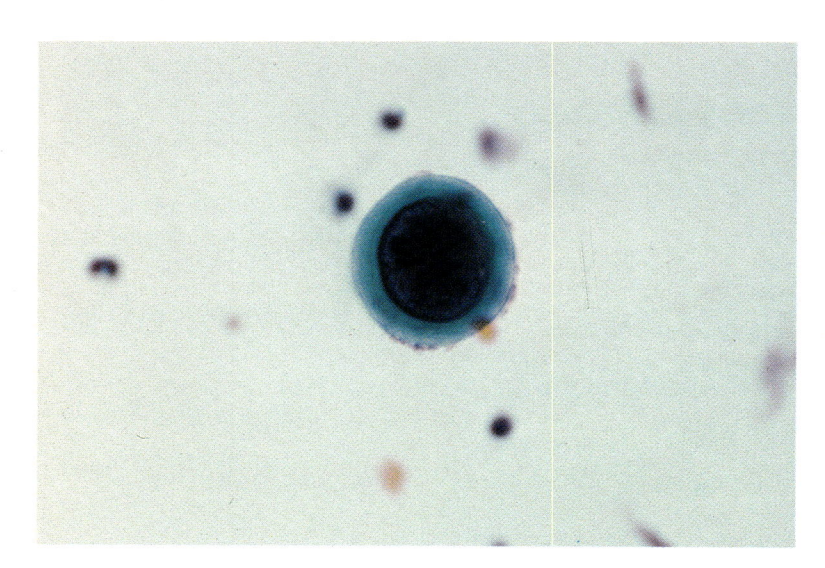

Fig. 4.43 Squamous cell carcinoma of lung

Papanicolaou ×720: pleural fluid

Malignant squamous cells are not often seen in serous effusions, even from a lung primary. When present, they usually show two features. Firstly, they are rarely keratinized even when the primary carcinoma is well differentiated. Secondly, they appear as single forms or at most, in very small groups. With the Papanicolaou stain, the cytoplasm is usually basophilic and opaque but may have a paler periphery. The nucleus is hyperchromic and the chromatin coarse.

Fig. 4.44 Squamous cell carcinoma of lung
MGG ×720: pleural fluid

A cell-within-a-cell formation is shown in this micrograph. The cell is recognized as being of squamous origin by its cytoplasm. In an MGG-stained smear, cytoplasm with some keratin appears colourless or pale blue. The coarse chromatin of the malignant squamous cell is usually arranged in criss-crossing strands.

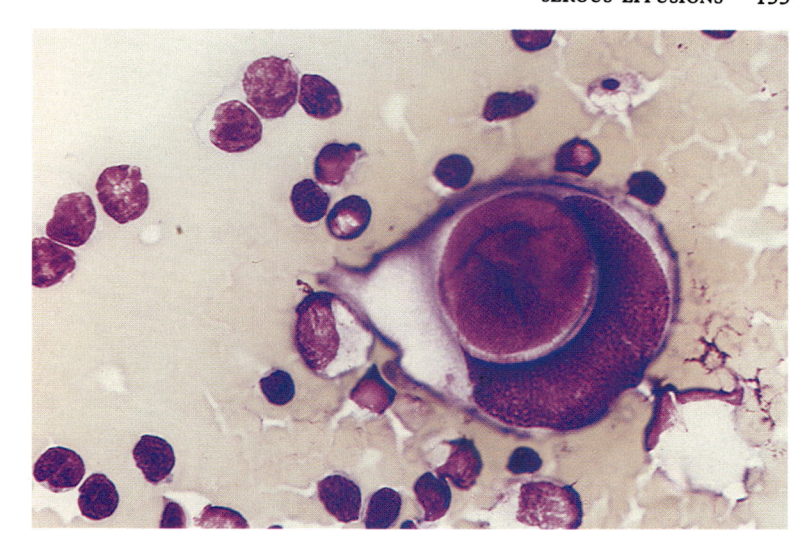

Fig. 4.45 Squamous cell carcinoma of lung
Papanicolaou ×720: pleural fluid

One variant of squamous cell carcinoma contains a spindle cell component: spindle cell (squamous) carcinoma. The tumour cells are fusiform, or spinde-shaped and resemble sarcoma cells. The pleural fluid from this patient contained many well preserved spindle forms and necrotic 'ghost' round tumour cells.

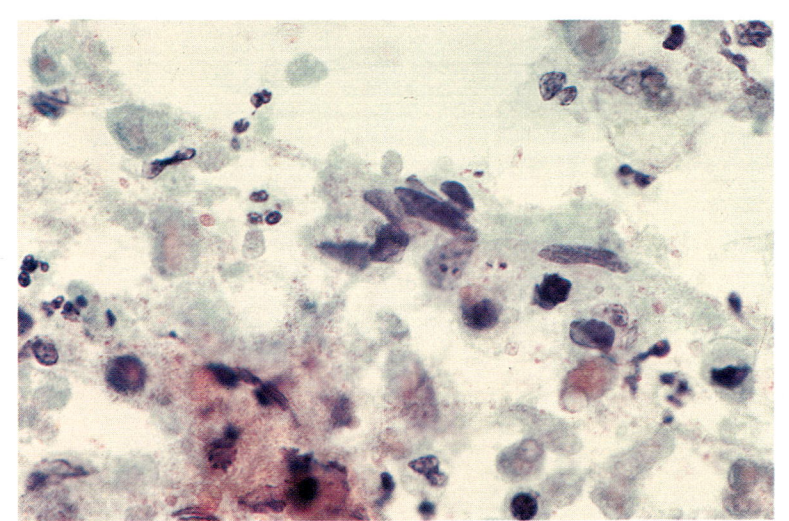

Fig. 4.46 Transitional cell carcinoma
MGG ×720: ascitic fluid

This micrograph shows a large multinucleated malignant cell with copious amphophilic cytoplasm, coarsely stranded chromatin and prominent nucleoli. The appearance was considered to be suggestive of a squamous origin. The cell was present in the ascitic fluid of a patient with a history of transitional cell carcinoma of the prostatic urethra. There was no evidence of another primary and the cell is assumed to be urothelial in type.

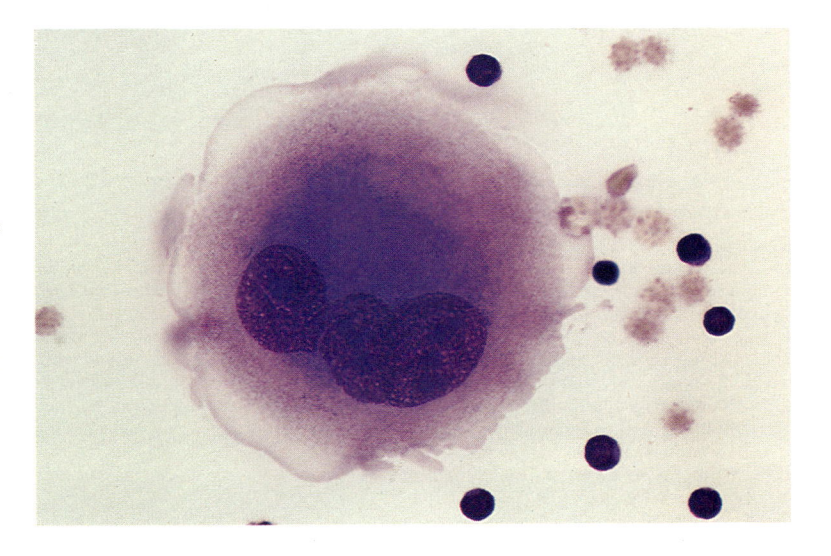

Sarcoma

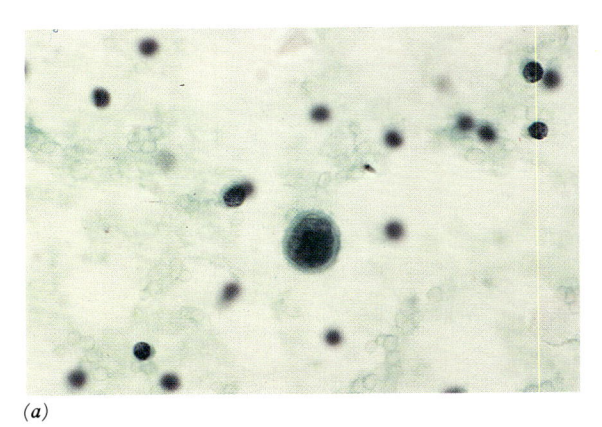

Fig. 4.47 Undifferential sarcoma

Papanicolaou ×525 (a) pleural fluid (b) same smear; another field

Two fields are illustrated from the pleural fluid of a 9-year-old boy from the Indian subcontinent, suspected to have tuberculous pleurisy. A few anaplastic malignant cells, discrete and cohesive, were seen in the fluid and a diagnosis of round cell sarcoma of childhood (not lymphoma) was submitted. Computerised axial tomography (CAT) revealed a mediastinal mass and an open lung biopsy was obtained. The tumour was non-reactive with cell markers for lymphoma and rhabdomyosarcoma. The histology was not consistent with nephroblastoma and the urine did not contain vanillymandelic acid (VMA) which is secreted by neuroblastomas. The tumour was classified as undifferentiated sarcoma.

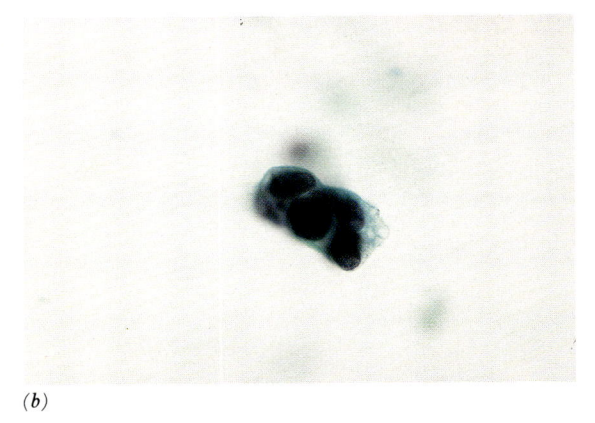

Lymphoproliferative and myeloproliferative disorders

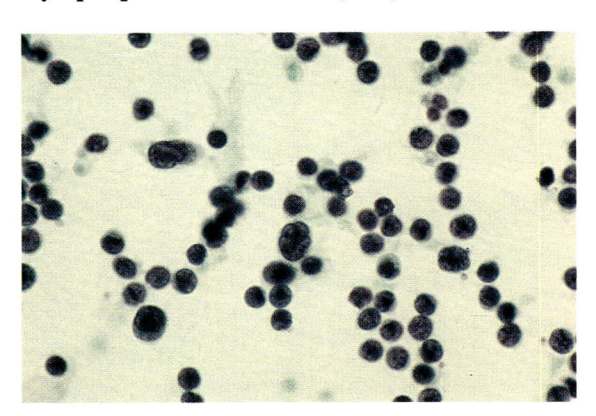

Fig. 4.48 Sezary's syndrome

Papanicolaou ×525: ascitic fluid

The neoplastic cell of Sezary's syndrome, a leukaemic variant of mycosis fungoides, is a malignant T-lymphocyte with little cytoplasm and an irregular nucleus characterized by deep convolutions reminiscent of the cerebrum, hence it is referred to as a cerebriform cell. Three typical Sezary cells accompanied by small lymphocytes are illustrated in the ascitic fluid of a man who presented with ascites, lymphadenopathy and erythrodermal lesions which started on the abdominal wall and gradually spread. A few abnormal T-cells were noted in the peripheral blood at this stage. The disease progressed with the development of a T-cell leukaemic blood picture.

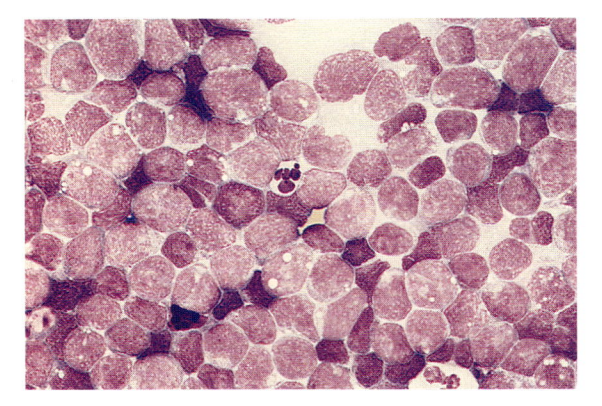

Fig. 4.49 T-cell acute lymphoblastic leukaemia

MGG ×525: pericardial fluid

The blast cells in the pericardial fluid of a 13-year-old girl are medium sized and moderately monomorphic. The cytoplasm is agranular; the nuclei almost fill the cells and do not show indentation and convolutions; one or two nucleoli are present but are inconspicuous. The cells are similar in size to myeloblasts with which they may be confused; nor can they be distinguished from centroblasts. The T-cell origin of the primitive blast cells was established by appropriate immunocytochemical and histochemical studies.

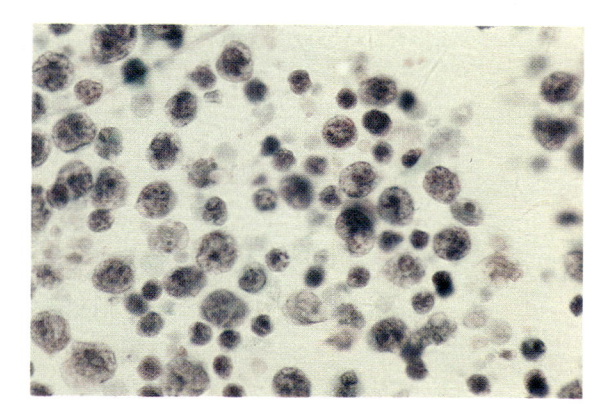

SEROUS EFFUSIONS

Fig. 4.50 Malignant lymphoma: centroblastic-centrocytic
Papanicolaou ×525: peritoneal dialysis fluid

This micrograph illustrates a typical cellular presentation of a centroblastic-centrocytic lymphoma in a fluid specimen. The fluid contains a virtually pure culture of discrete neoplastic cells; several have nuclear clefts characteristic of follicle centre cells. A continuous spectrum of size from small lymphocyte to large blast forms is seen. Nucleoli are evident in the larger blast cells and are small and inconspicuous in the smaller cells. The diagnosis of centroblastic-centrocytic malignant lymphoma was initially made by cytological examination of peritoneal dialysis fluid which the patient wisely brought in for examination, as it was milky in colour. Lymph node histology confirmed the diagnosis and demonstrated a follicular pattern.

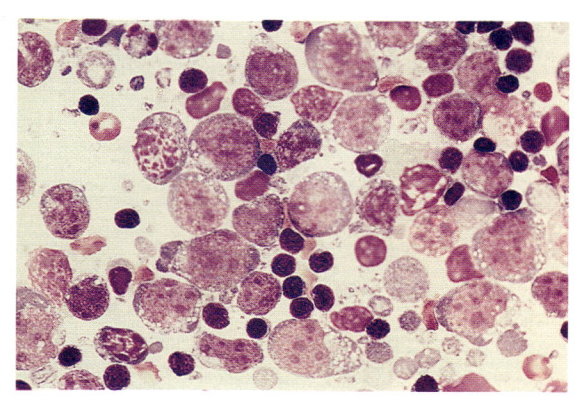

Fig. 4.51 Malignant lymphoma: centroblastic
MGG ×525: pleural fluid

Centroblastic lymphoma cells are large, and like all marrow-derived cells, are discrete. Their cytoplasm is basophilic, and usually moderately pyroninophilic. It often contains immunoglobulins which are PAS-positive. The nuclei are usually round, although a small dent may be seen in a few. Each nucleus contains several prominent nucleoli of varying sizes; some nucleoli are closely apposed to the nuclear membrane. Note that this specimen contains two distinct cell populations: malignant blast cells and benign mature lymphocytes. Compare this appearance with the centroblastic-centrocytic lymphoma (Fig. 4.50) in which all stages of transition from lymphocyte like to lymphoblast can be appreciated.

A centroblast with an intensely pyroninophilic cytoplasm and a single large central nucleolus is known as an immunoblast.

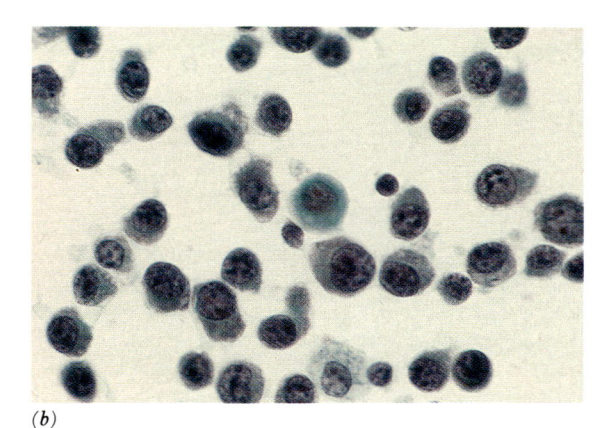

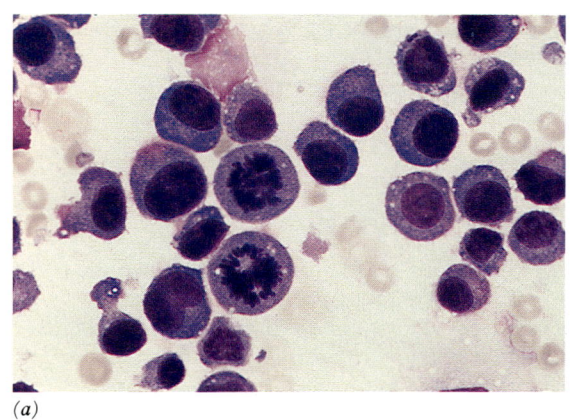

(a)   *(b)*

Fig. 4.52 Multiple myeloma
(a) MGG ×525: pleural fluid (b) Papanicolaou ×525: same specimen; another smear

The myeloma cells in (a) display a gradually progressive range in size, starting from a normal sized plasma cell. Two neoplastic cells are in mitosis. The larger myeloma cells are comparable in size to the normal mesothelial cell in the centre of (b). The close family resemblance of the myeloma cell with its deeply basophilic cytoplasm and eccentric nucleus to a normal plasmacytoid cell is immediately appreciated in the MGG smear (a). In the Papanicolaou-stained smear (b), the plasma cell origin is less obvious, and the myeloma cells might easily be mistaken for carcinoma cells. (Compare with Fig. 4.36a).

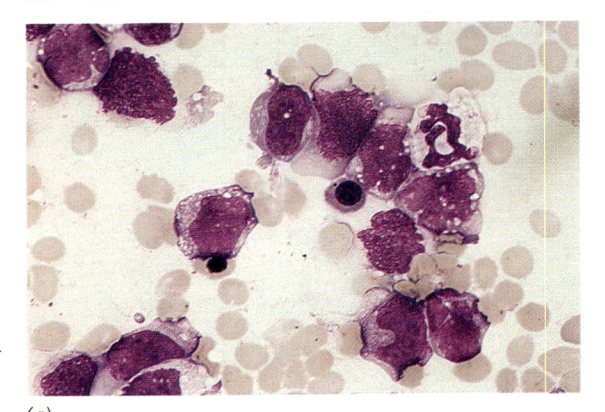

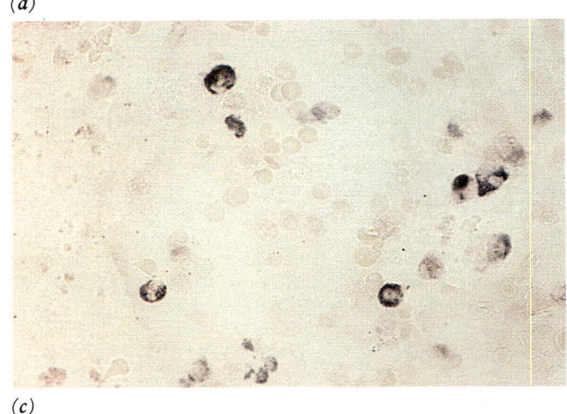

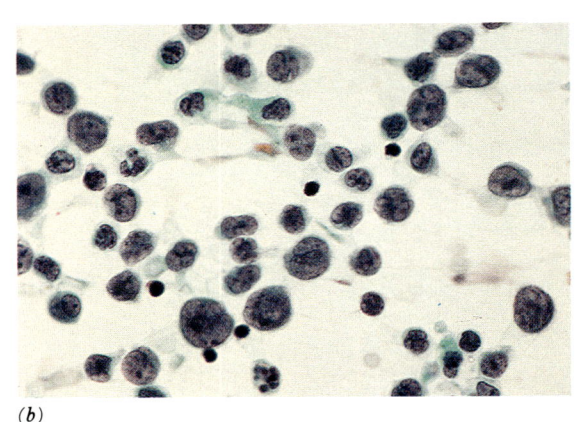

Fig. 4.53 Acute myeloid leukaemia

(a) *MGG ×525: pleural fluid* (b) *Papanicolaou × 525: pleural fluid; another case* (c) *Sudan black B ×333: same specimen as (b); another smear*

A large population or a pure content of leukaemic cells is seen in an effusion when the serous membrane is infiltrated. Two cases of pleural effusion associated with acute myeloid leukaemia are illustrated. The cells in (a) are large, but lack the basophilia of myeloblasts. The cytoplasm is more ample and in a few cells has a suggestion of fine granular stippling. Four to five nucleoli are discernible. The large cells have the appearance of promyelocytes. Several nuclei have irregular indentations found in cells referred to as parapromyelocytes. The two small acidophilic cells with condensed central nuclei are normoblasts. One degenerate polymorph is seen (upper right).

The primitive variable sized cells in (b) appear smaller; this is in part due to wet fixation in alcohol. Little or no cytoplasm is evident and the nuclei are indented or grossly convoluted. The appearance is similar to that seen in high grade T-cell lymphomas. The myeloid origin of the leukaemia cells was established by demonstrating Sudan black B-positive granules (c); these are not present in cells of lymphoid origin.

MESOTHELIOMA

A primary tumour of the mesothelial lining, known as mesothelioma, may be benign or malignant. The latter is induced by asbestos, usually of the crocidolite group.

A benign mesothelioma develops from the pleura as a localized mass, often pedunculated, and is typically of the fibrous type (fibroma of pleural origin); epithelial and mixed or biphasic forms are uncommon.

A malignant mesothelioma involves the visceral and parietal surfaces of the pleura, is usually diffuse and often encases the lung. The majority have a biphasic structure although monomorphic forms also occur. The extremely rare peritoneal malignant mesothelioma is also associated with exposure to a cancer-inducing asbestos.

The diagnosis of malignant mesothelioma in a pleural effusion is a particularly difficult one. The fibrous component of the commonest biphasic variety is rarely exfoliated. Well differentiated epithelial type tumour cells may be difficult to distinguish from benign reactive mesothelial cells. The more obviously malignant forms often closely resemble metastatic adenocarcinoma cells. The problem is not necessarily resolved by the use of special staining techniques. Both types of cancer cells may be rich in glycogen which stains red with PAS. The presence of diastase resistant PAS (D-PAS) positive epithelial mucin distinguishes a mucin-secreting adenocarcinoma but a negative reaction does not discriminate between a mesothelioma and a non-secretory adenocarcinoma. Abolition of alcian blue staining by prior treatment with hyaluronidase discriminates between a mesothelioma which synsethizes hyaluronic acid and a mucous carcinoma; a negative reaction with alcian blue cannot discriminate between a mesothelioma from which hyaluronic acid is absent and a non-mucinous carcinoma. Demonstration of cytoplasmic carcino-embryonic antigen (CEA) virtually excludes mesothelioma, but as the antigen is not expressed by all carcinomas, even this method is of limited value.

However, malignant cells in a pleural effusion which do not express CEA, are D-PAS- and hyaluronidase/alcian blue-negative *and* show morphological features of mesothelial cells are highly suggestive of a malignant mesothelioma.

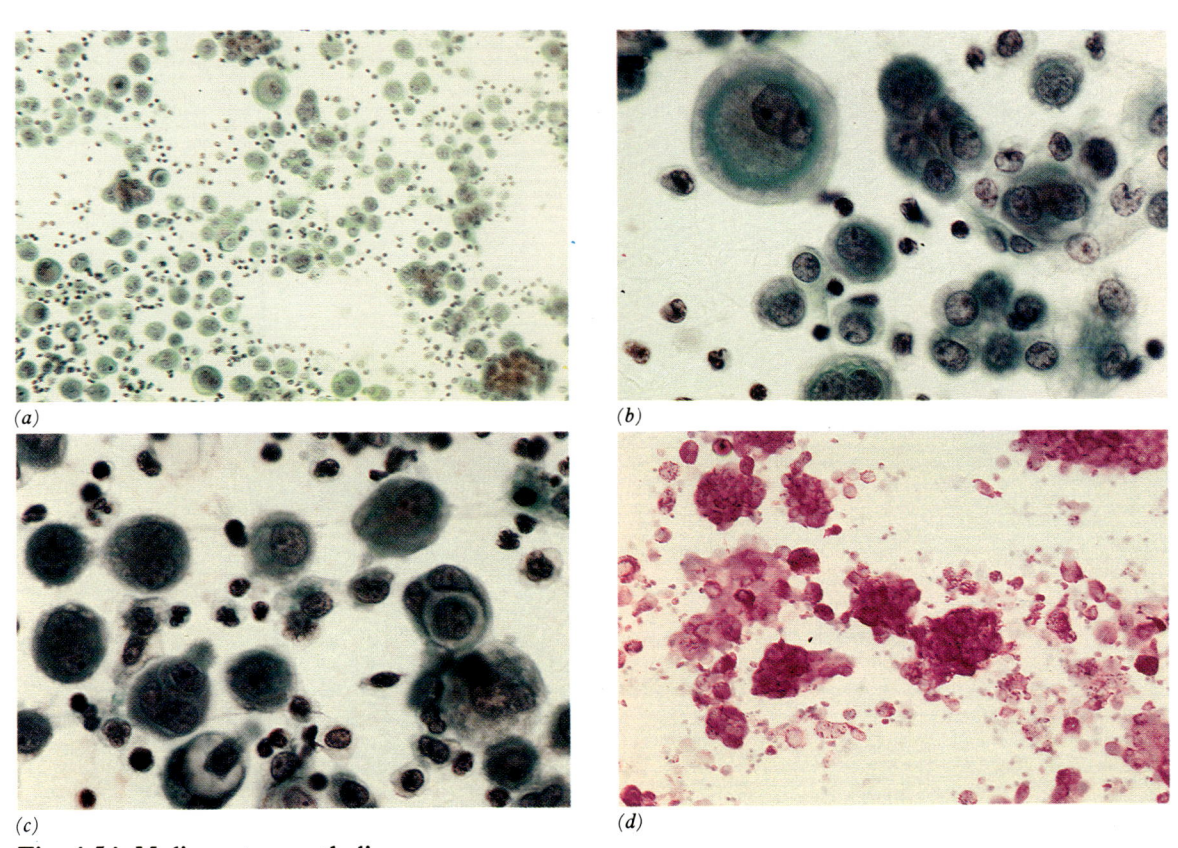

Fig. 4.54 Malignant mesothelioma

(a) Papanicolaou ×133: pleural fluid (b) ×525: same field (c) ×525: another part of same field (d) PAS ×133: same specimen; another smear

A pleural fluid from a case of malignant mesothelioma often contains abundant epithelial-type cells which occur singly, in small groups and in large mulberry-like clusters (a). The field in (b) shows leucocytes and large cells which clearly belong to one family. They display a wide range in size, and in the number of nuclei. The chromatin is finely stippled in some nuclei and coarsely granular in others. The nucleoli vary in size and some are prominent. Compare the tumour cells with benign mesothelial cells (Fig. 4.3). The similarities of shape and cytoplasmic features suggest a common origin. The two bird's eye forms seen in (c) are rarely found in benign mesothelial cells. The malignant cells in this effusion contained much glycogen (d) and were negative with D-PAS and alcian blue.

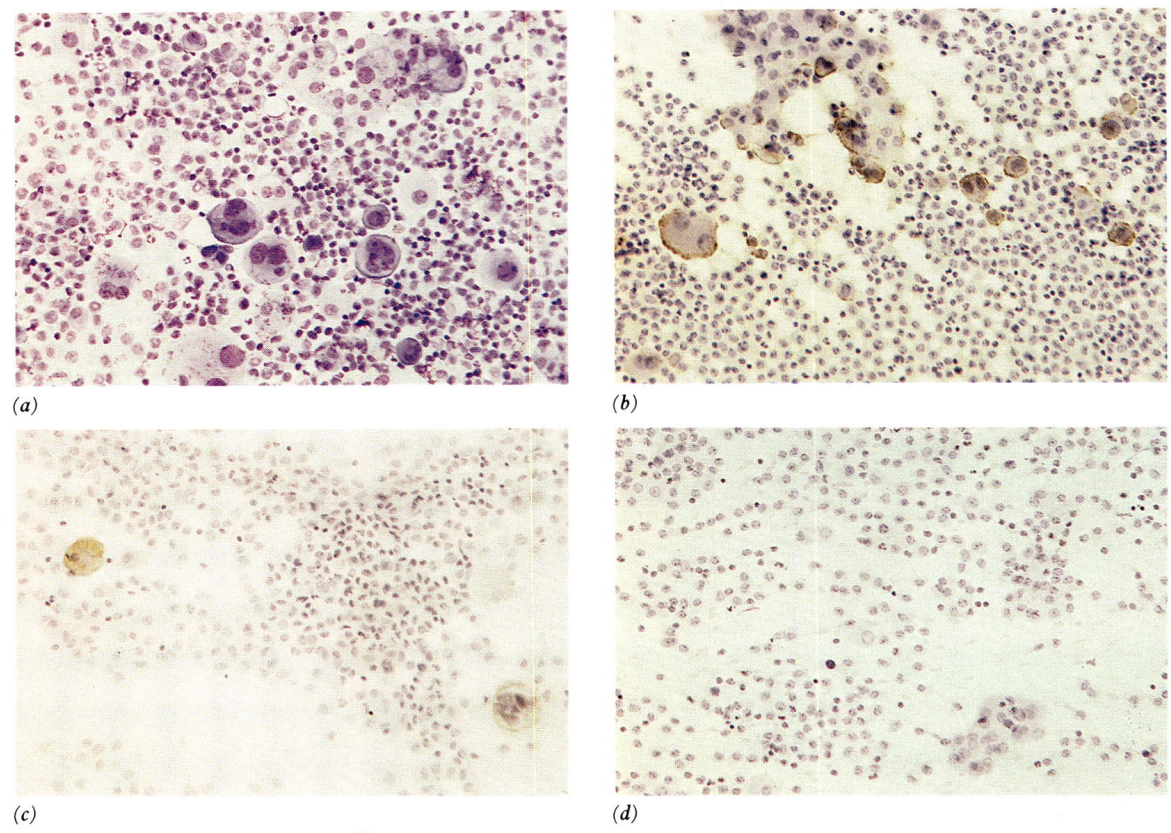

Fig. 4.55 Malignant mesothelioma

(a) MGG ×133: pleural fluid (b) Indirect immunoperoxidase LP 34 ×133: same specimen; another smear (c) Indirect immunoperoxidase Cam 5.2 ×133 same specimen; another smear (d) Indirect immunoperoxidase CEA ×133 same specimen; another smear

The application of immunocytochemistry to a pleural fluid sample is illustrated in a histologically diagnosed case of malignant mesothelioma. The tumour cells in the fluid showed variation in size and the number of nuclei, and the cytoplasmic features suggested a mesothelial origin (a). A few were reactive with two monoclonal antibodies to cytokeratin, LP 34(b) and Cam 5.2(c). As not all cells of a family express antigens, it is by no means uncommon to see random reactivity in an immunocytochemical preparation. Staining for CEA was uniformly negative (d).

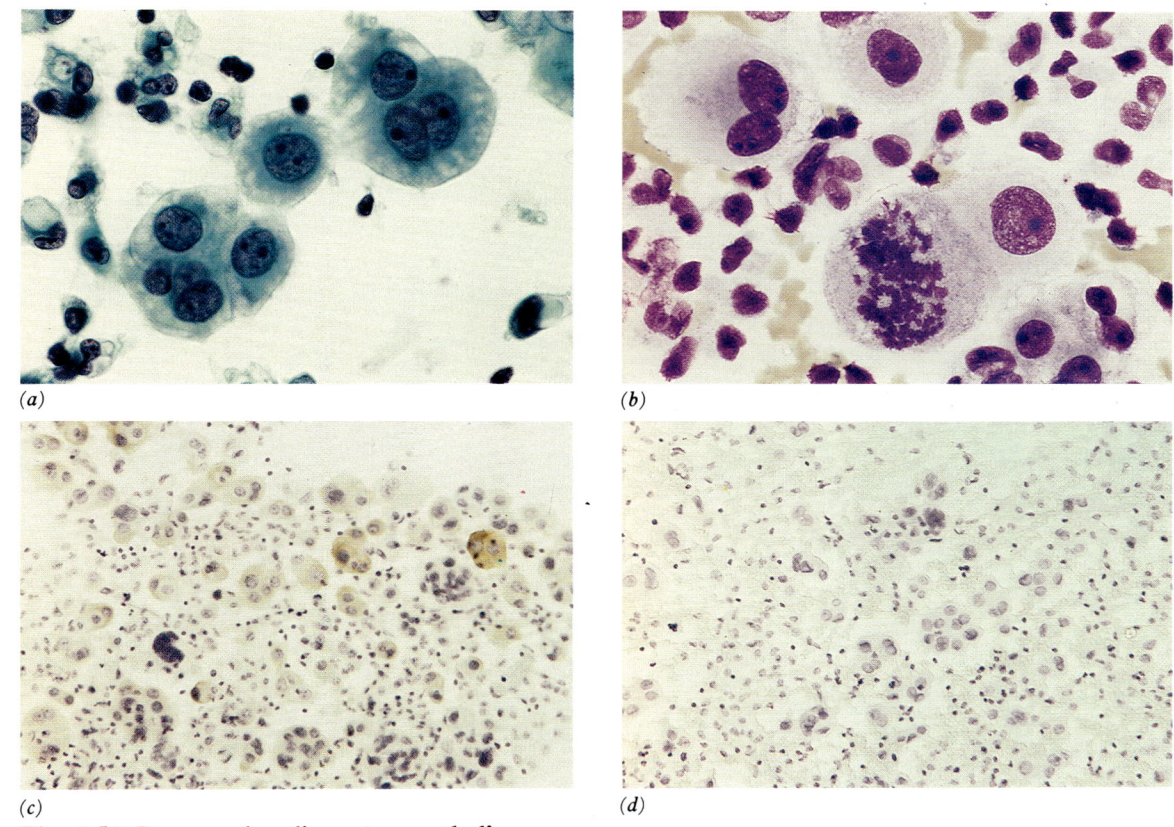

Fig. 4.56 Presumed malignant mesothelioma

(a) Papanicolaou ×525: pleural fluid (b) MGG ×525: same specimen; another smear (c) Indirect immunoperoxidase HMFG 1 ×133: same specimen; another smear (d) Indirect immunoperoxidase CEA ×133: same specimen; another smear

These micrographs illustrate the pleural fluid of a patient with a history of exposure to asbestos. Chest X-ray showed a grossly thickened pleura. The fluid contained a single population of epithelial type cells with malignant characteristics (a). One of several mitotic figures seen in the specimen is shown in (b). The cells reacted with a monoclonal antibody to human milk fat globule (HMFG) which characterizes epithelial cells (c). None of the tumour cells expressed CEA (d). Alcian blue staining was negative. The morphological appearance and the immunocytochemical reaction were considered to be consistent with malignant mesothelioma.

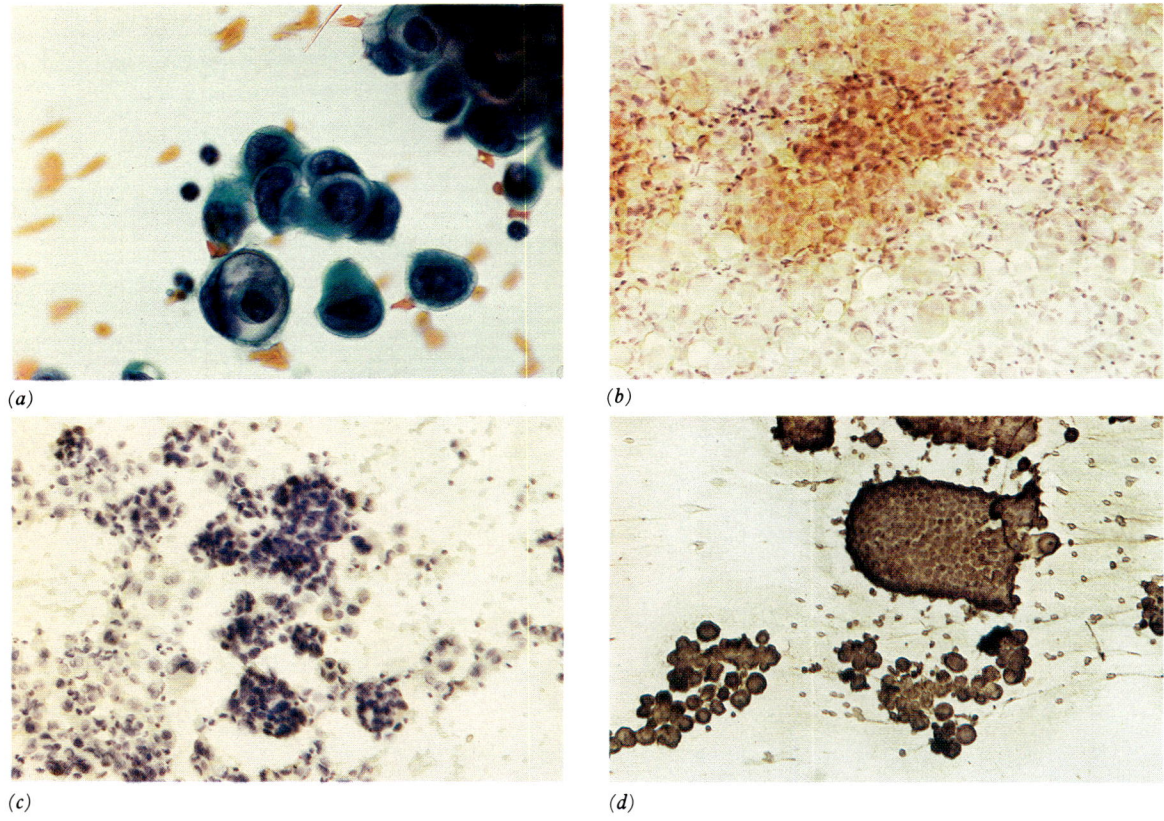

Fig. 4.57 Metastatic adenocarcinoma

(a) Papanicolaou ×525: ascitic fluid; adenocarcinoma of breast (b) Indirect immunoperoxidase HMFG 2 ×133: same specimen; another smear (c) Indirect immunoperoxidase CEA ×133: same specimen; another smear (d) Indirect immunoperoxidase CEA ×133: pleural fluid; another case; adenocarcinoma of lung

The immunocytochemical reactions of two cases of metastatic adenocarcinoma are shown for comparison with malignant mesothelioma. The ascitic fluid of a woman with disseminated breast carcinoma contained malignant cells with the typical morphology of adenocarcinoma cells (a). The cells were strongly reactive with the monoclonal epithelial anitbody HMFG 2 (b). Breast carcinoma cells vary in their ability to express CEA. Some tumours may be strongly positive for this antigen, others may be uniformly negative; in yet others, strongly reactive cells adjoin negative cells. The metastatic malignant cells in the ascitic fluid of this case were negative for CEA (c). The lung carcinoma metastatic to pleural fluid is, on the other hand, very strongly positive for this antigen (d).

5. Cerebrospinal fluid

Cerebrospinal fluid (CSF) may be lumbar puncture fluid from the central canal of the spinal cord, fluid from the ventricles of the brain or occasionally from a shunt inserted to relieve hydrocephalus.

The colour and volume of the CSF should be noted and a cell count performed on lumbar CSF. A normal CSF contains up to five mature lymphocytes per cubic millimetre; the cell count is often raised in pathological conditions. Ventricular and shunt fluids may contain fragments of tissue and a cell count is seldom feasible. The cells are concentrated for study in a cytocentrifuge or membrane filter preparation and stained by the Papanicolaou or Romanowsky methods. In smears made from centrifugated deposit, the notch of the lymphocyte may be accentuated and the cell may appear histiocytoid.

Aspiration or imprint smears from the brain may be obtained at operation. The use of these specimens is usually confined to specialist units attached to neurosurgical units.

Fig. 5.1 Leptomeningeal tissue
Papanicolaou ×183: shunt CSF

The leptomeningeal covering of the brain and the spinal cord consist of delicate connective tissue lined by cuboidal cells. A small fragment of the leptomeninges is illustrated in this micrograph of a specimen of CSF drained from the sub-arachnoidal space. A sparse number of spindle-shaped nuclei are seen in a matrix of fine cyanophilic tissue.

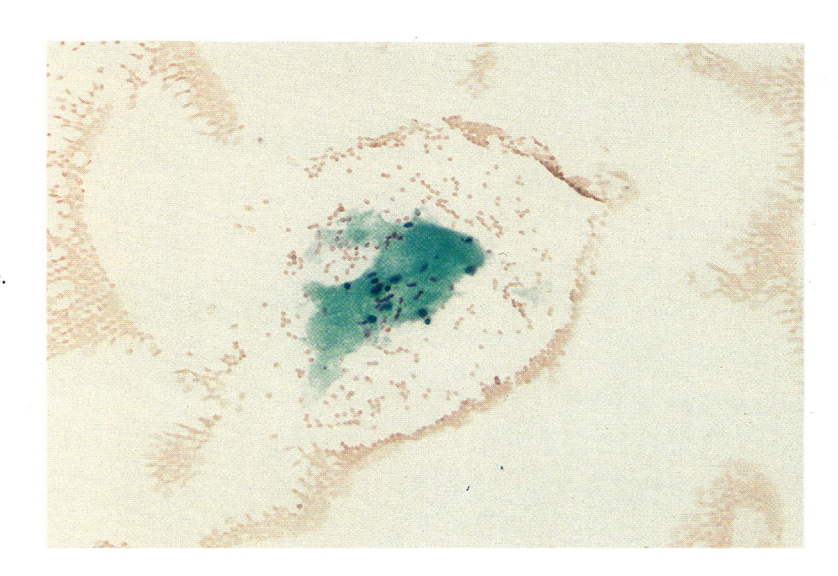

Fig. 5.2 Capillaries
Papanicolaou ×183: ventricular CSF

Aspiration of ventricular CSF may dislodge a fragment of the choroid plexus, a vascular structure arising from the walls of the ventricle. Fine blood vessels may also be seen when glial tissue has entered the needle. Several branching capillaries containing red blood cells are seen in this micrograph.

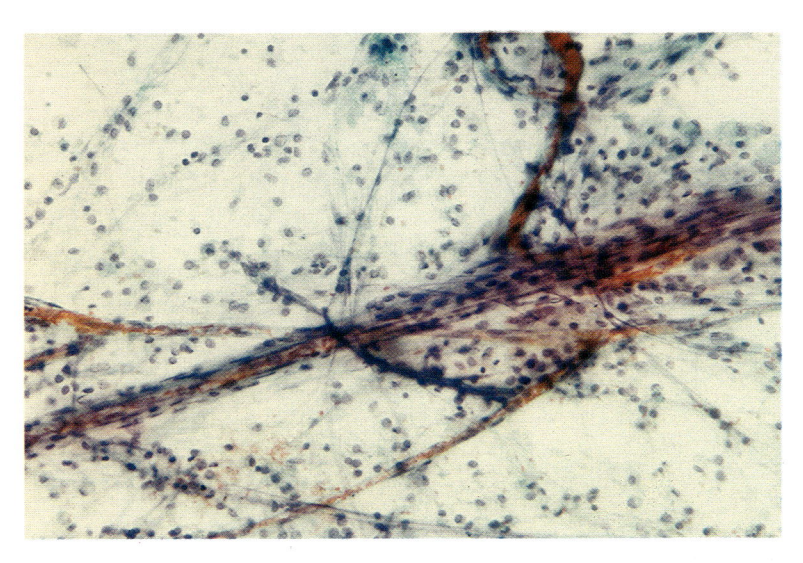

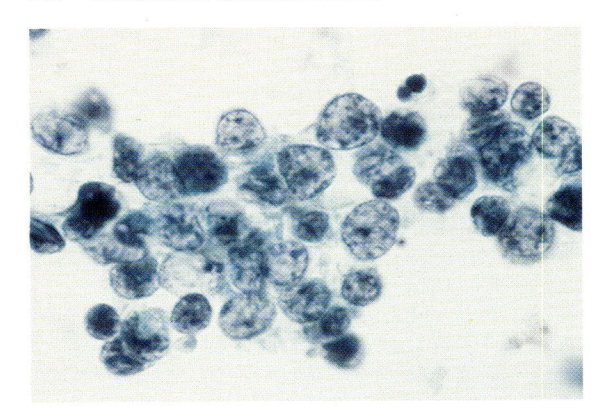

Fig. 5.3 Ependymoma

Papanicolaou ×832: lumbar CSF

The ventricles and the central spinal canal are lined by a single layer of specialised glial cells, referred to as ependymal cells. Tumours derived from these cells are known as ependymomas and constitute one variety of glial tumours or gliomas.

An ependymoma may develop in the brain or in the spinal column, the most common being a papillary tumour of the fourth ventricle. The tumours occur mainly in children and adolescents.

The tumour cells illustrated were recovered in great numbers from the lumbar CSF of a young boy several months after treatment of a histologically proven central ependymoma. The cells are small and have little cytoplasm. The nuclei are round, monomorphic and finely granular. The cells are loosely attached to each other and arranged round small spaces in a pseudo-acinar manner.

(a)

(b)

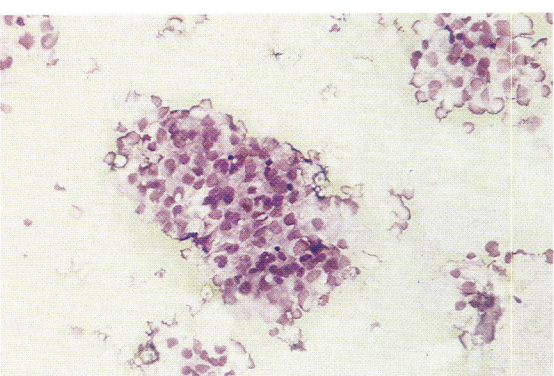

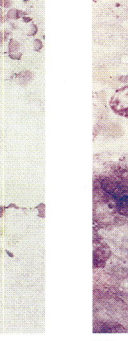

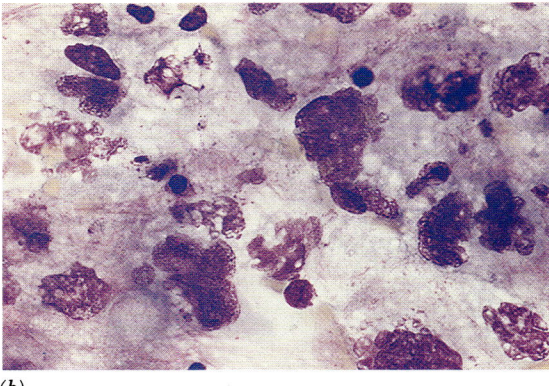

Fig. 5.4 Astrocytoma

(a) MGG ×133; imprint smear (b) MGG ×525: aspiration smear; another case (c) Papanicolaou ×525: same specimen as (b); another smear

Two cases of primary malignant tumours of glial tissue are illustrated in these micrographs. Normal glial tissue contains relatively few nuclei dispersed in delicate fibrillary material. The number of glial cells and consequently nuclei are increased in gliosis, and distinction between a low grade glioma and reactive gliosis may be difficult by histology and is rarely feasible by cytology.

The tissue in micrograph (a) is highly cellular, the nuclei are crowded together and display some variation in size and shape. The appearance therefore is highly suggestive of glioma; the definitive diagnosis of astrocytoma was established on tissue sections.

The nuclei illustrated in (b) and (c) are grossly aberrant and pleomorphic, and malignancy is self-evident. The fibrillary network in which they are dispersed is characteristic of glial tissue and a cytodiagnosis of a high grade glioma is possible on this aspirate of an area of cystic degeneration in the tumour, which was classified as an astrocytoma grade 4 by histology.

(c)

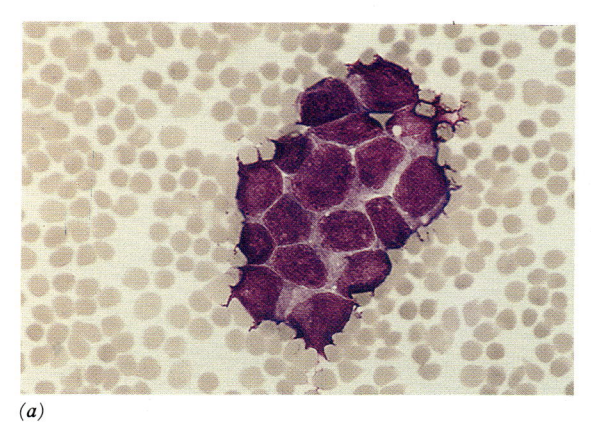

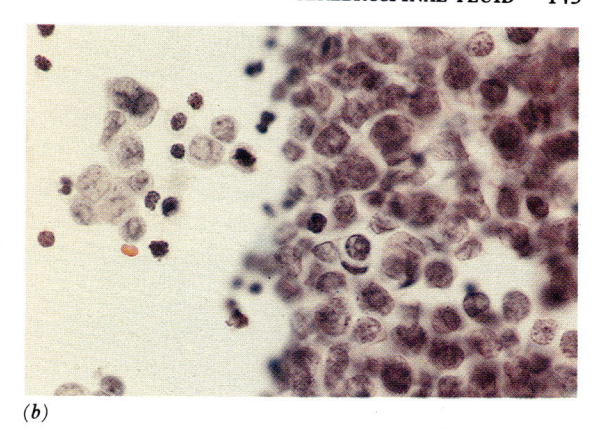

Fig. 5.5 Pinealoma

(a) MGG ×525: lumbar CSF (b) Papanicolaou ×525: lumbar CSF; another specimen from the same case

Another tumour of children, adolescents and young adults arises from the pineal gland (a specialised endocrine gland) the function of which is not fully understood. Histological variants include germinomas and teratomas. The case illustrated is the poorly differentiated small celled variety and occurred in a young boy. Micrograph (a) illustrates a group of cohesive cells with variable sized nuclei and little cytoplasm. Small multiple nucleoli are faintly discernible. Another specimen of fluid obtained some months after treatment contained similar cells (b). These appear smaller because they have been fixed in alcohol. The cell size approximates to that of lymphoblasts. The granularity of the nuclei is better appreciated in the Papanicolaou preparation.

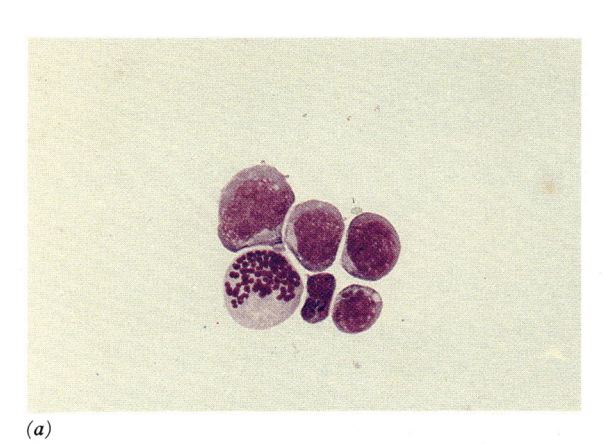

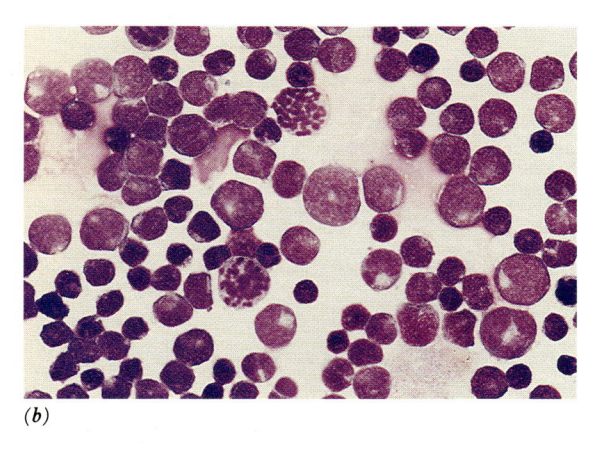

Fig. 5.6 Non-Hodgkin's malignant lymphoma

MGG ×525 Lumbar CSF (a) post-nasal lyphoma (b) lymphoblastic lymphoma

Involvement of the central nervous system by disseminated lymphoma is not uncommon and CSF cytology is often performed as part of the initial staging and subsequent assessment procedures. Distinction between benign reactive lymphocytes and a low grade lymphoma can be difficult; high grade tumours are more easily identifiable and CSF cytology plays an important and generally, primary, role in establishing central involvement.

The cell count is always raised in these cases and may be very high. Two cases of high grade lymphoma are illustrated in these micrographs. The cells in (a) are primitive and large. Anisocytosis and anisonucleosis are marked. Multiple macronucleoli are seen in the top left nucleus, below it is an abnormal mitotic figure. A mixed population of small lymphocytes and poorly differentiated large lymphoma cells are seen in (b). Several of the large nuclei are convoluted. Note the two abnormal mitoses.

In cases in which distinction between discrete carcinoma cells, lymphoma cells, or tumour cells of glial origin is not clear, the problem may be resolved by immunocytochemical typing of the cells.

Fig. 5.7 Metastatic carcinoma

MGG ×720 (a) squamous cell carcinoma of the lung (b) adenocarcinoma of the breast (c) adenocarcinoma from an unknown primary

Metastatic disease of the central nervous system is said to be more common than primary tumours. The commonest source of secondary deposits is a bronchogenic carcinoma, the breast being the second most frequently encountered site. Lumbar CSF may contain numerous tumour cells when the meninges are involved (carcinomatous meningitis). Micrograph (a) illustrates poorly differentiated malignant squamous cells from a lung primary. Unlike glial tissue, the four cells seen are clearly demarcated from each other and appear to be of epithelial origin. Adenocarcinoma cells with smooth borders, high nuclear-cytoplasmic ratios and prominent nucleoli seen in (b) were recovered from the lumbar CSF of a woman with disseminated breast carcinoma. The cohesive cluster of large vacuolated carcinoma cells with eccentric nuclei are characteristic of a mucus-secreting adenocarcinoma (c). The patient presented with symptoms of a space-occupying lesion in the cranium and a diagnosis of metastatic adenocarcinoma was established by lumbar CSF cytology. The primary was not established, but was suspected to be of colonic origin.

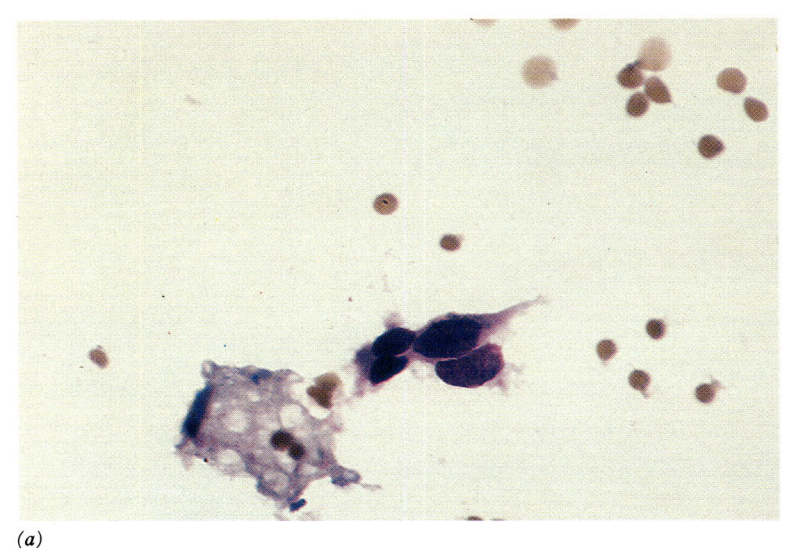

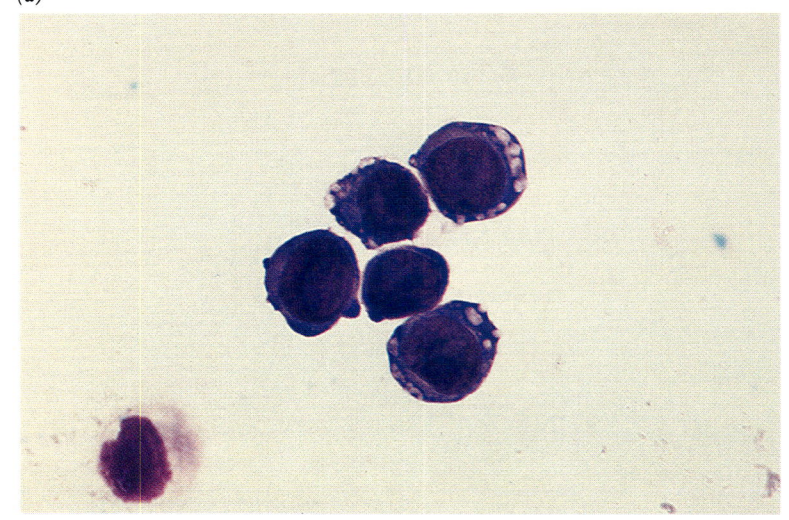

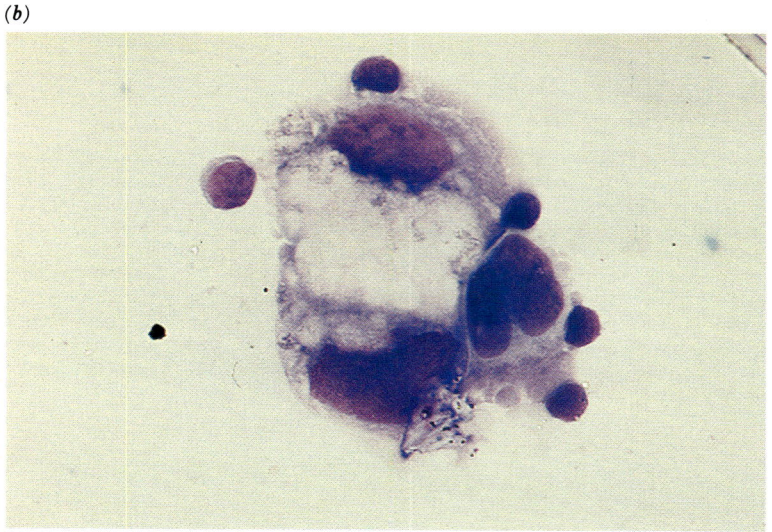

(a)

(b)

(c)

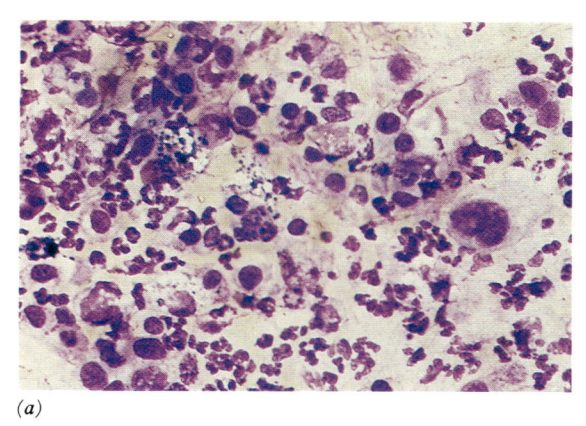

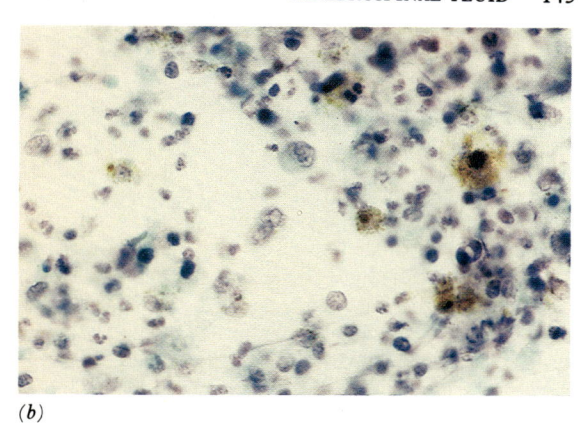

Fig. 5.8 Melanoma

(a) MGG ×525: ventricular CSF (b) Papanicolaou ×525: same specimen; another smear

Discrete tumour cells are seen interspersed amongst inflammatory cells in these micrographs. The neoplastic cells are variable in size and nuclear cytoplasmic ratio, and a large convoluted nucleus is seen opposite 3 o'clock in (a). Abundant intracellular pigment, blue black in the MGG preparation (a) and golden brown in the Papanicolaou smear (b) is seen. The differential diagnosis lies between iron pigment or melanin. The latter was demonstrated by the Masson-Fontana stain and the tumour identified as a melanotic melanoma.

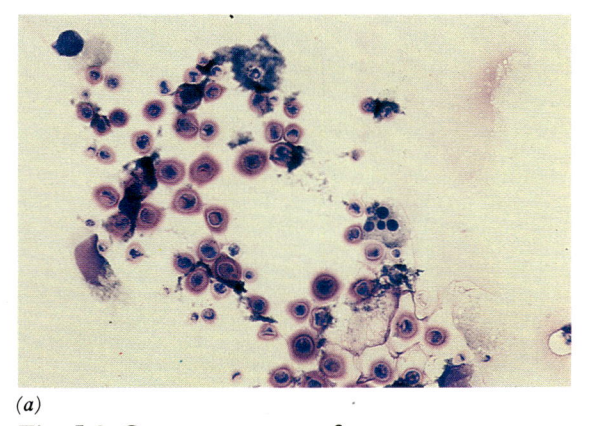

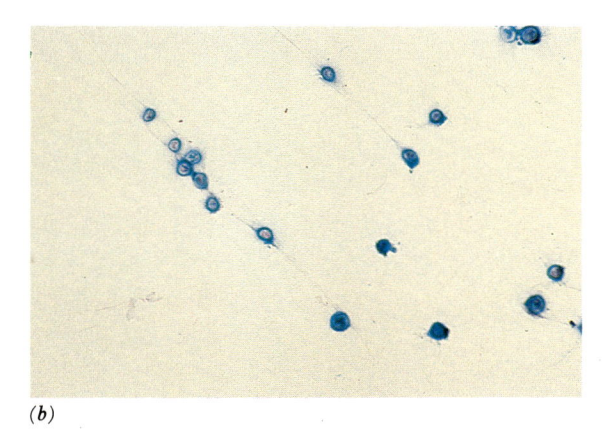

Fig. 5.9 Cryptococcus neoformans

(a) MGG ×525: lumbar CSF (b) Alcian blue ×525: same specimen; another smear

The yeast, *Cryptococcus neoformans*, usually enters the patient through the respiratory tract where it may produce a cryptococcoma (see p. 79). It has a predilection for the central nervous system and fungal meningitis occurs. The yeast is surrounded by a capsule composed of mucopolysaccharides; this stains violet with MGG (a) and is alcian blue-positive (b). The yeast within the capsule is seen as a blue-black ring in the MGG preparation and as a pale pink structure with alcian blue.

6. Oesophago-gastrointestinal tract

The role of cytopathology in the field of gastro-enterology has been extended in the last decade by the introduction of the flexible fibre-optic endoscope. It is now possible to visualize the entire gastrointestinal tract and acquire permanent documentation of the lesion under investigation by the use of a camera attachment.

The instruments have single or double channels through which diagnostic material may be obtained for biopsy histology and brush cytology and it is customary to obtain both types of specimens. The diagnostic rate for oesophageal and colonic carcinomas is high and equal by both methods. Biopsy histology is more successful than brush cytology in the diagnosis of gastric carcinoma of the fundus and the body. The cardia and the antrum beyond the incisura are not easily reached by the biopsy forceps but are generally accessible to the brush. The overall diagnostic rate for gastric carcinoma is improved by the combined use of cytology and histology.

Opinion varies as to the optimal sequence of collection of the specimens. In some centres brush specimens are collected prior to biopsy as it is considered that the bleeding caused by the biopsy forceps has an adverse effect on the smear. As against that, a brush rolled over an ulcer crater covered with slough or over an infiltrating carcinoma may not contain diagnostic cells, whereas a specimen obtained after prior biopsy has removed the slough or breached the surface over an infiltrating carcinoma may be more informative. The brush specimens illustrated in this section were obtained as a matter of policy, after biopsies which generally numbered four to six, and the blood was not found to interfere with the quality of the preparation or the interpretation.

A Romanowsky stain is not suitable for a gastrointestinal brush specimen on account of the mucin present. To avoid dehydration which damages morphology in an alcohol-fixed, Papanicolaou-stained smear, it is essential to spread and fix the smears one at a time. It is generally possible to make three or four good smears from a brush.

The technique of endoscopic retrograde cholangiopancreatography (ERCP) is used to visualize the pancreatic duct system by fluoroscopy after injection of contrast medium. The endoscope is introduced into the pancreatic duct through the ampulla of Vater and pancreatic juice obtained prior to injection of the dye may be used for cytological and biochemical analysis.

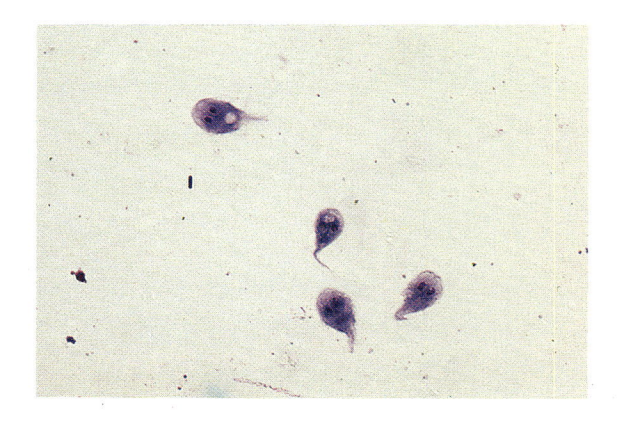

Fig. 6.1 Giardia lamblia

MGG ×525: pancreatic juice; ERCP

The gastrointestinal tract is a potential portal of entry for a wide variety of pathogens, viral, bacterial and parasitic. *Giardia lamblia*, an actively motile, multiflagellated, unicellular protozoon parasitizes the duodenum and the jejunum where it divides by simple binary fission. Infection is acquired by ingestion of water contaminated with faeces containing the ovoid cystic forms. The trophozoite released in the human intestine is pear-shaped with two nuclei and a central parabasal body, and resembles a human face.

G. lamblia is endemic in the tropics and in some parts of the United States and infects mainly children who suffer from a watery diarrhoea. In heavy chronic infestation, the jejunal mucosa may be covered with a host of parasites and malabsorption may occur. In recent years, giardiasis has emerged as a significant cause of traveller's diarrhoea. This is seldom acute and some subjects may remain asymptomatic for long periods.

The trophozoites illustrated were recovered from pancreatic juice collected in the course of ERCP, and are likely to be from the duodenum traversed by the endoscope.

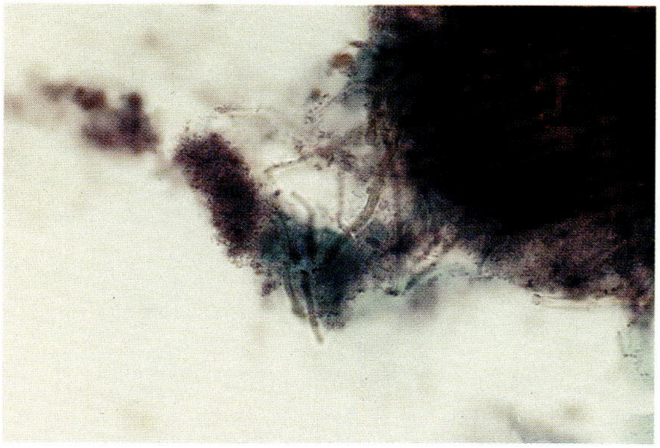

OESOPHAGO-GASTROINTESTINAL TRACT 147

(a) 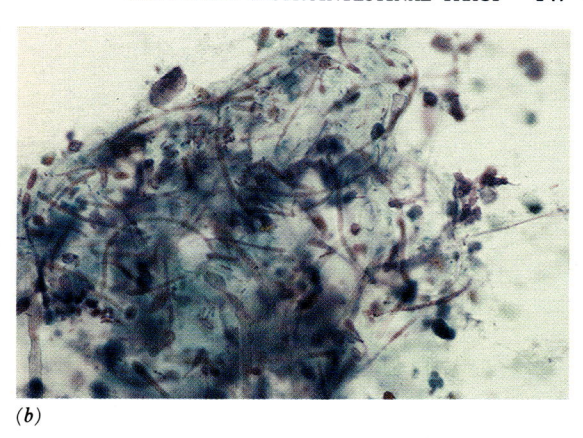   (b)

Fig. 6.2 Bacteria: Candida spp
Papanicolaou ×525 (a) oesophageal brush (b) gastric brush

Candida may be present in an oesophageal brush specimen in immunocompromised subjects and patients on antibiotic therapy, and bacteria and the fungus may be seen in cases of oesophagitis, ulcer or carcinoma.

The acidity of the normal stomach inhibits bacterial growth and a healthy stomach is sterile. In hypochlorhydria and achlorhydria, the stomach may be colonized by the opportunistic *Candida albicans*, and a chronic ulcer may show a polymicrobial invasion. Both Candida and bacteria are most frequently seen in association with gastric carcinoma.

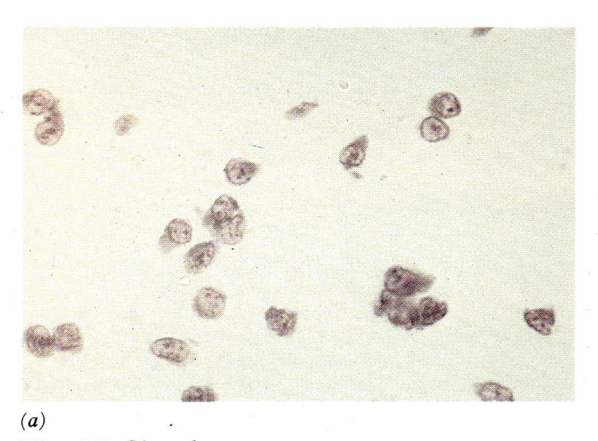

(a) 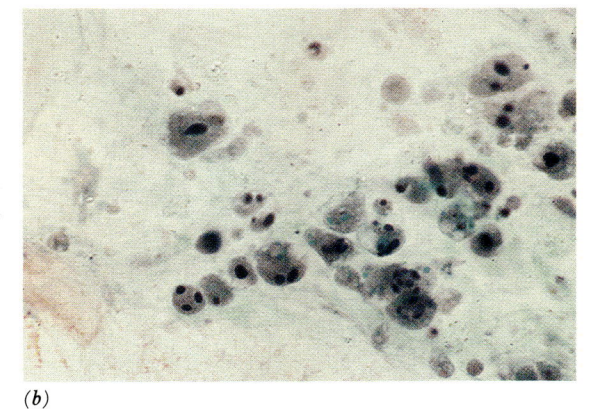   (b)

Fig. 6.3 Slough
Papanicolaou ×525: gastric brush (a) macrophages (b) necrotic epithelial cells

The crater of a gastric ulcer is usually covered with slough. Microscopically, this consists of inflammatory cells, macrophages (a) and a background of pale-staining proteinous debris overlaid with necrotic epithelial cells (b).

The necrosed cells show advanced karyopyknosis, karyorrhexis and karyolysis. A similar appearance is seen in cytological specimens of chronic pancreatitis and inflammatory diseases of the large bowel.

OESOPHAGUS

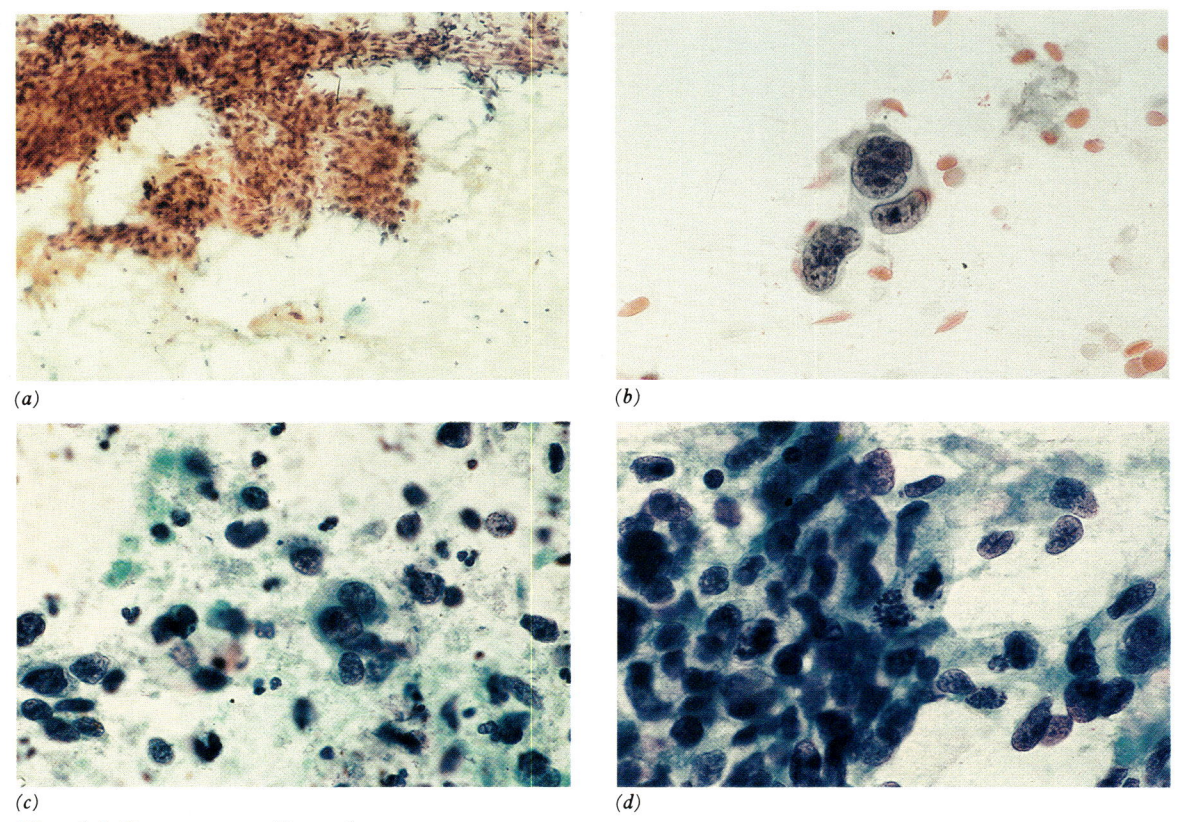

Fig. 6.4 Squamous cell carcinoma

Papanicolaou: oesophageal brush (a) ×133: well differentiated (b) ×525: another case; moderately differentiated (c) ×525: another case; poorly differentiated (d) ×525: another case; anaplastic

The oesophagus is lined by stratified squamous epithelium which changes abruptly to gastric mucosa at the cardio-oesophageal junction. The lower third may contain ectopic foci of gastric mucosa. The majority of oesophageal malignant tumours are of the squamous cell type. The well differentiated squamous cell carcinoma contains round or bizarre shaped cells identical in appearance to the keratinized carcinoma cells of the genital tract or bronchogenic squamous cell carcinoma. Micrograph (a) shows a well differentiated malignant cell in the lower half of the field and a sheet of cohesive, flattened tumour cells in the upper half. The moderately differentiated carcinoma cells in (b) are free of keratin. The nuclei are variable in size and markedly variable in shape. The nuclear chromatin is aggregated into small and coarse granules and is irregular in distribution; the chromatin pattern is different in each of the four nuclei. The nucleoli are prominent to the same degree as in moderately differentiated squamous cell carcinomas in other organs. The cells in (c) are poorly differentiated and display a greater degree of anisocytosis. Although distinctive cytoplasmic features of squamous cells are lacking, the lack of cell cohesion, the irregularity of cell shape, the absence of depth of focus or of intracellular mucin and the coarseness of the nuclei favours a presumptive diagnosis of a squamous cell origin. Note the scattered necrotic tumour cells. Total anaplasia is evident in the sheet of cells in (d). The nuclei vary in size and in shape from round to fusiform. The scant cytoplasm lacks recognizable limiting membranes and nucleoli are inconspicuous. The four mitotic figures present in one high power field are indicative of a rapid rate of cell proliferation.

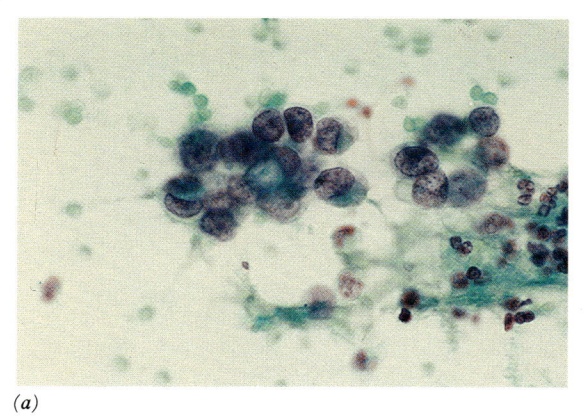

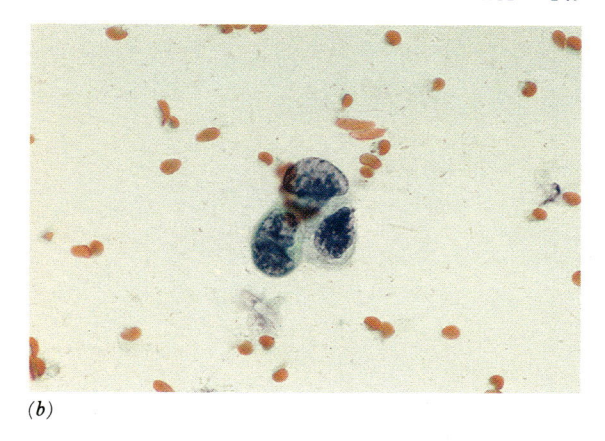

Fig. 6.5 Adenocarcinoma

(a) Alcian blue ×525: oesophageal brush (b) Papanicolaou ×525: gastro-oesophageal anastomosis brush; another case

Adenocarcinoma of the oesophagus is rare, and usually occurs in the lower third in an ectopic focus of gastric mucosa. More commonly it is an upward extension of a gastric primary.

Micrograph (a) of a brush smear from the lower third of the oesophagus illustrates adenocarcinoma cells. The cluster to the right shows an acinar arrangement. One cell in the cluster to the left contains a sharply delineated mucous vacuole, the mucin in the other cells is diffuse. The patient presented with symptoms due to an oesophageal stricture. In view of the rarity of adenocarcinoma in this area, a suggestive appearance of an adenocarcinoma can be altered to a definitive diagnosis by the use of appropriate special stains to demonstrate mucin. The primary tumour in this case originated in and involved the stomach. The adenocarcinoma cells in (b) were recovered from a recurrence of a gastric carcinoma at the site of anastomosis 23 years after a gastrectomy.

STOMACH

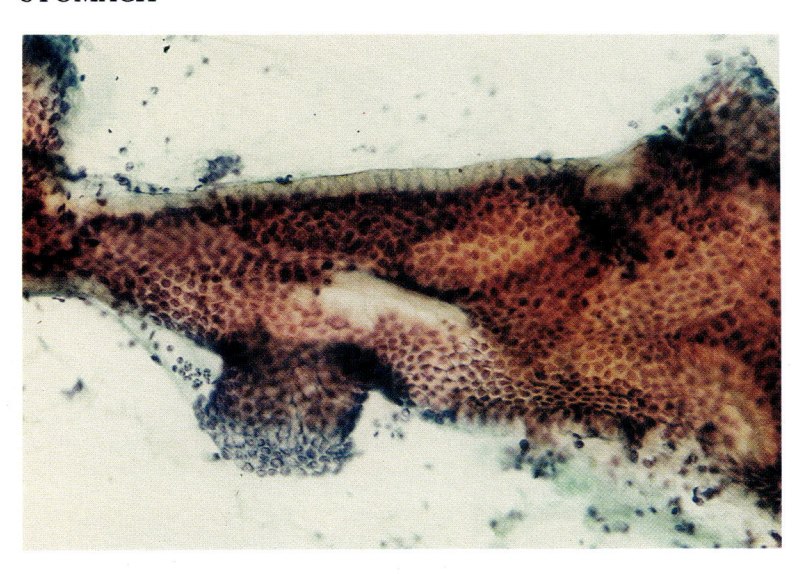

Fig. 6.6 Normal gastric mucosa

Papanicolaou ×183: gastric brush

This micrograph illustrates a fragment of normal gastric mucosa. The surface cells form a regular palisade and have abundant pale-staining cytoplasm with basally located nuclei. The same cells are seen deeper down lining the gastric pits or fovea. Foveal cells contain neutral mucin which stains strongly with PAS, but reacts weakly with alcian blue. The other cells that make up the gastric mucosa, the hydrochloric acid-secreting parietal or oxyntic cells and the pepsinogen-secreting peptic or chief cells are not easily discriminated in a Papanicolaou-stained smear.

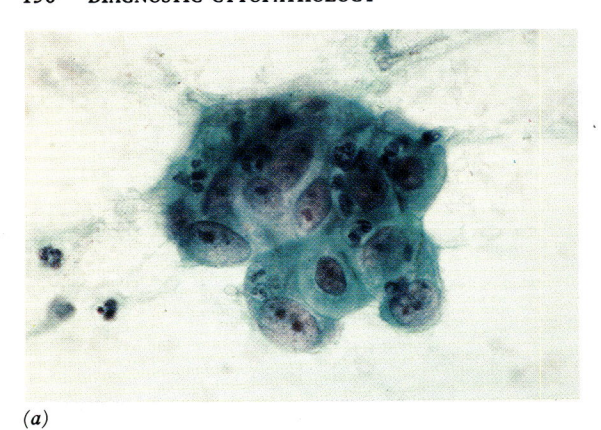

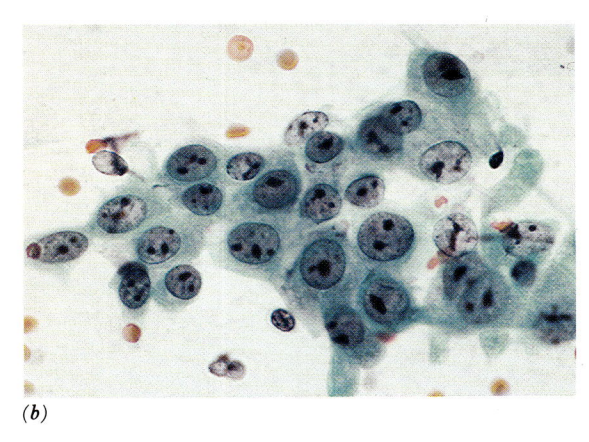

150 DIAGNOSTIC CYTOPATHOLOGY

(a)

(b)

Fig. 6.7 Regenerating gastric mucosa

Papanicolaou ×525: gastric brush (a) a case of chronic gastritis (b) another case

One of the major diagnostic problems met with in gastric cytopathology is presented by regenerating mucosal cells. These are seen particularly in hypersecretory chronic gastritis which is not a significant precursor of gastric carcinoma. The regenerating cells usually appear in sheets, have deeply basophilic cytoplasm, display some anisonucleosis and invariably contain prominent nucleoli which may be multiple and are often polymorphic. An occasional mitotic figure may be present. The features that aid in the correct identification of the benign proliferating cells are the relative flatness of the cell aggregate which is two-dimensional in the manner of lining cells, and, despite the anisocytosis, an overall impression of a more or less comparable nuclear-cytoplasmic ratio. In addition, the nuclei are vesicular and the chromatin pattern is not disorganised.

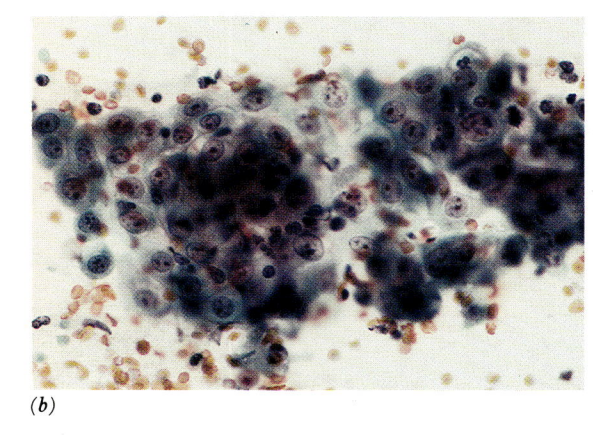

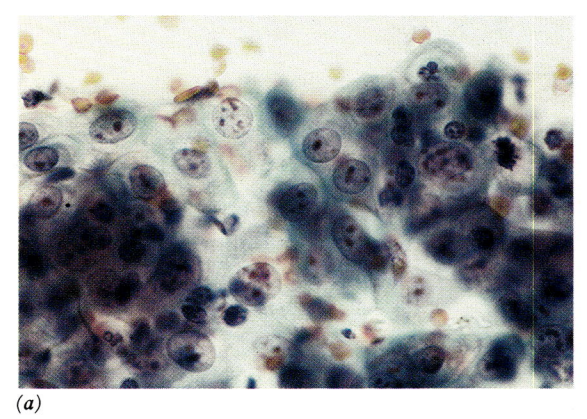

(a)

(b)

Fig. 6.8 Intestinal metaplasia

Papanicolaou (a) ×525: gastric brush (b) ×333: gastric brush

Chronic gastritis due to environmental causes is prevalent in populations at high risk of developing gastric carcinoma as in Japan, but occurs in sporadic cases in other parts of the world. The condition may result in atrophy of the gastric mucosa which is replaced by metaplastic epithelium of the intestinal type. The metaplasia may be complete and contain all the cell types seen in the small intestine or be incomplete and more closely resemble colonic metaplasia. Paneth and argentaffin cells are not identifiable in routine cytological smears and require special staining procedures for their demonstration. At a simple level, intestinalized gastric mucosa is seen to consist of goblet cells and absorptive cells. The goblet cell is larger, has a paler cytoplasm and contains mucous vacuoles; its distal border is often fuzzy and fine tags of cytoplasm extend beyond the luminal surface. The absorptive cell is smaller, has a deeper and more uniformly stained cytoplasm and does not contain intracytoplasmic secretory vacuoles. It is covered with fine, short microvilli and the line of attachment of the microvilli, although not as broad as the terminal bar of the ciliated cell, is sharp and imparts a clear definition to the luminal surface of the cell. Areas of intestinal metaplasia may also contain mitoses and a mitotic figure is seen opposite 1 o'clock (a). The cell arrangement is more disorganised than is the case with regenerating gastric mucosa cells. The benign nature of the cells is indicated by the extreme regularity of the nuclei, the uniformly low nuclear cytoplasmic ratio and the blandness of the nuclei (a). The relative flatness of the clusters is better appreciated at a lower magnification (b).

OESOPHAGO-GASTROINTESTINAL TRACT 151

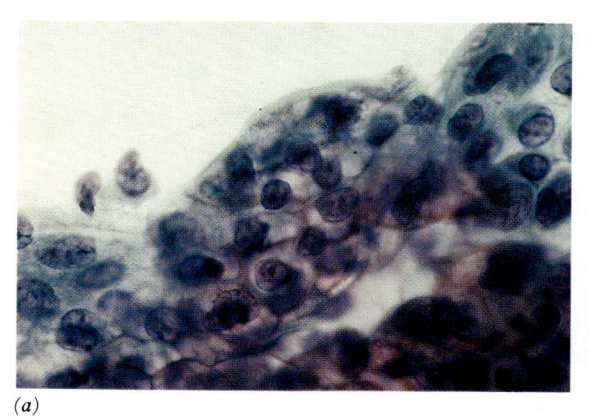

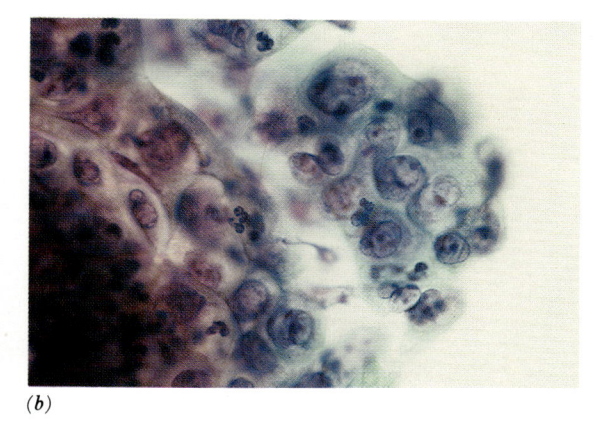

(a) (b)

Fig. 6.9 A case of pernicious anaemia

Papanicolaou ×525: gastric brush (a) intestinal metaplasia (b) dysplasia

The chronic gastritis associated with the pernicious anaemia syndrome is the result of injury to the intrinsic factor and the parietal cells by auto-antibodies. Like gastritis due to environmental causes, it leads to atrophy and subsequent intestinal metaplasia and is a significant precursor of gastric carcinoma. A sheet of benign intestinal metaplasia cells is illustrated in (a). An absorptive cell with a clear narrow end plate is seen interposed between two mucin-containing cells at the free edge of the sheet, the majority of the cells are of the goblet type. The cells are approximately the same size, the nuclei are regular and small.

Intestinal metaplasia may show cellular atypia and become dysplastic. The cells illustrated in (b) were seen in the same smear. They are larger and more variable in size. The nuclei show considerable variation in size and the nuclear cytoplasmic ratio is high. The chromatin content is increased and there is some disorganization of the chromatin pattern. The nucleoli are larger and more prominent. The cellular atypia is consistent with mild dysplasia.

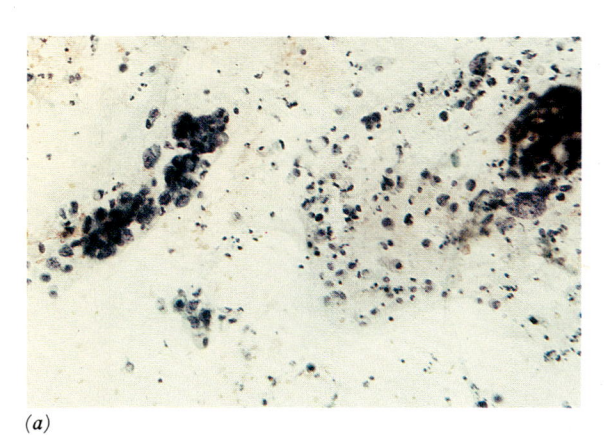

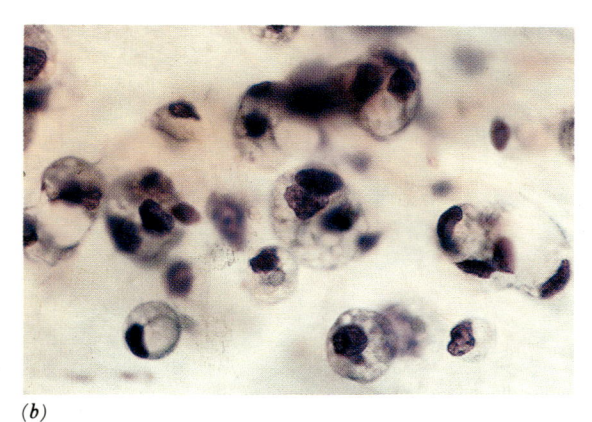

(a) (b)

Fig. 6.10 Signet-ring carcinoma in a case of pernicious anaemia

Papanicolaou gastric brush (a) ×133 (b) ×525: another field

A large number of neoplastic cells, some discrete, others in cohesive sheets are seen against a background of pale pink free mucin (a). At high magnification (b) the cells are seen to be distended with mucin. In some cells the mucous vacuoles are small and multiple; in others, the nucleus is pushed to one pole by a single, large secretory globule and the cell has acquired a signet ring appearance. The nuclear cytoplasmic ratio is low and the nuclei compressed by mucin are small and intensely hyperchromic. Sparse, scattered, signet-ring carcinoma cells are easily overlooked or mistaken for histiocytes. High power examination of cells caught in amorphous material is advisable to avoid a false negative report. If required, the acidic mucin in the cells may be confirmed with mucicarmine or alcian blue.

152 DIAGNOSTIC CYTOPATHOLOGY

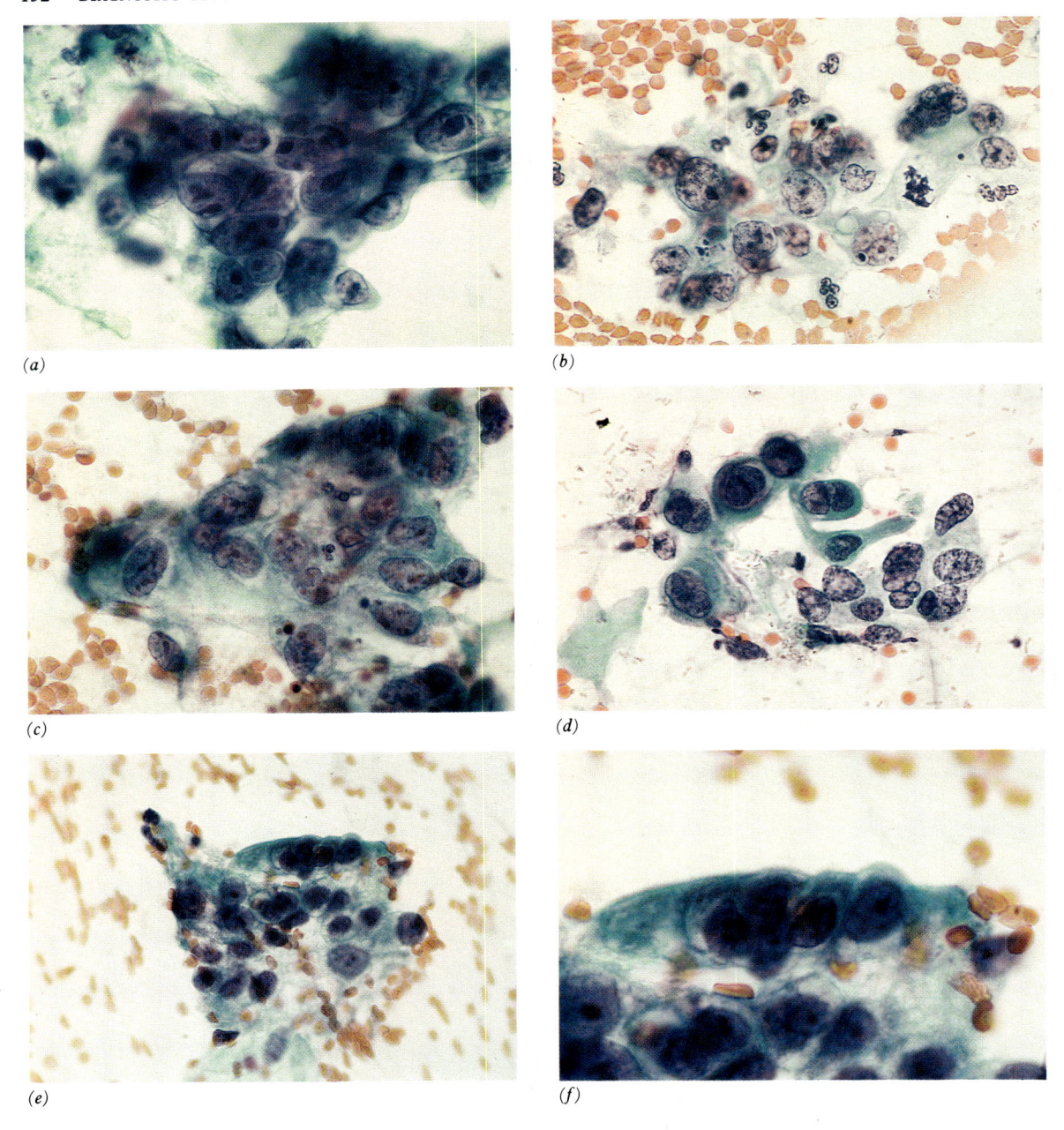

(a)

(b)

(c)

(d)

(e)

(f)

Fig. 6.11 Adenocarcinoma of the stomach (*illustrations opposite*)

Papanicolaou: gastric brush (a) ×525 (b) ×525: another case (c) ×525: another case (d) ×525: another case (e) ×333: another case (f) ×832: same field as (e)

The common cytological features of malignancy met with in endoscopic gastric brush cytology are illustrated in these micrographs by five cases. The first point to note is that although all the cases are of adenocarcinoma, the three-dimensional globular clusters characteristic of spontaneously exfoliated glandular cells are not a feature of a brush smear. The cell arrangement in clusters and sheets with uneven ragged borders is similar to that seen in bronchial brush and lung aspirate smears. The familiar appearance of rounded adenocarcinoma cells is an artefact as much of the type of specimen as of the nature of the cell and should not be sought in a brush smear of an adenocarcinoma.

The malignant cells in these micrographs are pleomorphic, the variation in shape and size being most evident in the nuclei and the nuclear-cytoplasmic ratio. Reasonably well preserved nuclei, freshly obtained from a tumour by brush or aspiration are not remarkable for hyperchromasia; they may be moderately hyperchromic (a), normochromic (b) or hypochromic (c). Nucleoli are usually present in gastric carcinoma cells, but vary in size and prominence from case to case. In (a) they are a dominant feature, like a dilated pupil in the cornea. In (b) and (c) they are appreciably smaller and less conspicuous than in benign regenerating cells (Fig. 6.7). The staining reaction of the nucleoli is as variable in malignant cells as in benign cells. As a rule, the nucleolus in a hypochromic nucleus is more likely to be eosinophilic (c).

The cytoplasm also varies from case to case. It is intensely basophilic in (a), paler and more fragile in (b) and (c). Cytoplasmic vacuolization is not an outstanding feature of these cases, but at least one cell in (a), (b) and (c) contains a mucous vacuole. A centrally located eosinophilic dot of condensed mucin within a clear vacuole, and an abnormal mitotic figure are present in (b).

The cells in (d) evince advanced degenerative changes as indicated by the many stripped malignant nuclei, and the perinuclear vacuolization of the binucleate cell.

In most cases, carcinoma cells in a brush smear do not exhibit any kind of architectural organization. On occasion, a strip of luminal neoplastic cells may be recovered along with deeper cells (e). The luminal cells are aligned in a palisade and their polarity is maintained. The distal surface is neat and covered with a microvillous brush border (f).

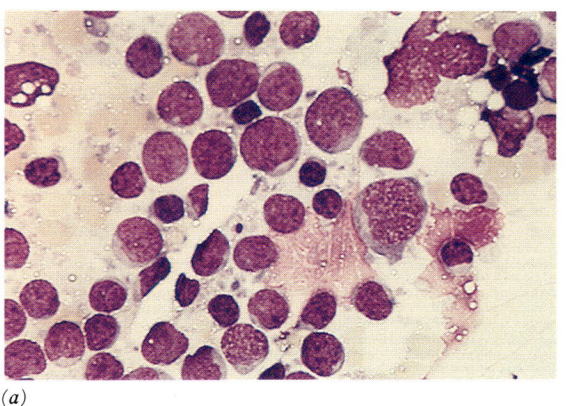

Fig. 6.12 Primary gastric lymphoma

(a) MGG ×525: gastric brush (b) Papanicolaou ×525: gastric brush; another case

These micrographs illustrate two cases in which a cytological diagnosis of non-Hodgkin's lymphoma was confirmed by histology; a full diagnosis of B-cell lymphoma was established by immunocytochemical study on the case shown in (b). The smears show a mixed population of discrete cells which include a few small lymphocytes with hyperchromic condensed nuclei and numerous immature lymphoid cells which show a progressive gradation in size (a) (b). Some of the nuclei are notched and several contain small multiple nucleoli.

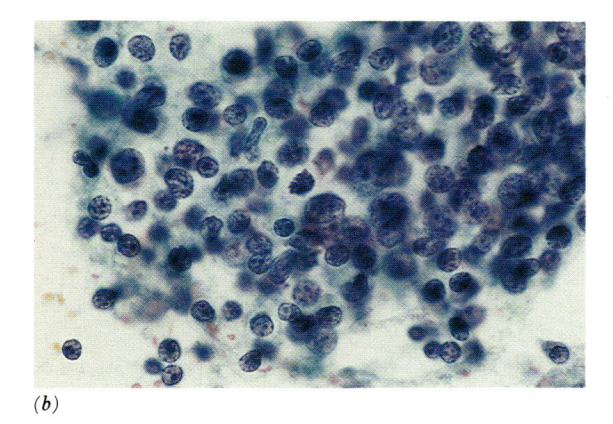

A presumptive cytodiagnosis of primary gastric lymphoma can be of value as this tumour is eminently treatable, may occur in the younger age groups and may present with the symptoms and appearance of a benign ulcer. Since, however, lymphocytes and plasma cells may occur in small numbers in a normal upper gastrointestinal brush smear, or in abundance in chronic gastritis, a cytological diagnosis of malignant lymphoma calls for careful morphological assessment and should always be confirmed by appropriate histological and immunological studies.

Fig. 6.13 Leiomyoma of stomach

Papanicolaou ×525: gastric brush

Another non-epithelial neoplasm of the stomach is a smooth muscle tumour which may be benign or malignant. Initially sub-mucous, it may project into the gastric cavity as a polypoid mass and erode the surface mucosa. Tumour tissue may be obtained in a brush smear at this stage. In the example of a leiomyoma illustrated, numerous smooth muscle cells are seen. The plump, fusiform nuclei are more or less alike in shape and size and mitoses are not evident. The nuclei of a poorly differentiated leiomyosarcoma are generally bizarre and pleomorphic and the diagnosis is self-evident. A well differentiated leiomyosarcoma shows relatively little nuclear deviation and the diagnosis of malignancy may have to be based on the number of mitotic figures seen per microscopic field in a histological specimen.

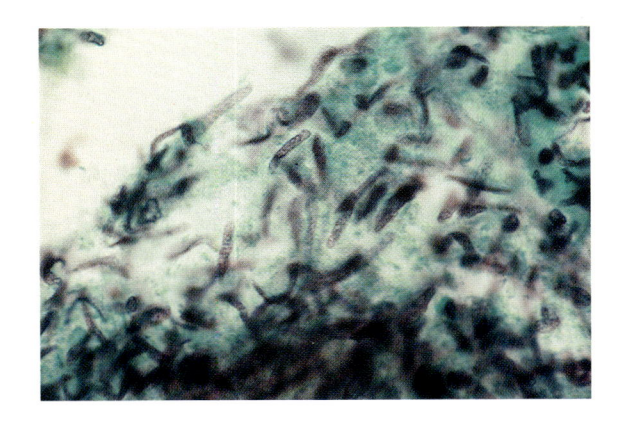

COLON

(a)

(b)

(c)

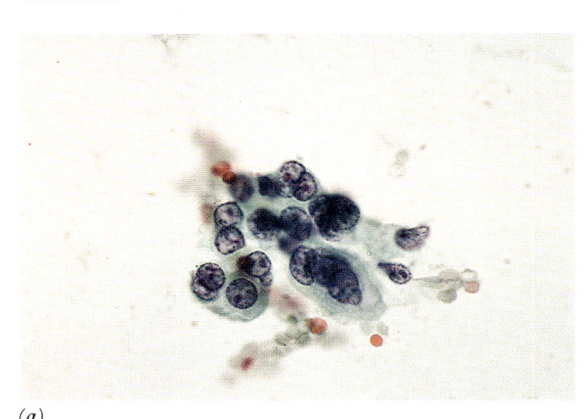

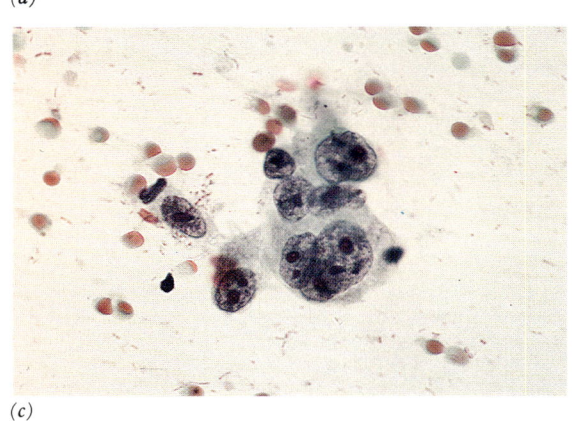

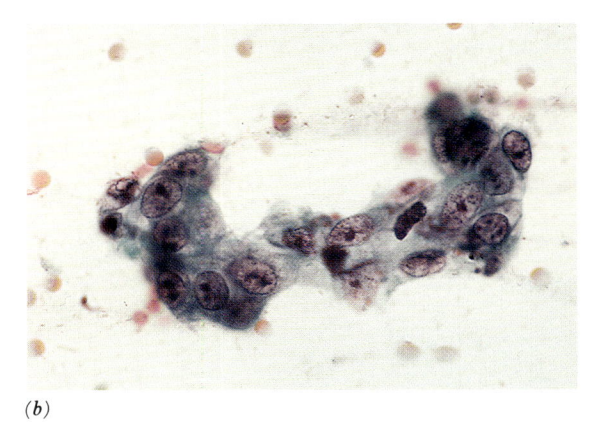

Fig. 6.14 Adenocarcinoma of the colon

Papanicolaou ×525: colonic brush (a) carcinoma of the caecum (b) carcinoma of the sigmoid colon; another case (c) carcinoma of the rectosigmoid colon; another case

Brush samples are obtainable from the entire colon up to the ileo-caecal valve. The majority of the primary colon carcinomas occur in the descending part. The tumours are adenocarcinomas and cytologically similar to gastric carcinomas. A well differentiated adenocarcinoma originating in the caecum is illustrated in micrograph (a). The cells are small, inter-cellular borders are well defined and nuclear variation is of a low degree; the nucleoli are small. A moderately differentiated carcinoma of the sigmoid colon has yielded cells which have more cytoplasm; the limiting membrane of the cells, however, is less well defined. The nuclei and nucleoli are larger than in (a). In a poorly differentiated tumour of the rectosigmoid, intercytoplasmic membranes are still less distinct, and the cytoplasm appears to form a syncytium. Anisonucleosis is marked and the nucleoli are prominent and variable in number and shape. Note the perinucleolar condensation of chromatin round the nucleoli in (c).

Fig. 6.15 Polyp with surface dysplasia

Papanicolaou (a) ×720: colonic brush (b) ×183: colonic brush; same field as (a) (c) ×720: colonic brush; same case; another field

Interest has centred in recent years on the early recognition and grading of dysplastic changes that occur in some lesions of the colon such as a villous adenoma, familial polyposis coli and long standing ulcerative colitis known to carry a high potential of malignant transformation. Whilst the high sensitivity of cytology in identifying dysplasia is universally acknowledged, distinction between severely dysplastic cells and cells brushed from the surface of an infiltrating lesion remains problematical. This may be achieved if adequate amount of tissue is present.

These micrographs illustrate a polypoid lesion of the sigmoid colon with severe dysplasia. The cells in (a) bear stigmata of malignancy; the nuclei are pleomorphic, the nuclear chromatin is stippled and the nuclear-cytoplasmic ratio is high. At a lower magnification (b), they are seen to form the surface of a non-malignant fragment of colonic tissue. A milder degree of dysplasia in hyperplastic mucosa is seen in (c). The cells are enlarged and nucleoli are prominent but the arrangement is orderly and polarity is maintained. Note the microvilli and the narrow end plate of the luminal absorptive cells.

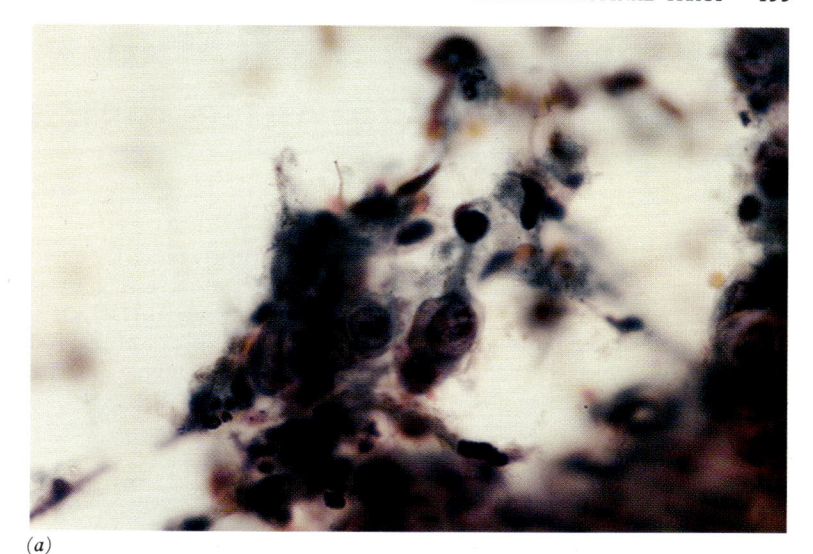

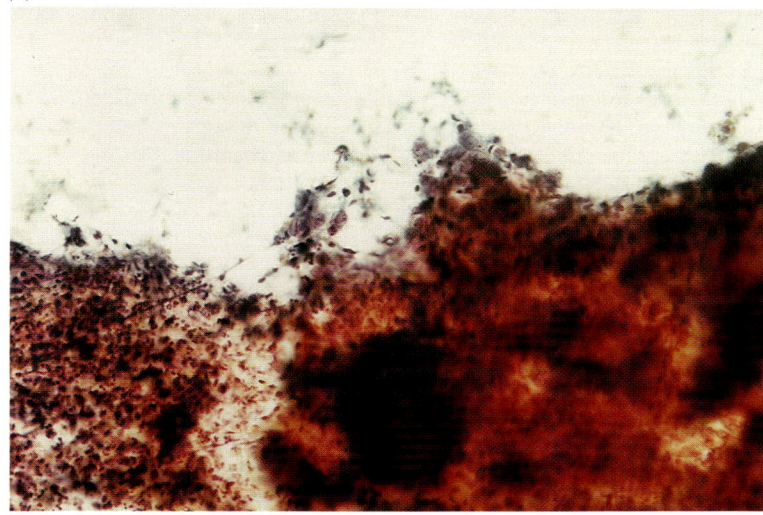

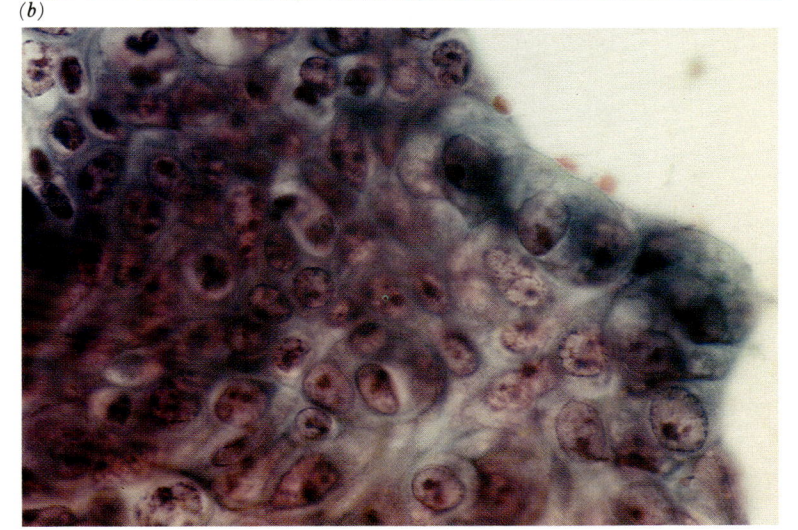

(a)

(b)

(c)

7. Fine needle aspiration cytology of sub-diaphragmatic lesions

The initial diagnosis of sub-diaphragmatic lesions, formerly requiring exploratory laparotomy, has been revolutionized by advances in interventional radiology and increasing use of cytopathology. A suspected malignancy is the chief indication for fine needle aspiration (FNA) which is a simple, safe and low cost procedure. It is particularly useful for the confirmation of metastatic disease of the liver and to establish a primary carcinoma of the pancreas which is generally inoperable at first presentation.

SAMPLING TECHNIQUES

The lesion is localized by one of several radiological procedures and aspirated through the abdominal skin and sub-cutaneous tissues with a fine 21–23 gauge needle under imaging control. This is generally ultrasonography, CT scan being the next common procedure employed. The preparation of the aspirated material is as for intrathoracic FNA specimens.

For correct interpretation of cell pathology and accurate localization of the lesion, certain points require careful consideration. Familiarity with the normal cells of the various intra-abdominal organs is essential. It is important to learn from the radiologist the ostensible site of aspiration; this, however, should be confirmed if possible, by assessment of the internal evidence in the specimen, e.g. hepatocytes in a liver aspiration and acinar cells in a pancreatic sample. This may not be feasible when the aspirate consists exclusively of metastatic tumour cells or a duct cell carcinoma, in the absence of informative cells originating in the host tissue. It is also important to bear in mind that depending on the location of the target organ and the direction of approach, benign cells from an overlying organ may enter the needle, 'contaminate' the specimen and become a possible source of incorrect interpretation; intestinal mucosa accidentally picked up in an aspiration of a retroperitoneal lymph node may be mistaken for a metastatic mucin-secreting carcinoma.

FNA of ovarian lesions is considered in Chapter 1 and of renal lesions in Chapter 8.

LIVER AND BILIARY SYSTEM

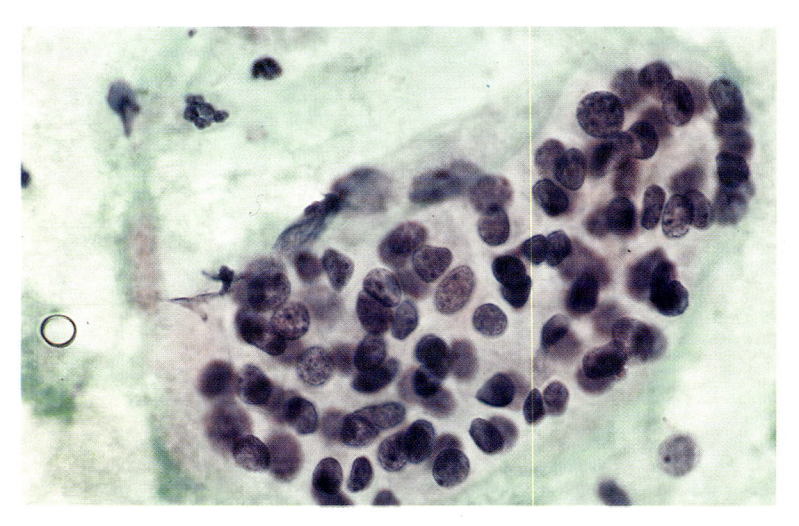

Fig. 7.1 Cholangiocytes
Papanicolaou ×720: FNA; liver

The liver synthesizes bile which is secreted into a system of fine canaliculi which drain into intrahepatic bile ducts, whence it is transported to the duodenum via the common bile duct. The lining cells of intrahepatic bile ducts, known as cholangiocytes, vary from cuboidal in the small ducts to low columnar in the larger ducts.

The cytoplasm of cholangiocytes is cyanophilic and sparse. The nuclei, about the size of a neutrophil, are round or oval, hyperchromic and granular. The nuclear cytoplasmic ratio is high and a small nucleolus may be present. Cholangiocytes usually occur in groups and sheets and the monomorphism of the nuclei is a striking feature.

Fig. 7.2 Hepatocytes: Kupffer cells: bile pigment

(a) Papanicolaou ×720: FNA; liver (b) MGG ×720: same specimen; another smear (c) Papanicolaou ×720: FNA; liver; another case

The parenchymal liver cell or hepatocyte is a large polyhedral cell with abundant cytoplasm. This is eosinophilic with the Papanicolaou stain (a) and violet with MGG (b); however, the intensity of cytoplasmic staining varies with the metabolic state of the cell and may not be uniform throughout. The healthy liver cell is rich in organelles and glycogen, and at times lipid, and the cytoplasm may appear finely granular.

The nucleus of the hepatocyte is round with evenly dispersed chromatin and the nuclear-cytoplasmic ratio is low on account of the large volume of cytoplasm. One or more prominent nucleoli are always present. The normal liver often contains a fair proportion of cells with double or quadruple the diploid complement of chromosomes. The tetraploid and polyploid cells may have large nuclei; in consequence, anisonucleosis is a frequently encountered feature of liver aspirates. Binucleate forms are often present (a), (b) and the occasional cell may contain three (a) or more nuclei. Variation in the size and number of liver cell nuclei is without any diagnostic significance.

Bile may be seen in the form of yellow or light brown intracytoplasmic granules of variable size (c).

The sinusoids between plates of liver cells are lined by flattened slender cells with scant pale cytoplasm and elongated nuclei (a) (b). These cells have a phagocytic function and are referred to as Kupffer cells.

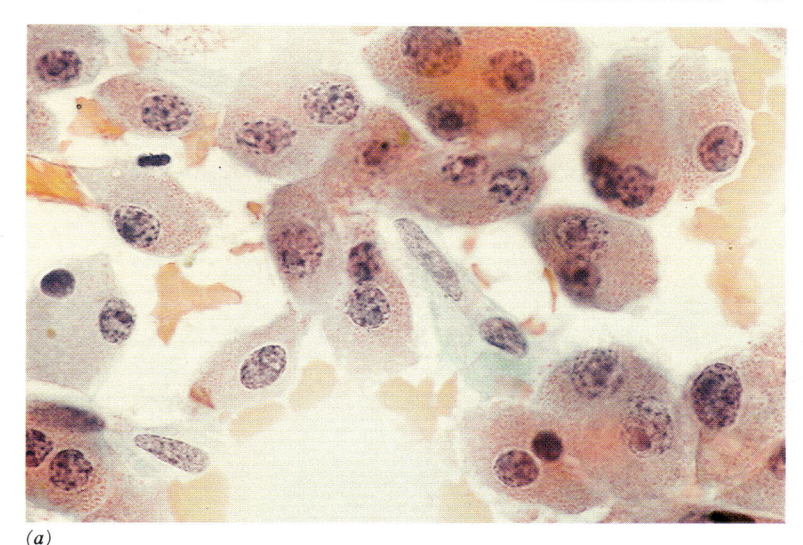

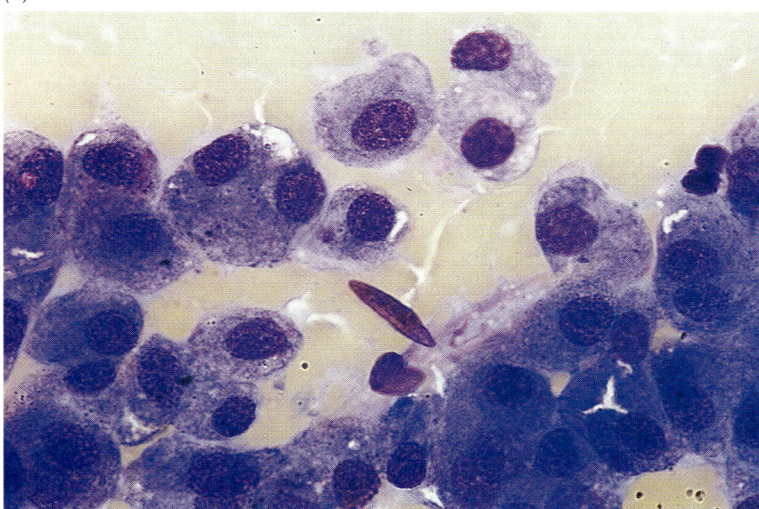

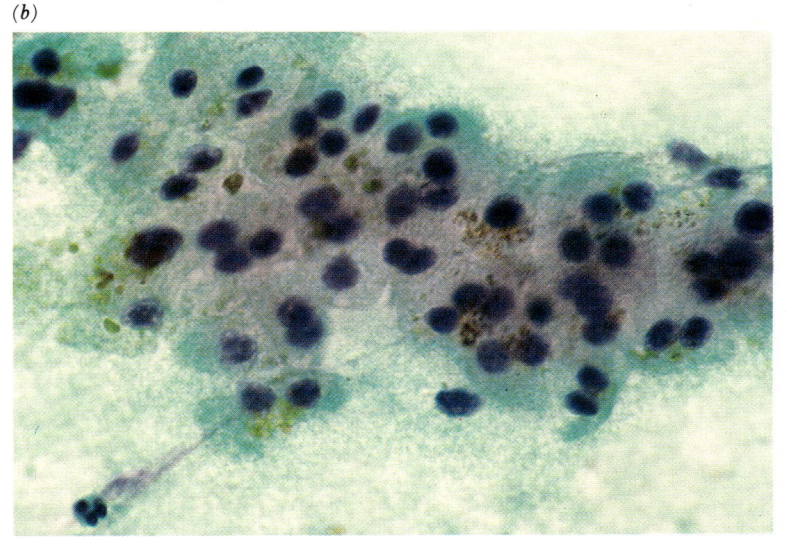

(a)

(b)

(c)

158   DIAGNOSTIC CYTOPATHOLOGY

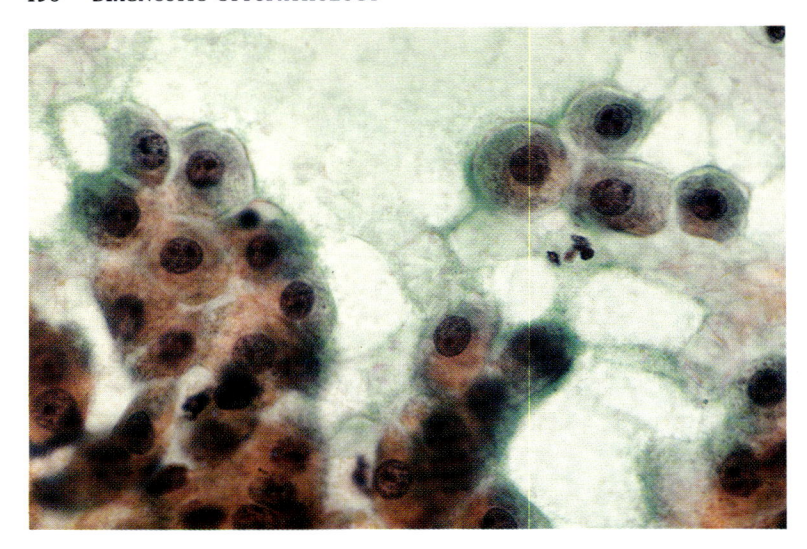

Fig. 7.3 Cirrhosis
Papanicolaou ×720: FNA; liver

The diagnosis of cirrhosis of the liver is a histological one and cytology has no contribution to make. Indeed, barring the very exceptional case in which clinical data and cytological appearance are carefully correlated to exclude malignancy in a nodular liver, cytodiagnosis of liver cirrhosis is unwarranted. The cells from a cirrhotic nodule may appear quite normal; in some cases, the nuclear variation of the healthy liver may be exaggerated. The normal looking cells illustrated in this micrograph came from a biopsy shared with histology which established the diagnosis.

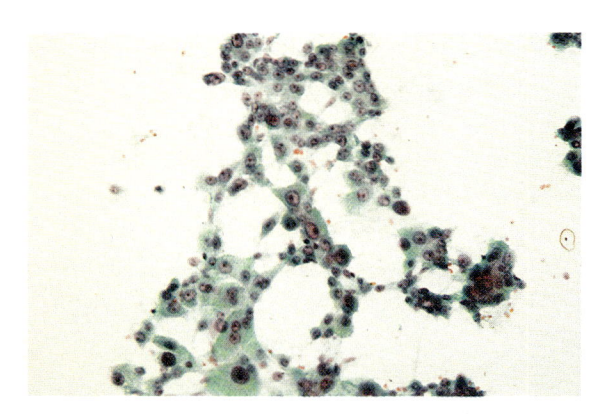

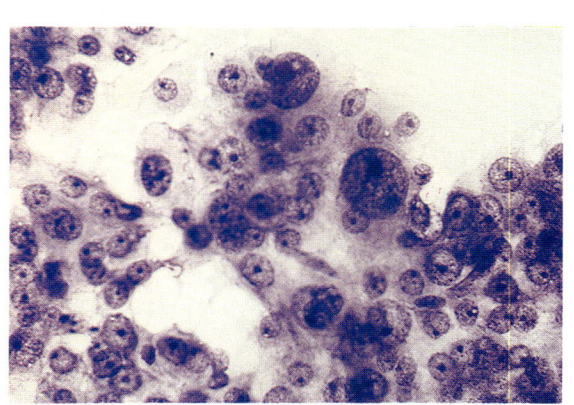

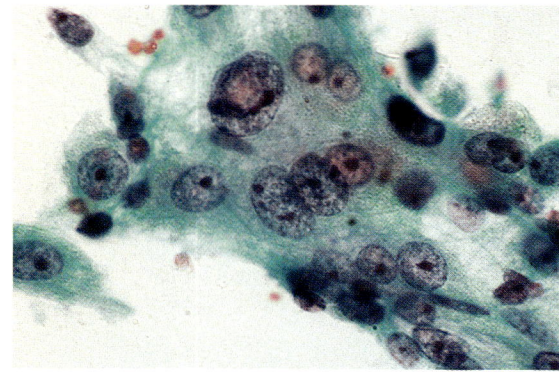

(b)

Fig. 7.4 Hepatocellular carcinoma in pre-existing cirrhosis

(a) Papanicolaou ×133: FNA; liver (b) ×525: same field
(c) MGG ×525: same specimen, another smear

Primary liver cell carcinoma is a common cancer in some African countries but is relatively rare in the West. It often develops in pre-existing cirrhosis, and is heralded by a sudden deterioration in the patient's condition. A case of hepatocellular carcinoma in a patient with an established diagnosis of liver cirrhosis is illustrated. Micrograph (a) shows anastomosing cords of recognizable liver cells arranged round spaces in a pseudo-acinar manner. Variation in the amount of cytoplasm per cell can be appreciated at low power. At a higher magnification (b), (c), a marked degree of anisonucleosis becomes evident. The distribution of the nuclei is irregular, several are closely packed and overlap each other. Compare these cells with benign hepatocytes in Figure 7.2 and note that the chromatin of the malignant cells is very finely stippled, the nuclei are hypochromic and the nucleoli are eosinophilic and more prominent. A hepatocellular carcinoma may contain PAS-positive material, but does not produce mucin. Plasma alpha-fetoprotein raised in the majority of primary liver cell carcinomas was high in the case illustrated.

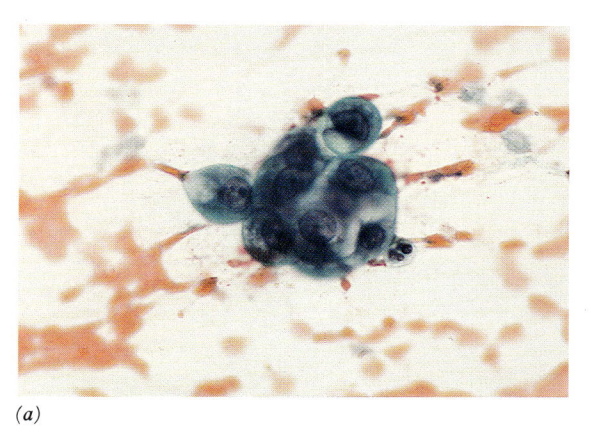

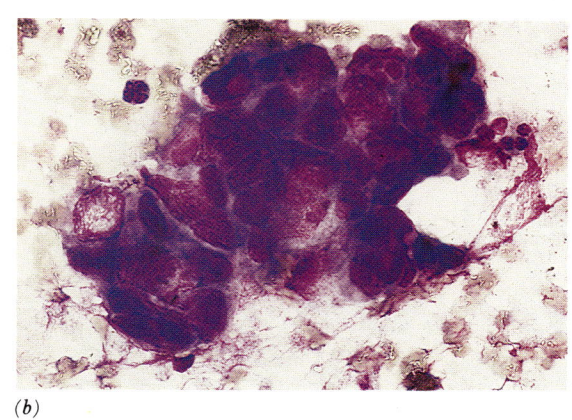

(a) (b)
Fig. 7.5 Cholangiocarcinoma: intra-hepatic duct cell carcinoma
(a) Papanicolaou ×525: FNA; liver (b) MGG ×525: same specimen; another smear

A primary carcinoma of intrahepatic bile ducts is even less common than a liver cell carcinoma. The malignant cholangiocytes are larger than benign duct lining cells and the appearance and arrangement of the cells is that of an adenocarcinoma. Most cholangiocarcinomas are mucin producing; this allows distinction from a hepatocellular carcinoma, but not from a metastatic, mucin-secreting adenocarcinoma. Neither a cytological nor a histological diagnosis of a primary intrahepatic bile duct carcinoma can be affirmed in the absence of firm clinical data and clear-cut radiological evidence. The case illustrated is one of recurrent disease in a previously diagnosed and treated cholangiocarcinoma of the liver.

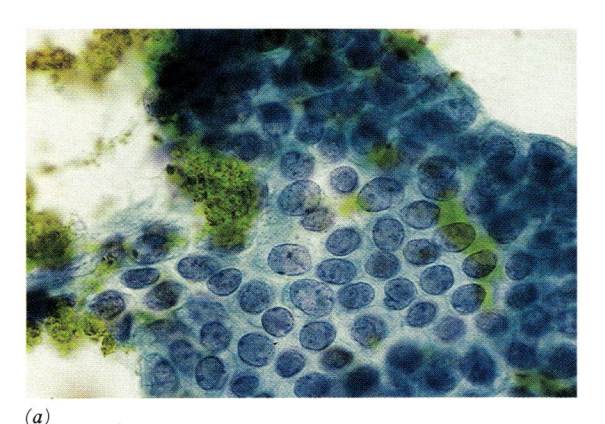

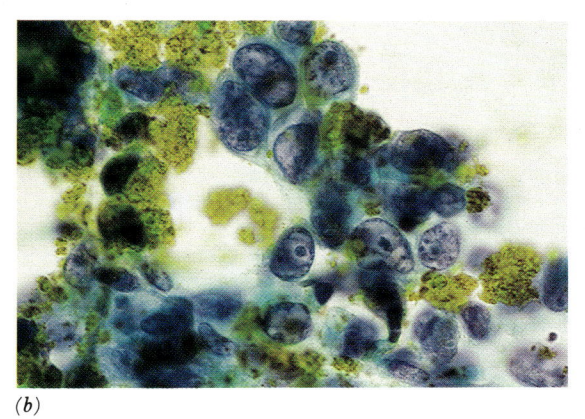

(a) (b)
Fig. 7.6 Cholangiocarcinoma: extra-hepatic bile duct carcinoma
Papanicolaou ×525: bile (a) benign ductal cells (b) malignant ductal cells

Percutaneous transhepatic cholangiography is a diagnostic procedure used to examine the extrahepatic biliary system. A needle introduced through the skin is guided into an intrahepatic bile duct under fluoroscopic control, dye injected and the biliary system examined radiologically. An indwelling catheter may be used to drain a dilated biliary tree into the duodenum or percutaneously and to relieve obstructive jaundice. The bile drained externally may be examined for the presence of neoplastic cells. It should however be reasonably fresh as cells left in bile deteriorate rapidly.

These micrographs illustrate cells in bile drained through a catheter. Abundant yellow bile pigment is seen in both micrographs. The cells in (a) are benign ductal cells in a sheet. The nuclei are evenly spaced, monomorphic and normochromic; the nuclear chromatin is sparse. The carcinoma cells in (b) are appreciably larger; the nuclei vary in size and shape and nuclear-cytoplasmic ratio is high. The nuclear chromatin is increased in quantity and disorganized in arrangement.

160 DIAGNOSTIC CYTOPATHOLOGY

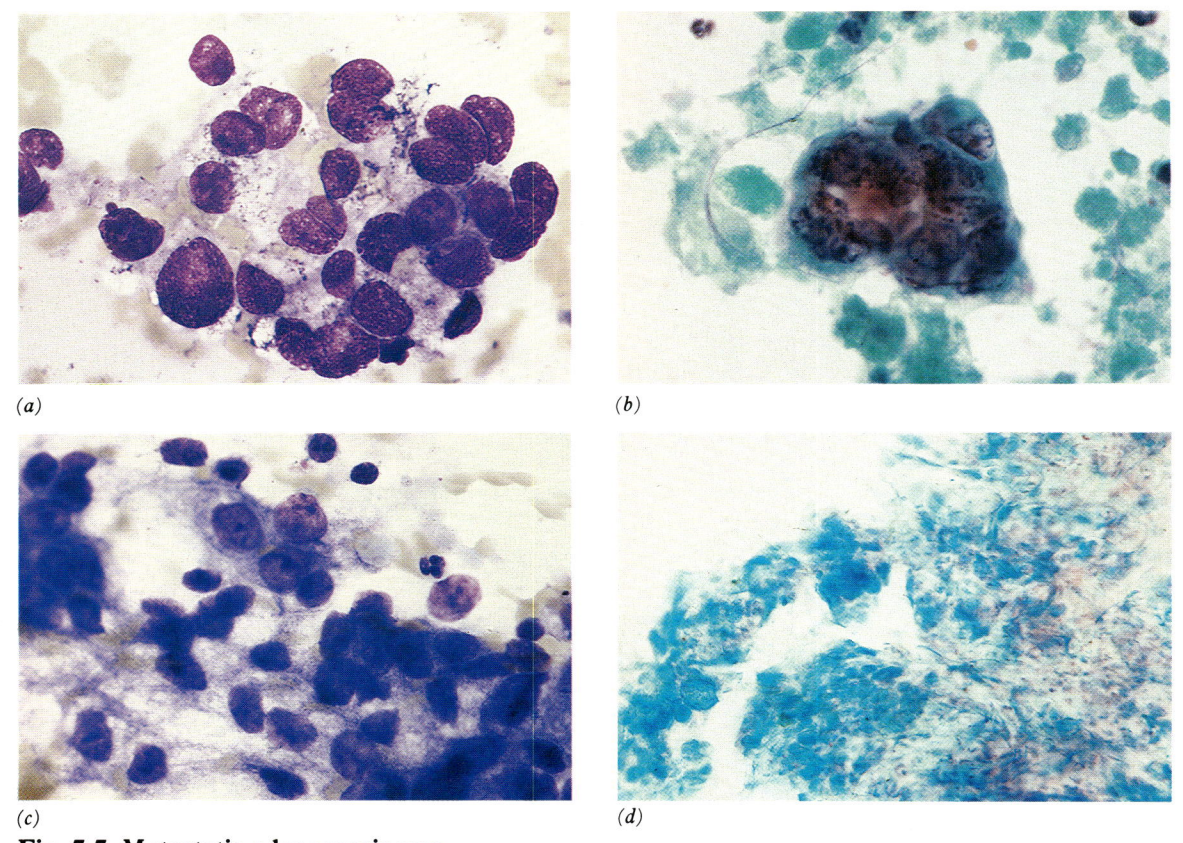

Fig. 7.7 Metastatic adenocarcinoma

(a) MGG ×525: FNA; liver (b) Papanicolaou ×525: FNA; liver; another case (c) MGG ×525 FNA; liver; another case (d) Alcian blue ×133: same specimen as (c); another smear

The liver is a common site of metastatic cancer. In a large proportion of cases, the primary is known, in some, a patient without an established diagnosis or without evidence of disease elsewhere may present with symptoms that direct attention to the liver. Evidence of one or more space-occupying lesions identified by ultrasonography or CT scan is the usual indication for aspiration cytology. Metastatic adenocarcinoma is the commonest malignancy seen and three cases are illustrated in these micrographs. In micrograph (a), the cells aspirated under ultrasound control display a marked degree of nuclear pleomorphism; the cytoplasm is fine in texture and contains small vacuoles. Adherent tumour cells aspirated under CT guidance are seen in (b). In this example of a metastatic adenocarcinoma, the cytoplasm is firm and deeply basophilic, and the nuclei are large and crowded and compressed together. Note the necrotic tumour tissue surrounding the malignant cluster. In the third case (c), also aspirated under ultrasound control, the nuclei appear to be embedded in an amorphous matrix. The appearance suggestive of free mucin was confirmed by staining a duplicate smear with alcian blue (d). An aspirate of a mucoid carcinoma is often viscous and may be gelatinous.

FNA CYTOLOGY OF SUB-DIAPHRAGMATIC LESIONS 161

Fig. 7.8 Metastatic malignant non-Hodgkin's lymphoma

*(a) MGG ×720: FNA; liver
(b) Papanicolaou ×720: same specimen; another smear (c) Papanicolaou ×720: ascitic fluid; same case*

The liver may be involved in disseminated malignant lymphoma. The neoplastic cells in these micrographs are small and discrete. A variable amount of cytoplasm can be appreciated in the air dried MGG preparaions and is seen to have plasmacytoid features (a); the alcohol-fixed cells in (b) appear to consist almost entirely of nucleus. The nucleoli are more obvious in the Papanicolaou smear (b), and vary in number from one to three or more. Tumour cell necrosis is a prominent feature. Cells identical to the liver cell aspirate (a), (b) were found in the ascitic fluid (c).

The case illustrated highlights some important practical points. The patient was a 5-year-old boy. The differential diagnosis includes other small cell malignancies of childhood, such as neuroblastoma, nephroblastoma and myosarcoma. A cytodiagnosis of malignant lymphoma was based on cell morphology taken in conjunction with the significant absence of any cell cohesion; the Papanicolaou and MGG stains were complementary. The biopsy histology report on the same case was nephroblastoma, and was doubtless due to compression of the cells in a small specimen. The cytohistological discrepancy was resolved by immunocytochemical studies done on cells in suspension in the ascitic fluid and a diagnosis of a high grade B cell lymphoma was confirmed.

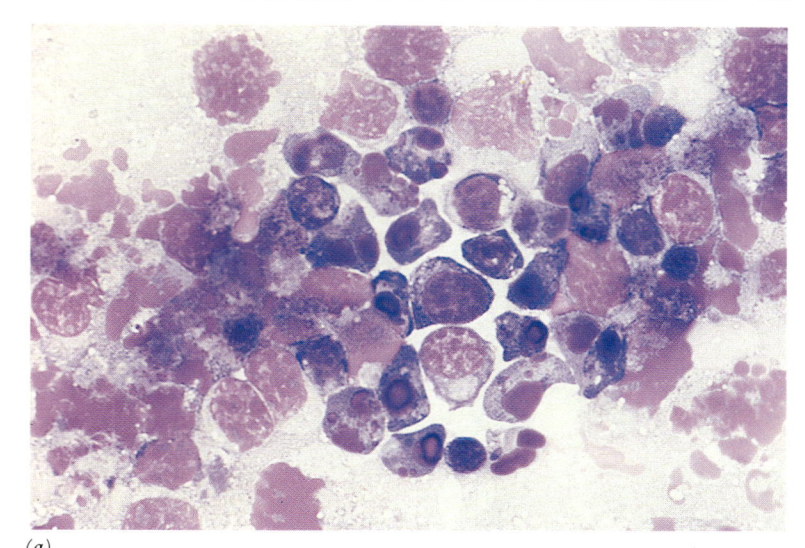

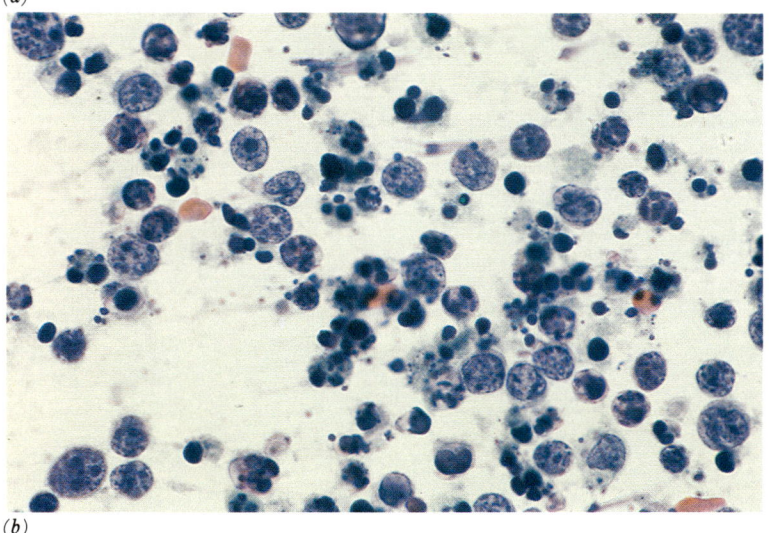

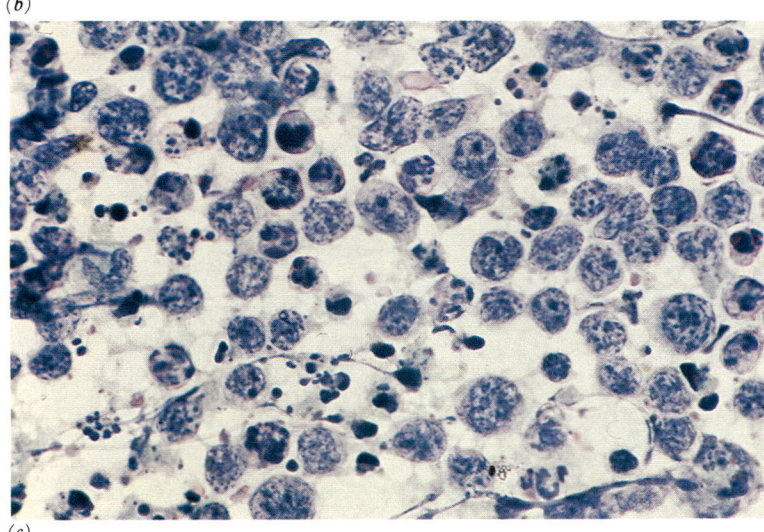

(a)

(b)

(c)

162 DIAGNOSTIC CYTOPATHOLOGY

PANCREAS

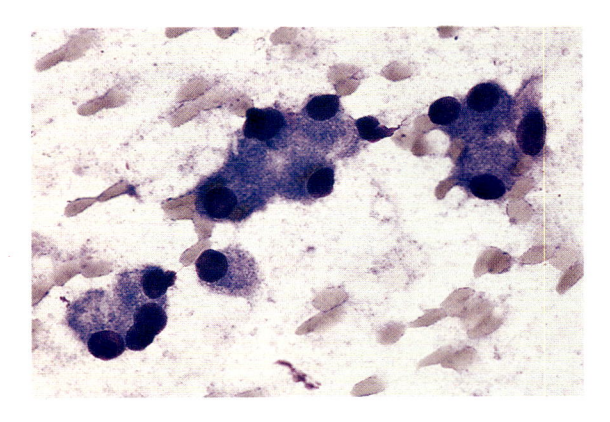

Fig. 7.9 Pancreatic acinar cells
MGG ×525: FNA; pancreas

An aspirate of the exocrine pancreas contains cells from the acini and the lining membrane of the ducts. The acinar cells, illustrated, are small, roughly pyramidal and have basal nuclei. The apices of acinar cells in an aggregate may be seen directed inwards towards a small central space. The cytoplasm is granular on account of abundant zymogen granules. These stain purple with Romanowsky stains, are eosinophilic with Papanicolaou and H & E and acquire a vivid red colour with phloxine tartrazine.

Acinar cells should be sought in a presumed pancreatic aspirate as they provide confirmatory evidence that the target has been sampled. The duct lining cells are identical in appearance to other ductal cells such as cholangiocytes and do not contribute to the identity of the organ.

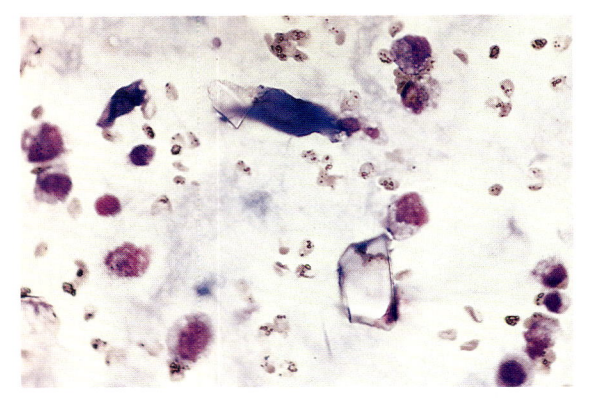

Fig. 7.10 Pseudocyst of pancreas
MGG ×333: FNA; pancreas

A pseudocyst, so-called because it does not have a lining membrane, is in most cases, a sequela of acute pancreatitis. It may present as a palpable mass or be detected in a symptomatic patient, as in this case illustrated, by ultrasonography. The cell contents consist of degenerate epithelial cells, red blood cells and amorphous debris. The transparent, plate-like crystals of cholesterol seen here indicate a long duration.

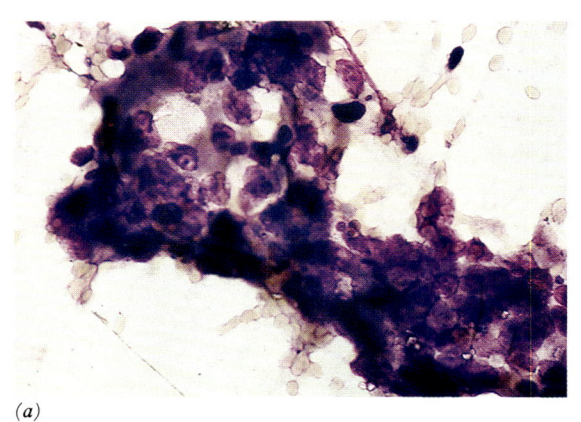

(a) 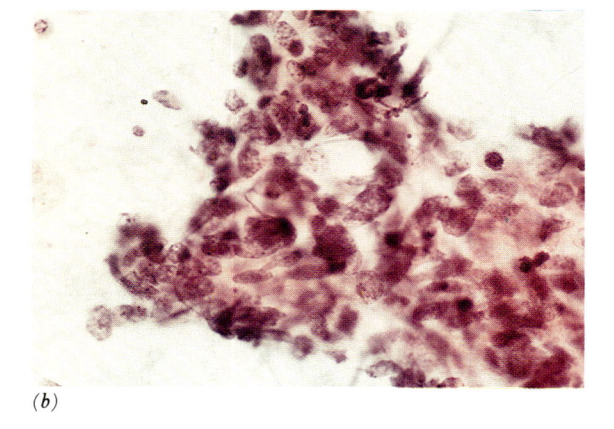   (b)

Fig. 7.11 Carcinoma of the pancreas
(a) MGG × 333: FNA; pancreas (b) Papanicolaou ×333: same case; another smear

The majority of pancreatic carcinomas are adenocarcinomas of the duct lining epithelium, an acinar cell carcinoma being rare. The tumours may assume a papillary formation, most contain some intracellular mucin, and occasionally a mucoid picture may be seen. This micrograph illustrates a poorly differentiated adenocarcinoma which was located in the head of the pancreas. The tumour cells form sheets, and an occasional rudimentary, acinus-like space is seen. The nuclei are crowded together with virtually no intervening cytoplasm, the nuclear chromatin is granular and nucleoli are insignificant.

MISCELLANEOUS

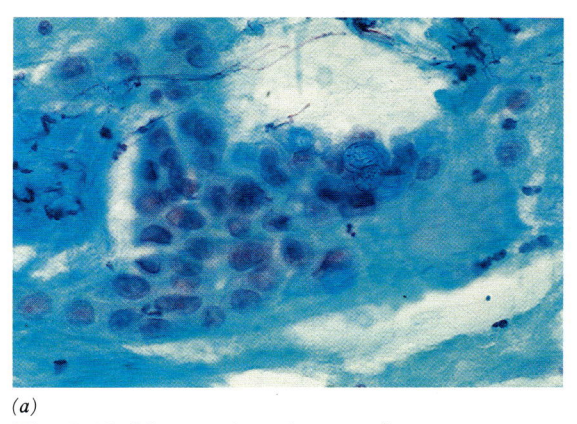

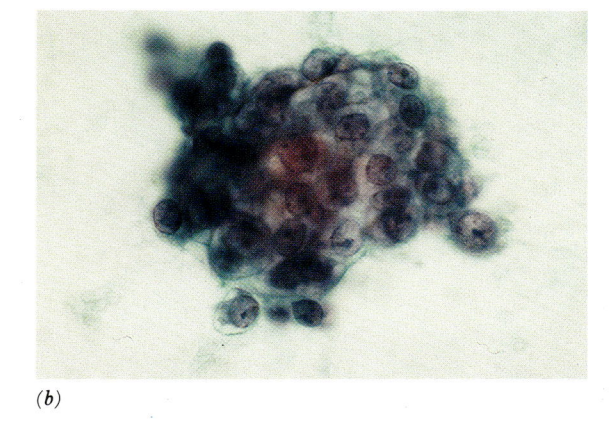

(a) (b)

Fig. 7.12 Metastatic colon carcinoma

(a) *Alcian blue ×333: FNA; adrenal* (b) *Papanicolaou ×525: FNA; peribladder mass; another case*

The two cases illustrated in these micrographs had a previous history of colon carcinoma, and developed abdominal masses after treatment. The nature of the lesions was definitively diagnosed by ultra-sound guided aspiration cytology. The large amount of extracellular mucin in which the tumour cells are embedded identifies a mucoid carcinoma (a). The cells in the extravesical mass are from a moderately differentiated adenocarcinoma and contain a few intra-cellular mucus vacuoles (b).

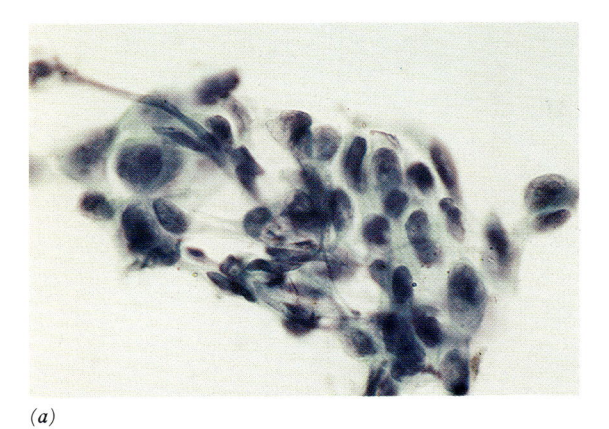

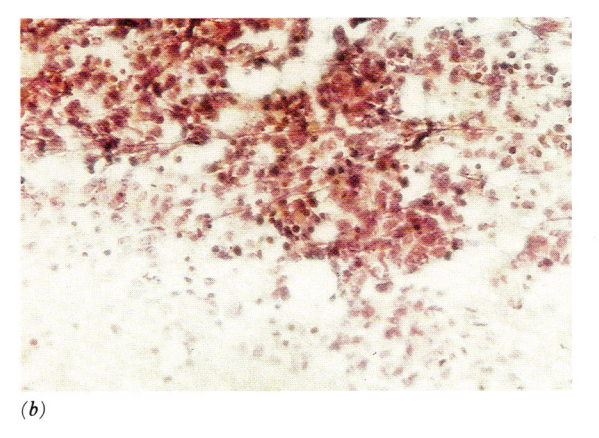

(a) (b)

Fig. 7.13 Metastatic squamous cell carcinoma

Papanicolaou ×525: FNA; psoas muscle (a) squamous cell carcinoma of the cervix uteri (b) squamous cell carcinoma of the lung; another case

A cold retroperitoneal psoas abscess is characteristically associated with tuberculosis of the spine. Abdominal pain and hip spasm are common presenting symptoms and a deep mass is usually palpable. The two cases illustrated were free of tuberculosis but suffered from malignant disease. The lesions were aspirated under CT guidance, and poorly differentiated squamous cells were identified in both samples. The cells in micrograph (a) are from a patient with squamous cell carcinoma of the cervix; those in (b) are from a male patient with bronchogenic squamous cell carcinoma.

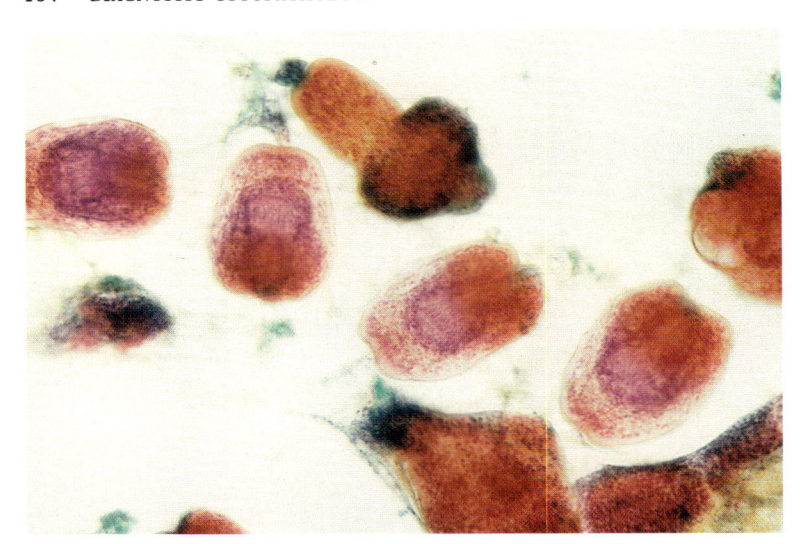

Fig. 7.14 Hydatid cyst
Papanicolaou ×720: FNA; left iliac fossa

Scolices of Echinococcus granulosus aspirated from an iliac cystic mass present in a young male patient from the Middle East are shown in this micrograph. The morphology of the scolices and mode of infection is discussed in Chapter 3.

8. Urinary system

The role of cytopathology in this field is limited mainly to the diagnosis of malignant disease, a few bengin disorders and a few parasitic infestations such as schistosomiasis and the occasional trichomoniasis of the male urethra may also be identified. The variety of inflammatory and autoimmune disorders, particularly of the kidney, are outside the scope of cytology.

SAMPLING TECHNIQUES

The different types of specimens that may be obtained and examined are normally voided and catheter specimens of urine, bladder washings, endoscopic brush and fine needle aspiration samples.

An early morning specimen of urine, formerly recommended, is unsuitable as the cells in the highly concentrated urine are too degenerate to be assessable. A fresh specimen voided at any time may be used, a mid-morning specimen passed preferably 30 minutes to 1 hour after a drink such as tea or coffee is often convenient for the patient and the laboratory. The specimen should be despatched to the laboratory without delay as cell deterioration can be fairly rapid.

Urine and bladder washings are centrifugated and smears made from the deposit. As urine is often hypocellular, it is desirable to concentrate the cells by using part of the specimen to make a millipore filter preparation. Crystals which form in vitro may render a urine cloudy and mask the cells in the smear; phosphates may be removed by the addition of 1% acetic acid and urates by gentle heating.

Brush and aspiration smears are prepared and processed as for other organ systems. Smears from all types of specimens listed above may be stained by the Papanicolaou and Romanowsky methods.

URINARY TRACT

Fig. 8.1 Transitional cells
Papanicolaou ×720: ureteric urine

The urinary tract is lined with transitional epithelium also referred to as urothelium. The morphology of normal transitional cells is illustrated in a fresh specimen of urine obtained through a ureteric ureter, as cells in bladder urine tend to be sparse and degenerate. The cells to the lower right are fairly small and vary little in size. They have a moderate amount of cytoplasm and round or oval nuclei with scanty chromatin and micronucleoli. The shape varies: cuboidal, pyramidal and cylindrical forms are seen. The variation in shape is an artefact created by the spread of the smear.
Substantially larger cells with abundant cytoplasm are seen to the top left of the field. The nuclei of these cells are identical in shape, staining reaction and chromatin content with the nuclei of the smaller cells but number from one to three per cell. The larger cells are derived from the surface layer of the urothelium, extend across two or three smaller subjacent cells and are known as umbrella cells.

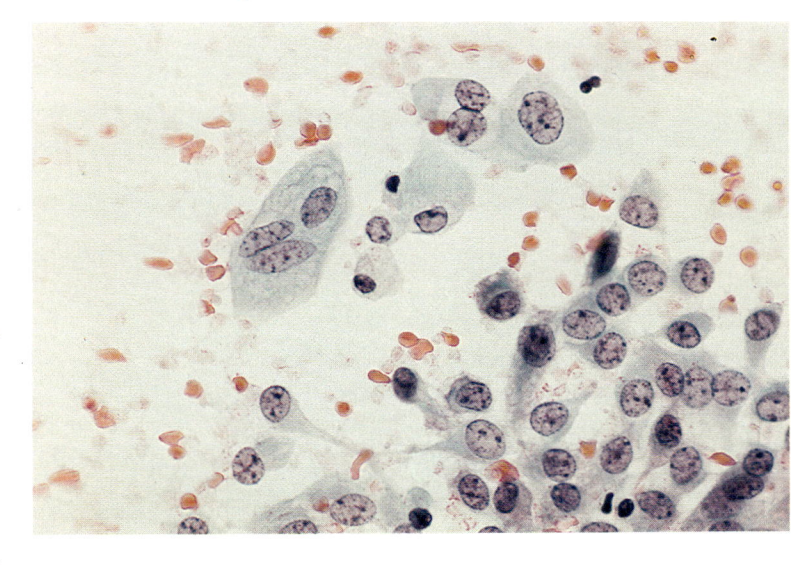

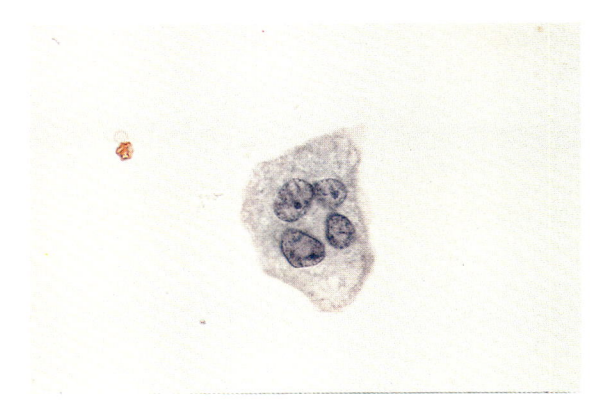

166 DIAGNOSTIC CYTOPATHOLOGY

Fig. 8.2 Umbrella cell
Papanicolaou ×525: voided urine
An umbrella cell with four nuclei is illustrated in this micrograph. Apart from the larger size, the distinctive feature of these surface urothelial cells is the exceptional thickness of their distal plasma membrane. The thick membranes render the epithelium impermeable to urine and protect it from the toxic effects of what is essentially a hypertonic toxic solution. The cytoplasm of the umbrella cell is slightly foamy.

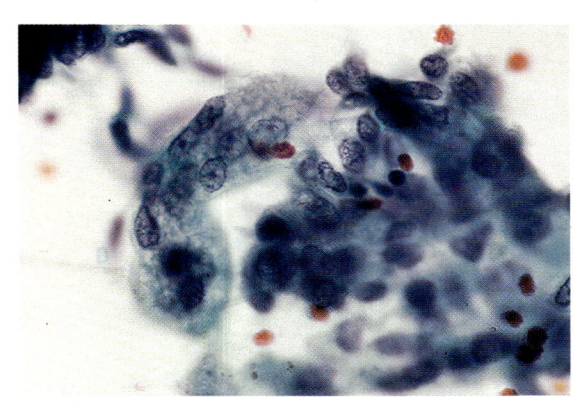

Fig. 8.3 Transitional cells
Papanicolaou ×525: ureteric brush
Diagnostic material may be obtained from the upper urinary tract with a fine endoscopic brush guided at cystoscopy into the ureter as far as the renal pelvis. Cells obtained by this method usually appear in sheets. Normal transitional cells are illustrated in this micrograph. The small overlapping cells in the right lower corner are deeper urothelial cells and two multinucleated umbrella cells are seen to the left.

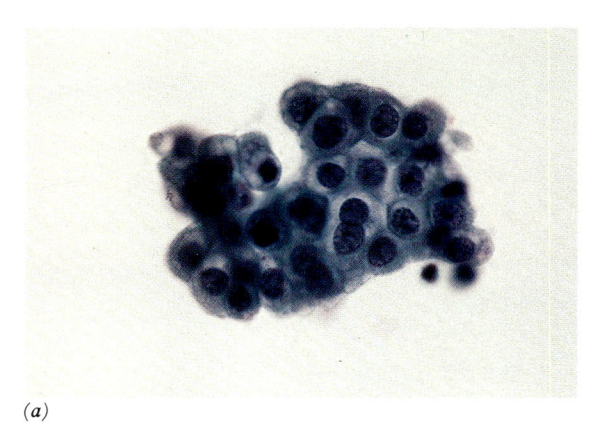

(a)

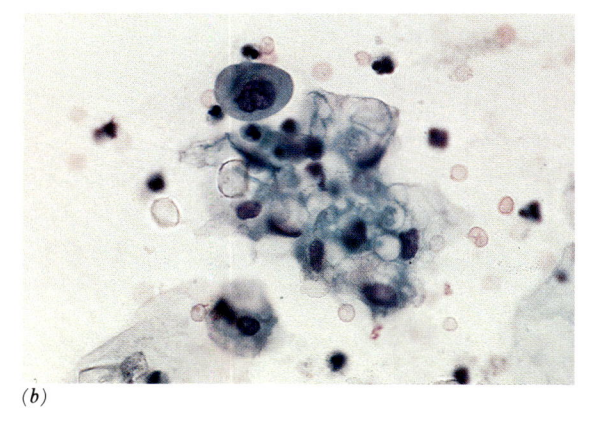

(b)

Fig. 8.4 Reactive transitional cells
Papanicolaou ×525 (a) voided urine (b) voided urine; other case
The cells illustrated in these micrographs were recovered from urine from two patients with large stones in the renal pelvis. The irritation to the renal pelvis epithelium caused by constant friction may induce reactive hyperplastic changes and abnormally excessive exfoliation. The cells in (a) are arranged in a honeycomb pattern. They are uniform in size, have round and regular nuclei and contain perinuclear haloes. The chromatin content is greater than in normal transitional cells and the cytoplasm beyond the vacuoles is dense and basophilic. The appearance is of hyperplastic cells overtaken by degenerative changes. These are more advanced in (b). Excepting one cell, the cytoplasm is filled with hydropic vacuoles. The nuclei are structureless, crenated and are pushed to the periphery of the cells which appear signet ring-shaped.

Changes produced in transitional epithelium by a renal stone may prove misleading and be a potential source of an incorrect interpretation of malignancy, particularly an adenocarcinoma.

URINARY SYSTEM   167

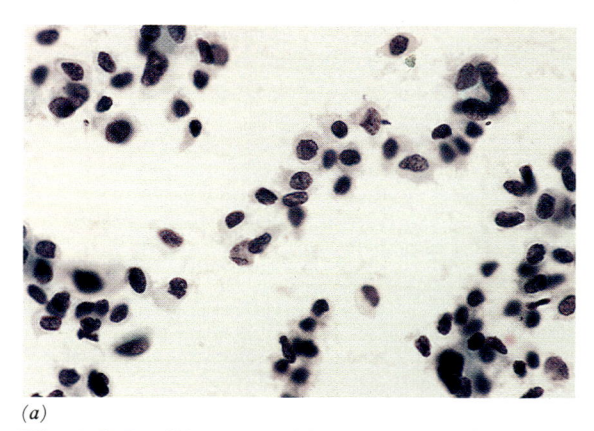

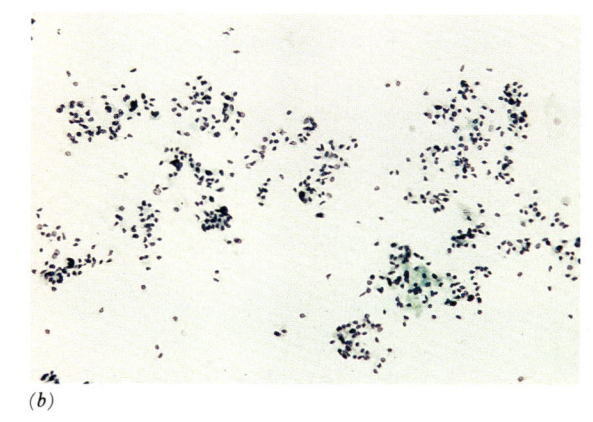

(a)   (b)

Fig. 8.5 Papillary transitional cell carcinoma
Papanicolaou (a) ×525: voided urine (b) ×133: same field; pattern of spontaneous exfoliation

The sensitivity of urinary cytology in the diagnosis of urothelial malignancy varies directly with the histological grade and type of tumour and is notoriously poor for low grade papillary carcinoma. The cells that cover the finger-like projections of these tumours are extremely well differentiated and virtually indistinguishable from benign transitional cells. Tumour cells from a grade 1 papillary carcinoma of the bladder mucosa are illustrated in micrograph (a). In shape, they resemble benign transitional cells (Fig. 8.1) and in size, are, if anything, smaller on account of the degenerative changes. The hyperchromasia of the nuclei is due to pyknotic degeneration and a cytodiagnostic assessment of nuclear pleomorphism and disorganised chromatin pattern is inapplicable.

The one significant feature seen here (b) is the degree and pattern of cell exfoliation. Urine which is normally hypocellular may in some cases of low grade papillary tumours contain showers of more or less normal looking cells. The majority of cells are discrete, but a few cell aggregates or microbiopsies are present. This appearance can be the basis of a correct diagnosis in the absence of cystitis or lithiasis. The criterion, however, is applicable only to normally voided urine and has no relevance to cases in which a significantly large population of normal looking cells is dislodged by iatrogenic causes such as catheterization or surgical exploration.

Fig. 8.6 Transitional cell carcinoma
MGG ×720: voided urine

Exfoliative urine cytology is of greater value in the diagnosis of higher grades of urothelial carcinomas when the standard criteria of malignancy can be applied. The cells in this case of a grade 3 carcinoma are large. The nuclei and the nuclear cytoplasmic ratio are significantly variable and nuclear pleomorphism is a notable feature. The degree and pattern of exfoliation is not relevant when frankly malignant cells are seen, and the number of neoplastic cells exfoliated is often small.

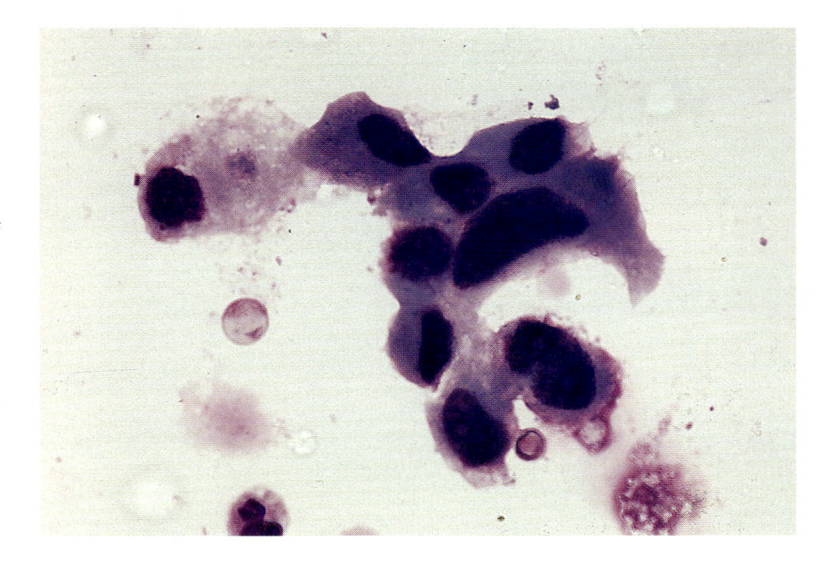

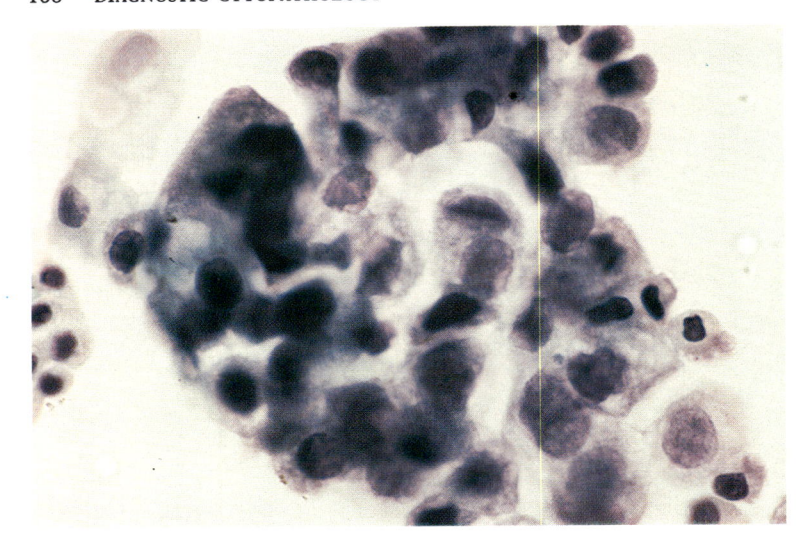

Fig. 8.7 Transitional cell carcinoma

Papanicolaou ×720: bladder washings

The yield of tumour cells may be increased by washing out the bladder with normal saline: this procedure is usually carried out at cystoscopy. Bladder washings contain numerous cells which are often aggregated in large sheets. In this example the cells and nuclei are large and there is significant variation in the size of the nuclei and the nuclear-cytoplasmic ratio.

Bladder washings collected at check cystoscopy are of particular value in patients being followed up after a treated transitional cell carcinoma. Neoplastic transformation of the urothelium occurs in subjects exposed to industrial toxins and is usually multifocal. A transitional cell carcinoma may remain in situ for a long period and this and some deeply infiltrating tumours may not be identifiable at cystoscopy or by retrograde urography. Washing out the bladder dislodges many cells, some of which may be informative and form the basis for further management.

(a)

(b)

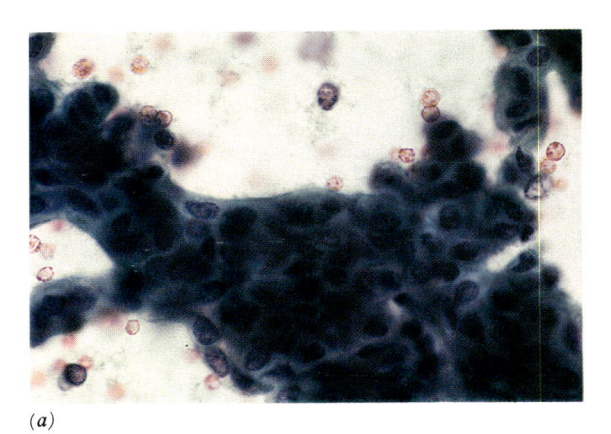

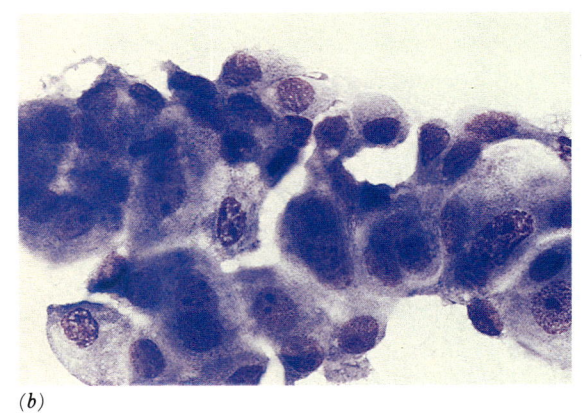

Fig. 8.8 Transitional cell carcinoma

(a) Papanicolaou ×525: renal pelvis brush (b) MGG ×525: renal pelvis brush; another case

Tumours in the upper part of the urinary tract may be sampled with a brush which removes large numbers of cohesive cells. These micrographs illustrate two cases of grade 2 carcinoma of the renal pelvis. The cells in (a) are small, but the nuclei are disproportionately large and crowded together. A moderate degree of anisonucleosis is seen. The cells in (b) being air dried, appear larger and variations in nuclear size and nuclear-cytoplasmic ratio are more obvious. Small but distinct nucleoli are seen.

Fig. 8.9 Transitional cell carcinoma

MGG ×720: FNA; renal pelvis

Another useful approach to a tumour in the renal pelvis is by percutaneous fine aspiration. A case of grade 2 transitional cell carcinoma sampled by this method is illustrated in this micrograph. An important point to bear in mind in the assessment of brush and aspiration specimens is that the cells obtained by these methods differ in appearance from cells exfoliated in urine. The arrangement of the cells may resemble that of adenocarcinoma cells and distinction between a urothelial and a renal cell carcinoma may on occasion be difficult.

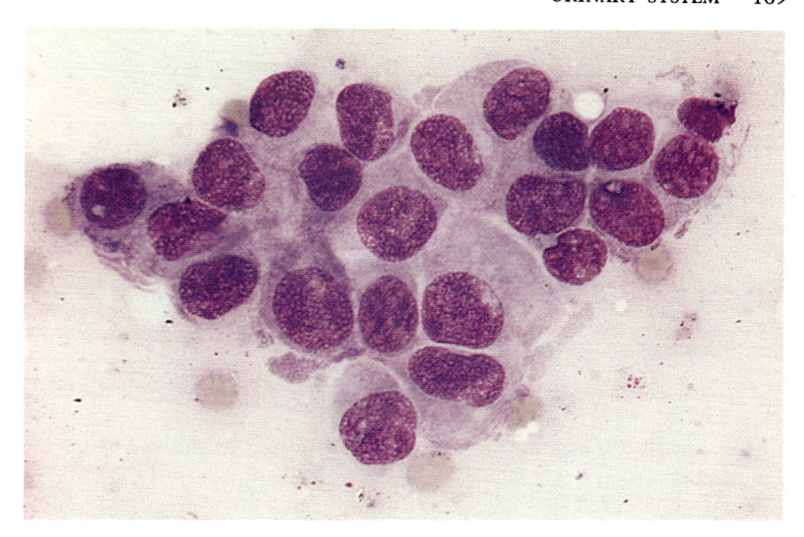

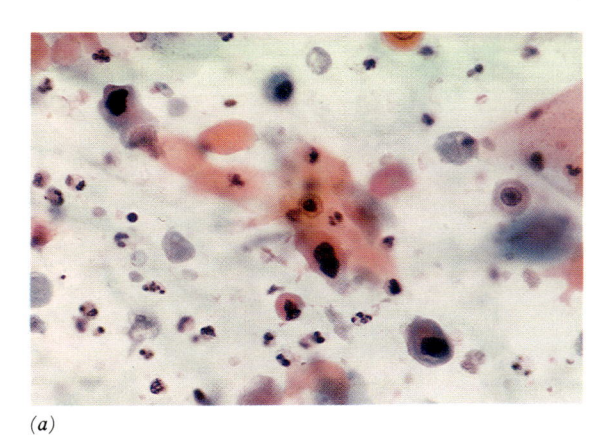

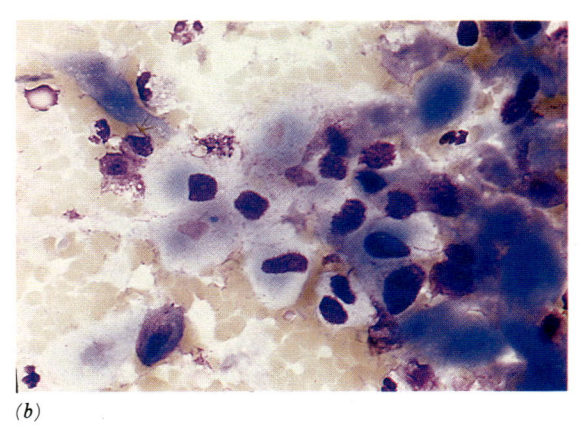

(a) (b)

Fig. 8.10 Primary squamous cell carcinoma of the bladder

(a) Papanicolaou ×525: voided urine (b) MGG ×525: same specimen, another smear

Squamous cell carcinoma of the bladder usually develops in a pre-existing metaplastic squamous epithelium which is formed in response to chronic irritation such as a stone or a parasitic infestation. It is the commonest type of bladder carcinoma in geographical regions in which schistosomiasis is endemic; elsewhere it constitutes less than 5% of urinary tract neoplasms. The male urethera contains foci of squamous epithelium which may, very rarely, become neoplastic.

The case illustrated in this micrograph, of an Englishwoman without renal tract lithiasis, a normal genital tract and no history of exposure to a provocative parasite, is a sporadic one. The malignant cells in the urine are well differentiated and bizarre shaped, have cytoplasmic bulbous expansions and India ink nuclei (a). The pale or azure staining of the cytoplasm with MGG is often seen in a keratinized cell.

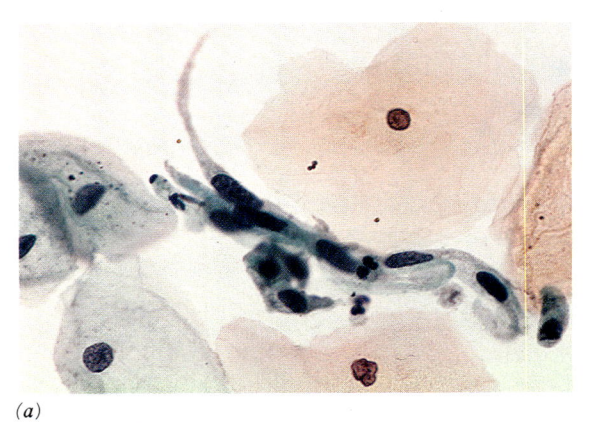

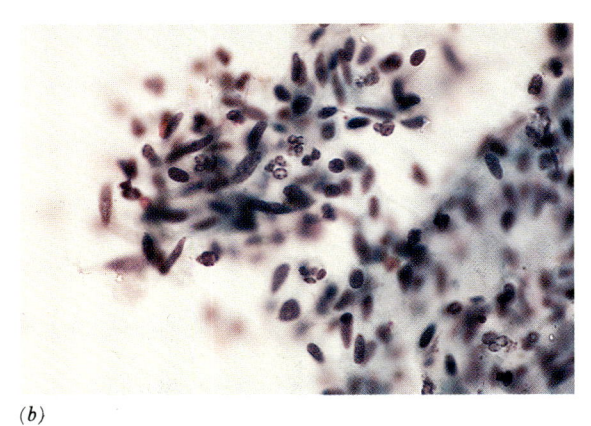

Fig. 8.11 Secondary squamous cell carcinoma of the bladder.

Papanicolaou (a) ×525: catheter urine (b) ×333: catheter urine; another case

Squamous carcinoma of the bladder in the female is more likely to be an extension of a primary genital tract tumour and investigation should include vaginal and/or cervical cytology. Two examples of secondary involvement of the bladder are illustrated in these micrographs. The poorly differentiated, fibre-shaped malignant squamous cells in (a) were recovered from a catheter specimen of urine. Biopsy histology of a puckered ulcerated area on the posterior wall of the bladder confirmed infiltration by a genital tract squamous carcinoma. The patient with a history of CIN and VAIN and subsequent invasive carcinoma of the vagina has been discussed on p. 31. Compare these cells with Figure 1.33. The sheet of poorly differentiated, spindle-shaped malignant squamous cells in (b) are from a woman with stage 4 carcinoma of the cervix and a vesico-vaginal fistula. To ensure against vaginal contamination, urine cytology in such a case should be done on a catheter specimen.

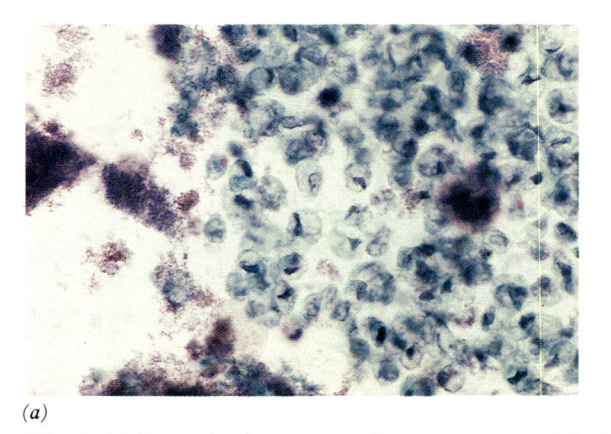

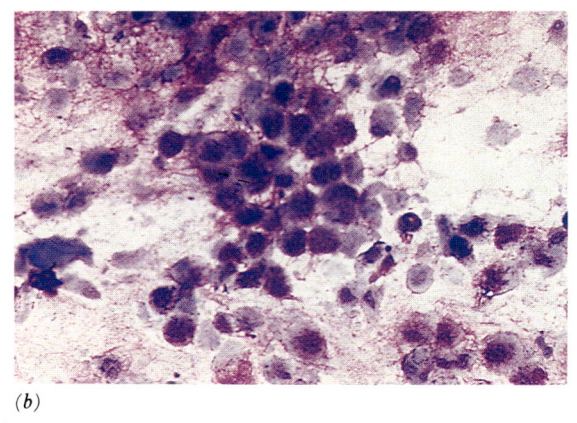

Fig. 8.12 Intestinal mucosa of reconstructed bladder

Papanicolaou ×525: voided urine; caecocystoplasty (b) MGG ×525: voided urine; ileal bladder, another case

Two examples of urine cytology of patients with bladders reconstructed from the intestine following total cystectomy are illustrated. The cells are of glandular origin and markedly degenerate. In (a) they have signet ring shapes and in (b) they are arranged in honeycomb against a background of homogenous material. Mucin secreted by the intestinal mucosa cells is often present in these specimens. Neoplastic transformation may occur.

Fig. 8.13 Viral cytopathia
Papanicolaou (a) ×720: voided urine
(b) ×720: voided urine; another case

Urothelial cells may show cytopathic effects in a number of viral infections. The variable appearances illustrated in these micrographs have been attributed to polyoma viruses. The cells in (a) were seen in the urine of a 5-year-old boy with a febrile illness of short duration, abdominal lymphadenopathy and a high erythrocyte sedimentation rate. Mononuclear and multinucleated forms are seen, the size of the cell being proportional with the number of nuclei. These are uniformly pale and homogenous and are ringed by a narrow band of chromatin on the nuclear membrane. The cells in (b) from the urine of a 3-year-old boy, also with a febrile illness but no lymphadenopathy, contain intranuclear inclusions which are punctate in the cell on the left and large and dense in the cell to the right.

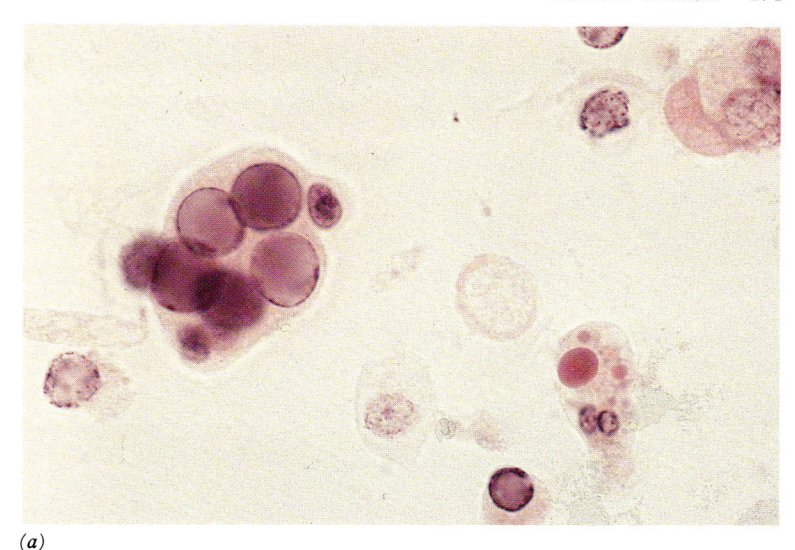

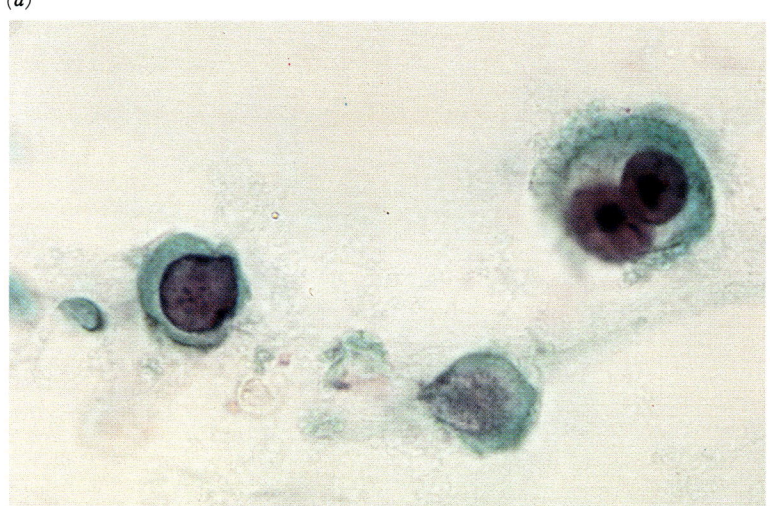

Fig. 8.14 Histiocyte with inclusion
Papanicolaou ×720: voided urine

The urine may occasionally have small structures which seem to be peculiar to it, and virtually identify the specimen. These are probably histiocytes and are characterized by the presence of smooth contoured eosinophilic or orange inclusions. The identity of these inclusions is not known and as far as can be determined, these bodies do not have pathological significance. Compare with viral changes in the preceding micrograph.

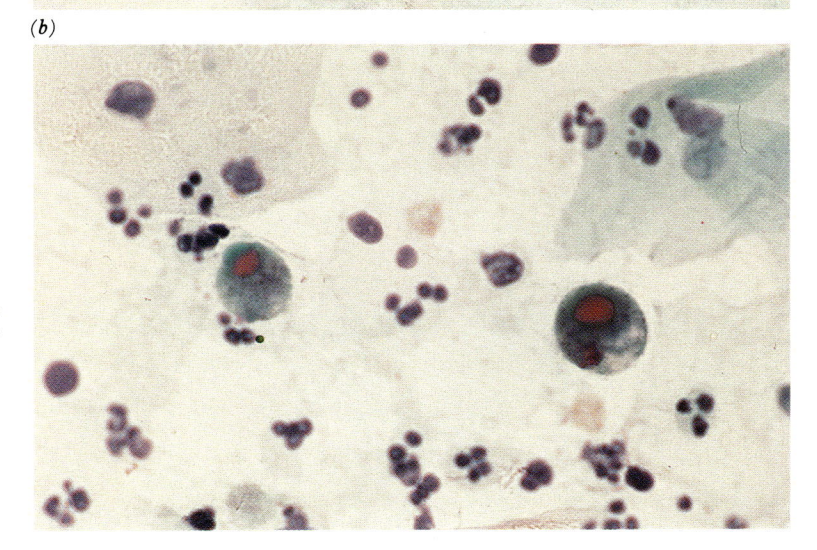

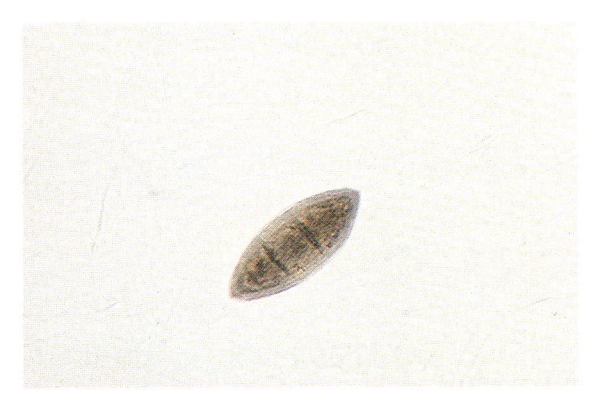

Fig. 8.15 Pollen

Papanicolaou ×525: voided urine

A contaminant which bears a superficial resemblance to a schistosome (see Fig. 8.16) but is, in fact, a pollen grain, may be seen in urine. It is distinguished from an ovum by its smaller size, the bipolar angular terminations of its capsule and its generalised granularity.

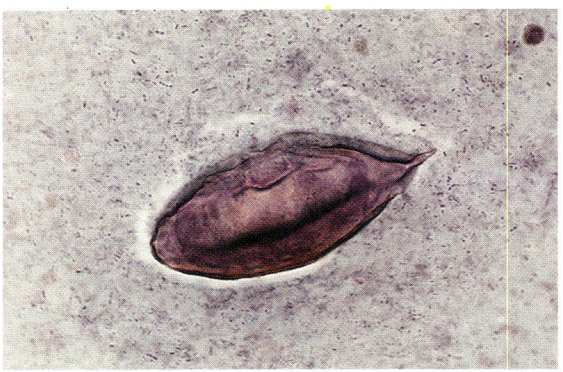

Fig. 8.16 Schistosoma haematobium

(a) Papanicolaou ×333: voided urine; ovum (b) MGG ×333: voided urine; ovum; another case (c) Papanicolaou ×333: same smear as (a); another field; miracidium

Schistosomiasis or bilharziasis is caused by three closely related trematodes, whose definitive host is a fresh water snail. Infection is acquired when cercarial larvae released by the snail into water penetrate the skin of the human host. The larvae enter the venous capillaries and make their way into the systemic circulation by a circuitous route through the right side of the heart, the pulmonary circulatory system, into the left ventricle.

From the mesenteric blood vessels, they enter the portal venous system where the adult worms reach maturity. *S. japonicum* and *S. mansoni* preferentially infest the digestive tract. *S. haematobium* travels to the capillaries of the bladder where the female deposits her eggs. These are embedded in the bladder mucosa which becomes inflamed and eventually responds by undergoing squamous metaplasia. The eggs may rupture through the mucosa and be passed in urine. The ova of the three species are distinguished by their size and the position of the spine. The ovum of *S. haematobium* is large and has a terminal spine (a), (b) at one pole. An embryo is faintly discernible in (a). Aggregates of inflammatory cells may accompany the ovum (b). On contact with fresh water, the embryo in the egg hatches into a miracidium, the surface of which is covered with numerous cilia (c). The miracidium penetrates the specific snail host and the life cycle is repeated. The miracidium illustrated in (c) was one of several in a voided specimen of urine; dilution with fresh water is assumed to have occurred at some stage.

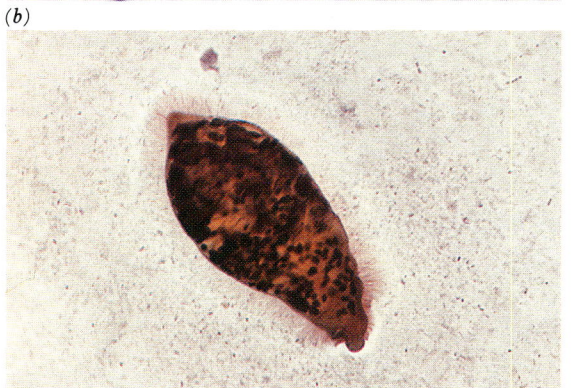

KIDNEY

Fig. 8.17 Benign renal cyst

Papanicolaou ×133: FNA; kidney

Fluid from a benign renal cyst is generally straw-coloured or, on occasion, slightly tinged with blood. The cell content varies in quantity and consists mainly of large foam cells with degenerate nuclei. Iron-laden macrophages or histiocytic cells with autofluorescent, yellow-green granules of lipofuscin (known as the ageing pigment) may also be seen. The appearance is non-specific and identical to the cellular presentation of some cases of duct ectasia of the breast (Fig. 2.7) or an inclusion cyst of the ovary (Fig. 1.49).

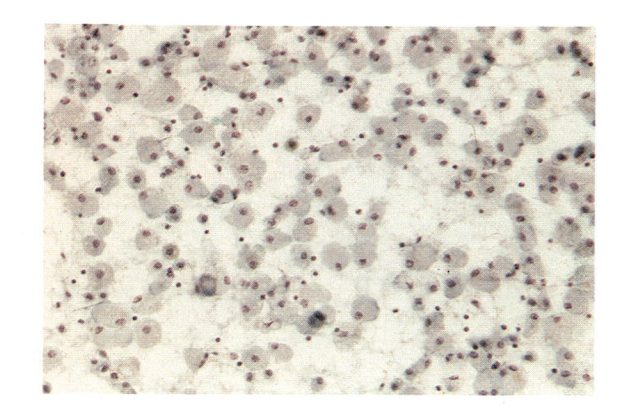

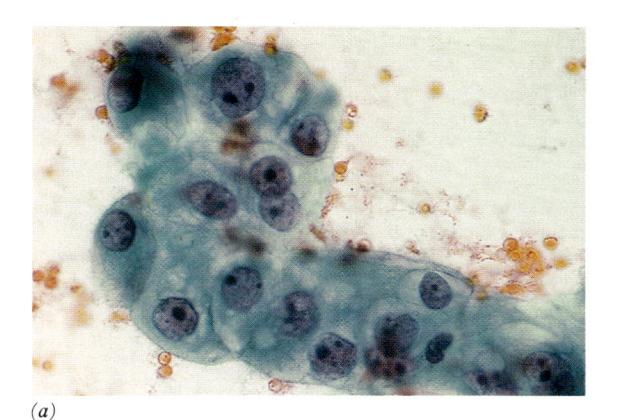

(a)   (b)

Fig. 8.18 Renal cell carcinoma

Papanicolaou (a) ×525: FNA; kidney (b) ×832: FNA; kidney; another case (c) same smear as (b); another field

Renal cell carcinoma also referred to as hypernephroma or clear cell carcinoma is an adenocarcinoma of the renal tubule epithelium. The tumour cells are large and polygonal in shape (a), (b). The cytoplasm is abundant, and vacuolated (a) and may be foamy (b). The nuclei are generally round and may be hypochromic (a); the chromatin content may be small and the nuclear cytoplasmic ratio low (a), (b). In some cases or in some areas of a renal cell carcinoma, the nuclei may appear deceptively bland (a). The diagnosis may prove difficult unless these features are taken into account. Smaller cells with non-vacuolated, uniformly staining cytoplasm and a relatively high nuclear cytoplasmic ratio (c) may be additionally present or constitute the main or sole population of another histological variant. Large prominent nucleoli are always present in both types of cells.

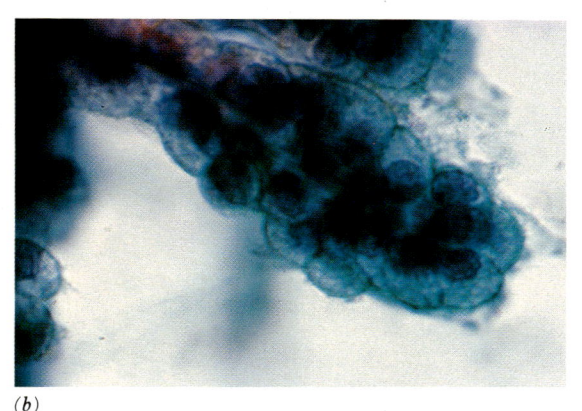

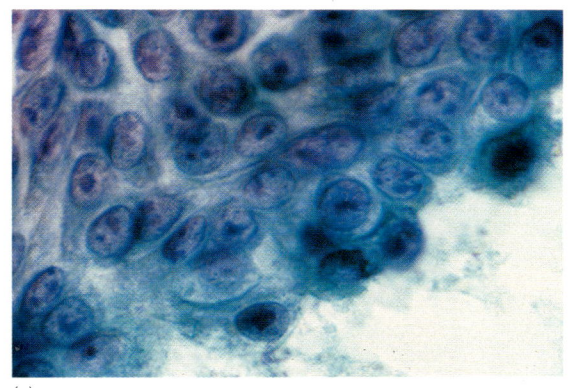

(c)

174 DIAGNOSTIC CYTOPATHOLOGY

(a)

(b)

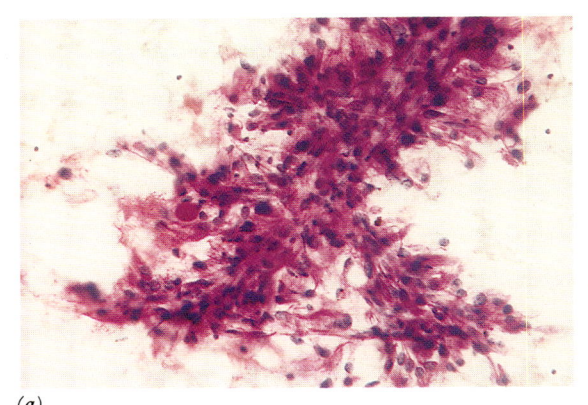

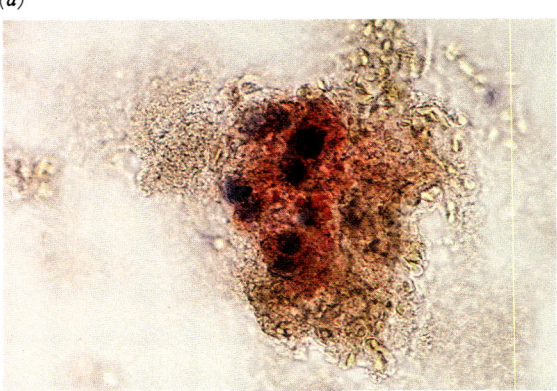

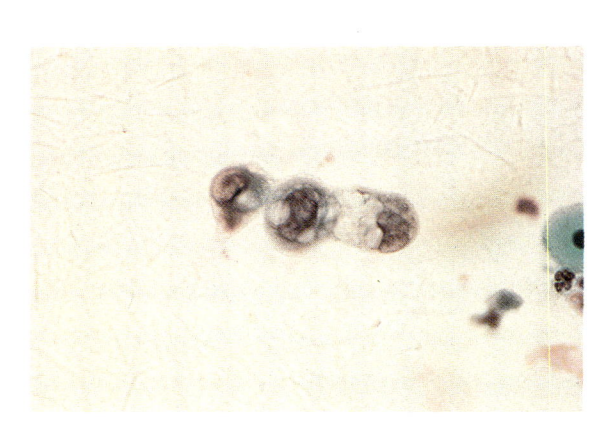

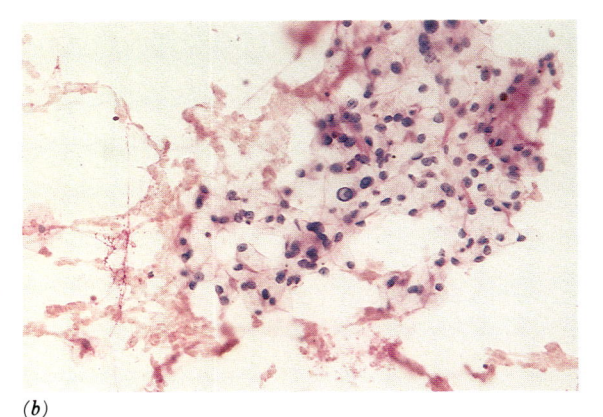

Fig. 8.19 Renal cell carcinoma

(a) PAS 133: FNA; kidney (b) D-PAS ×133: same specimen; another smear (c) sudan III (oil scarlet) ×333: same specimen; another smear

The clear or foamy appearance of the cytoplasm of malignant renal cells is due to accumulation of glycogen and lipid; mucin is not secreted by these cells. It is advisable to confirm these biochemical characteristics in a suspected renal cell carcinoma for three reasons. Firstly, a needle aspiration may not contain ancillary evidence by which the target organ can be identified; secondly, the specimen may be contaminated by benign intestinal mucosa, even when the approach is from the flank; thirdly, a renal cell carcinoma may appear deceptively bland on account of its low nuclear cytoplasmic ratio and hypochromic nuclei. Micrograph (a) demonstrates the positivity with PAS of both the cells and the connective tissue in which they are embedded in an aspirate of a renal cell carcinoma. Prior digestion with diastase has removed the glycogen from the cells but not the mucopolysaccharides from the connective tissue (b). Abundant intra- and extra-cellular lipid droplets are confirmed by a fat stain in (c).

(c)

Fig. 8.20 Renal cell carcinoma

Papanicolaou ×525: voided urine

Malignant renal cells may be seen in urine when the tumour has ruptured through the renal pelvis. The cells in this micrograph are copiously vacuolated, have smooth outlines and the arrangement of adenocarcinoma cells. The nuclei are variable in size and a nucleolus is seen in the cell to the left. As will be seen, the cells and particularly the nuclei are extremely degenerate. This is usually the case with exfoliated malignant renal cells and a urine cytology diagnosis of a renal primary is, in most cases, tentative.

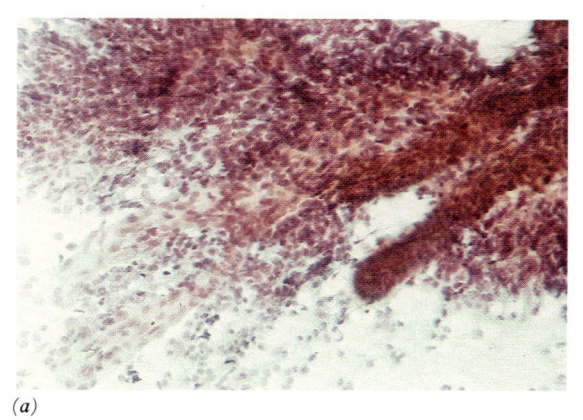

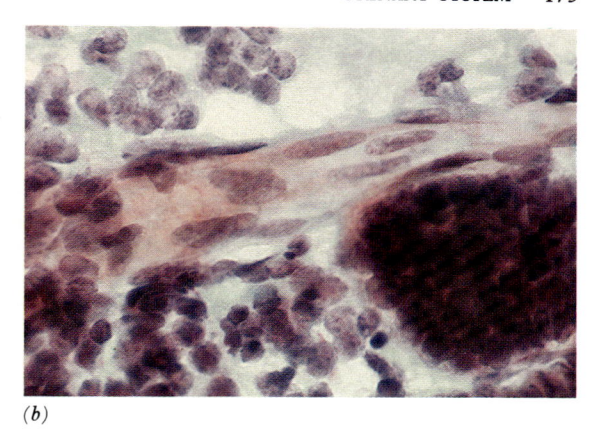

Fig. 8.21 Nephroblastoma
Papanicolaou (a) ×133: FNA; kidney (b) ×525: same smear; another field

This embryonal tumour, also known as Wilm's tumour, is one of the most aggressive and important tumours of early childhood. The neoplastic transformation is believed to occur in embryonic renal blastema in the pre-natal period and the tumour contains both sarcomatous and carcinomatous elements (a). Cellular detail is seen in (b). The sarcomatous element consists of pleomorphic plump and slender fusiform or spindle-shaped nuclei in a pink-staining matrix. This is flanked above and below by small, round, undifferentiated cells with virtually no cytoplasm and finely granular nuclei. The epithelial element, seen in the lower right corner also consists of small round cells which are organised into a tubular structure.

Wilm's tumour can be identified in an FNA specimen without difficulty when all the components of the tumour are present. In the absence of a sarcomatous element, the differential diagnosis would include neuroblastoma. In the absence of tubular structures, an undifferentiated rhabdomyosarcoma and a high grade lymphoma need to be taken into account.

Wilm's tumour may occasionally develop in renal tissue rests outside the kidney.

Fig. 8.22 Metastatic squamous cell carcinoma
Papanicolaou ×720: FNA; kidney

The kidney is not infrequently involved in malignant lymphoma and may be the site of a metastatic carcinoma. In considering the latter, care needs to be taken to confirm that the secondary deposit is not in the adrenal which is a commoner site of metastatic disease. This may not be possible by ultrasound or cytology when the upper pole of kidney appears to be involved. In the case illustrated in the micrograph, extremely well differentiated malignant squamous cells were aspirated from a mass circumscribed within the kidney. The patient was a known case of squamous cell carcinoma of the lung.

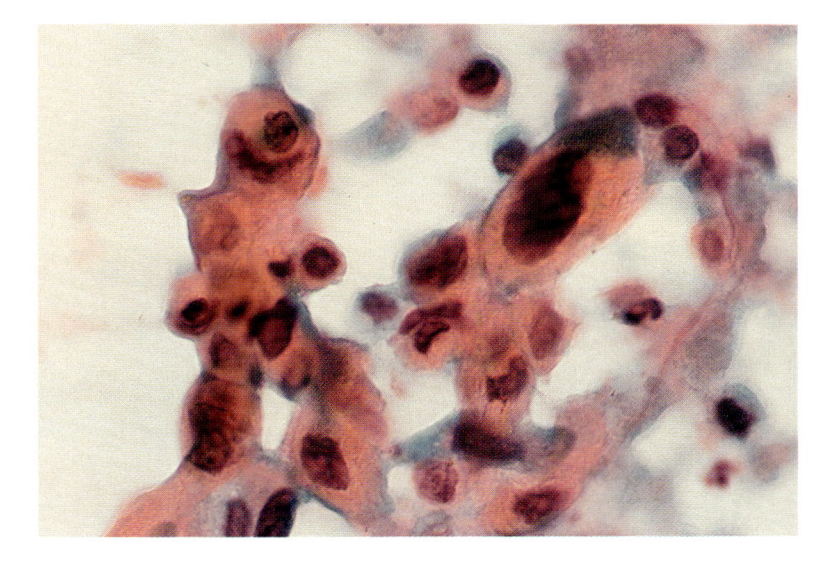

9. Male genital system

The widest application of cytopathology of the male genital system is in fine needle aspiration of the prostate. Testicular tumours are only occasionally sampled for cytology as the complexity of their structure and prognostic assessment requires detailed examination of greater amounts of tissue than are obtained with a fine needle. The presence of tumour markers and their focal variation is also better assessed in sections. A specimen commonly submitted for cytology is hydrocoele or spermatocoele fluid.

An important practical point for consideration is that spermatozoa do not adhere firmly to a glass slide, even an albuminized one, and are likely to float off on to other slides processed in the same batch. This may be avoided by using separate jars of fixative and stains for smears of fluid from the scrotal sac.

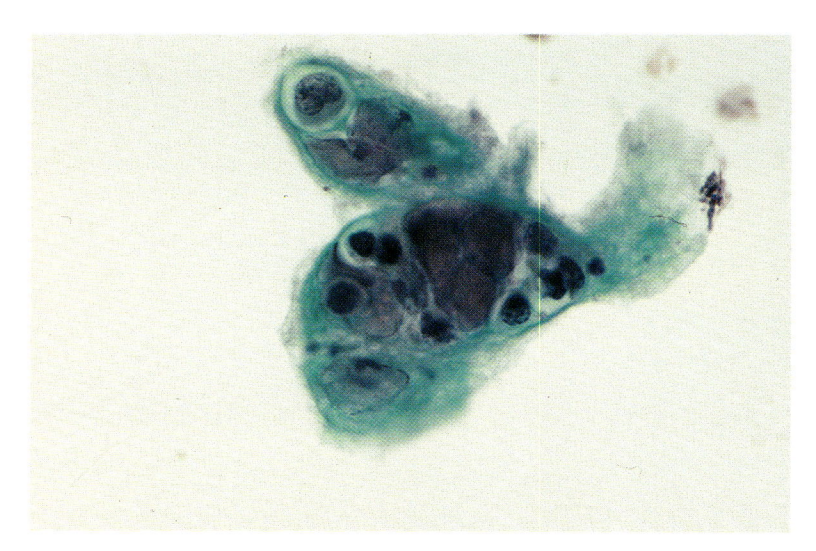

Fig. 9.1 Herpesvirus simplex (HVS)

Papanicolaou ×720: penile scrape

A herpetic lesion on the penis, usually caused by the sexually transmitted HVS type 2 may be easily and rapidly diagnosed by cytology. An intact vesicle is ruptured, the droplet of fluid and a scrape of the floor of the vesicle used to make a single smear. Squamous cells with characteristic cytopathic effects, described in Chapter 1, are observed. A secondarily infected herpetic lesion is unsuitable for study.

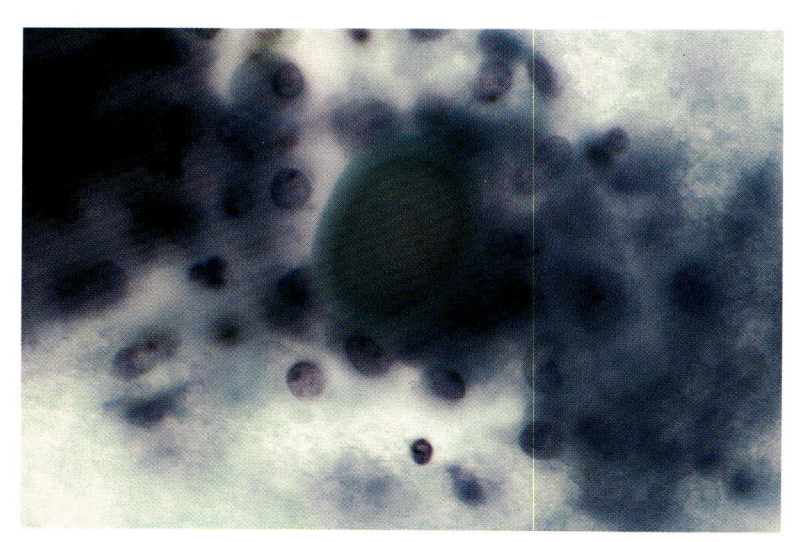

Fig. 9.2 Corpora amylacea

Papanicolaou ×720: voided urine; millipore filter

The elliptical organised structure with concentric rings seen in the centre of the field is a corpora amylacea and is the form in which prostatic secretion is stored. These structures may be seen in the prostate gland of the adult male, and increase in number with advancing years, and may become calcified. The structure illustrated was seen in the urine of a 65-year-old male with benign nodular hyperplasia of the prostate and urinary frequency. Exfoliation of corpora amylacea in urine is uncommon, does not denote a papillary tumour and is without diagnostic significance.

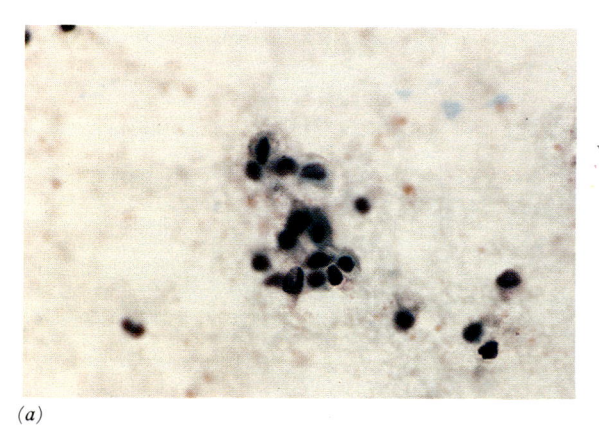

(a) 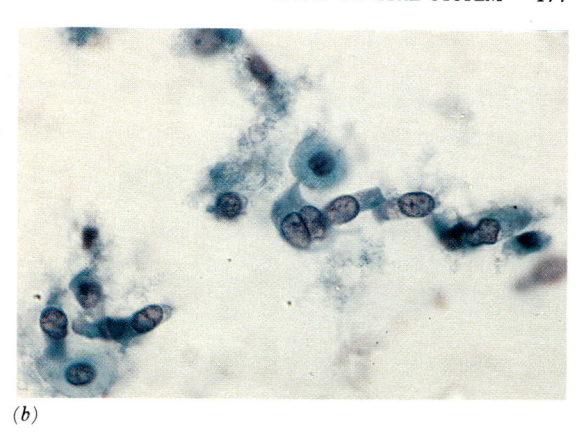 (b)

Fig. 9.3 Prostatic cells

Papanicolaou ×525 (a) prostate fluid (b) prostate fluid: another case

Prostatic epithelial cells are usually present in a needle aspirate. FNA is better avoided in a case of suspected prostatitis and material may be obtained via the urethera after prostatic massage. The appearance of the cells varies with the degree of secretory activity which is under the influence of androgenic hormones. Inactive prostatic epithelial cells are small, cuboidal and have darkly-staining condensed nuclei (a). The active cells are larger and columnar in shape, the cytoplasm may be finely vacuolated; the basally situated nuclei are vesicular (b).

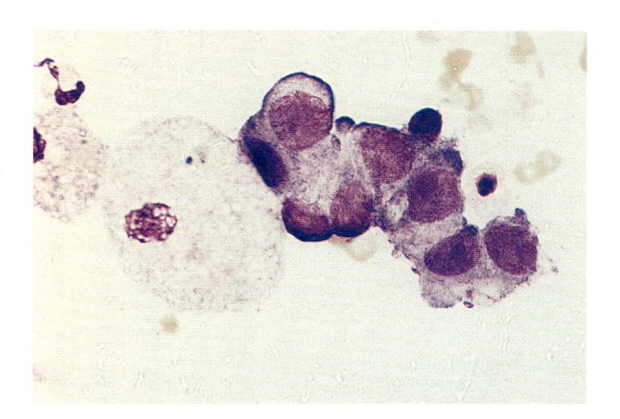

Fig. 9.4 Adenocarcinoma of the prostate

MGG ×525: Franzen needle aspirate; prostate

This micrograph illustrates malignant cells from a well differentiated adenocarcinoma of the prostate. The cells are large and display anisocytosis and anisonucleosis. Most of the nuclei are eccentric in position and some lie on the outer contour of the cell; nucleoli are often large in prostatic carcinoma and are seen in three nuclei.

The cohesiveness of the cells varies with the degree of differentiation and diminishes with increasing anaplasia.

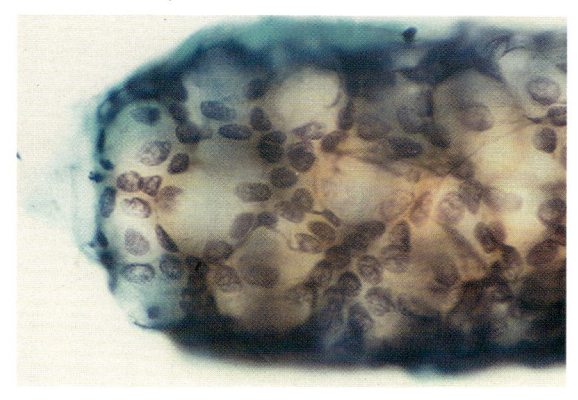

Fig. 9.5 Rectal mucosa

Papanicolaou ×525: Franzen needle aspirate; prostate

The Franzen needle used for aspiration biopsy of the prostate is introduced per rectum and it is quite common to see benign rectal mucosa in a prostatic aspiration smear. It is important to distinguish it from prostatic tissue and thereby avoid an incorrect diagnosis of a mucin-secreting adenocarcinoma. The colonic mucosa is often arranged in acini and may be identified by the large goblet cells with distended vacuolated cytoplasm and small nuclei.

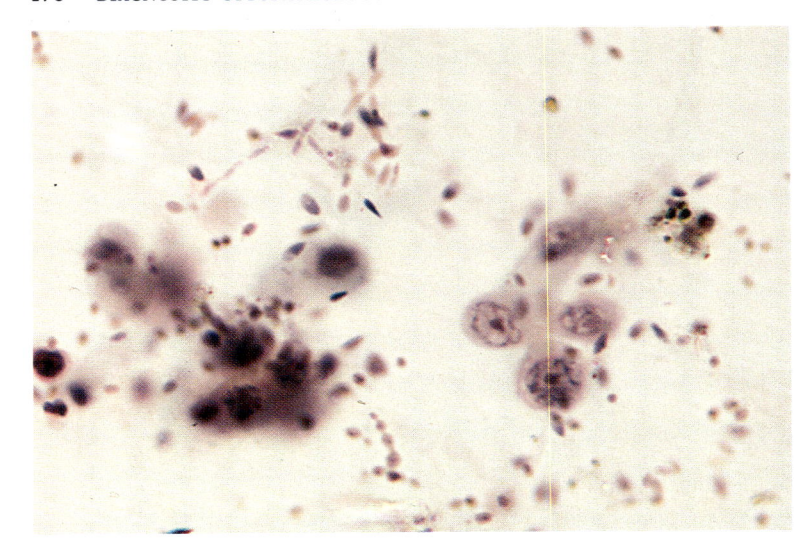

Fig. 9.6 Carcinoma of the prostate

Papanicolaou ×720: voided urine

The adenocarcinoma cells in this micrograph were seen in the urine of a patient with a known carcinoma of the prostate. These tumours may release cells into the urethra, but this occurrence is relatively uncommon. Compare these cells with the exfoliated renal cell carcinoma cells in Figure 8.20 and note the resemblance. Distinction between a prostatic carcinoma, a primary adenocarcinoma of the bladder and a renal cell carcinoma is seldom possible by exfoliative cytology and the presumptive diagnosis should be correlated with the clinical, radiological and biochemical findings. Note the spermatozoa and the fungal pseudohyphae, the latter are contaminants.

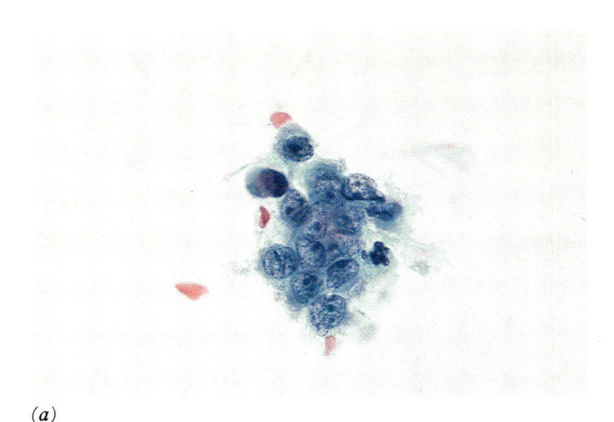

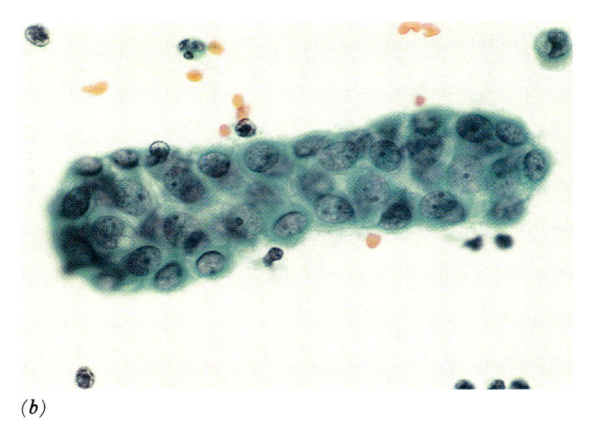

(a)   (b)

Fig. 9.7 Hydrocoele

Papanicolaou ×525: (a) FNA: scrotum (b) FNA; scrotum; another case

Aspiration of a fluid from a hydrocoele, which is an accumulation of fluid in the scrotal sac serves a double function, being both diagnostic and therapeutic. The scrotal sac, an extension of the peritoneum is lined with mesothelium. The cellular presentation of a hydrocoele is variable. In some cases, all the cells show hydropic degeneration and are foamy; in others, better preserved mesothelial cells are also present. Less commonly, the mesothelial cells are hyperplastic and arranged in acinar (a) or tubular (b) structures. This cytological appearance may be associated with papillary excrescences on the inner surface of the mesothelial lining.

Fig. 9.8 Malignant teratoma undifferentiated (MTU) of the testis

(a) Papanicolaou ×720: FNA; testis
(b) MGG ×720: same specimen; another smear

Malignant tumours of the testis include seminomas and teratomas or a combination of the two. The teratomas are thought to be derived from multipotent cells. Many histological variants have been classified. A well differentiated teratoma may contain an assortment of recognizable adult tissue, whereas an undifferentiated tumour may be totally anaplastic. The tumours occur in younger age groups, and a case of a malignant teratoma in a 35-year-old man is illustrated in these micrographs. The cells are seen in a solid sheet and are poorly differentiated. The large nuclei are surrounded by a narrow rim of cytoplasm and contain polymorphic macronucleoli. The malignant nature of the cells is obvious but it must be appreciated that cytology does not contribute much more than the recognition of malignancy. Immunocytochemical studies for human chorionic gonadotropin (HGG) and alpha feto-protein (AFP) are possible but interpretation may be rendered difficult by the blood and cell necrosis that is often seen. The diagnosis of malignant teratoma undifferentiated was established by histological examination of the orchidectomy specimen.

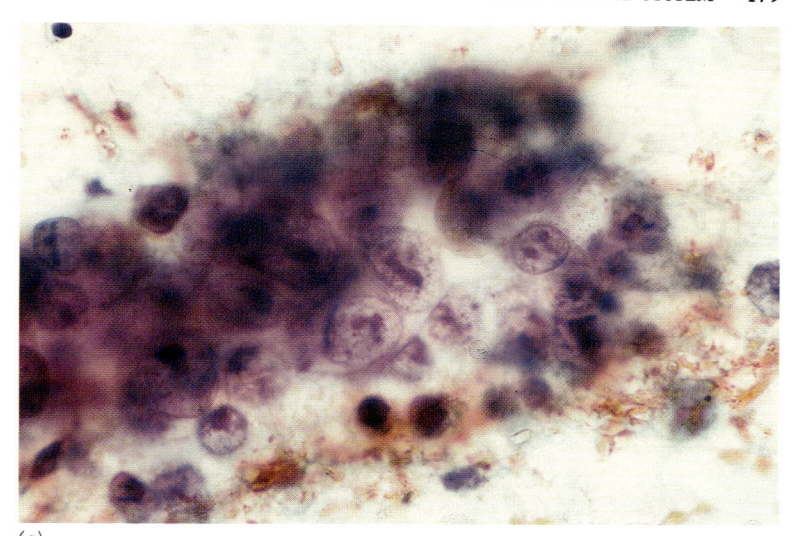

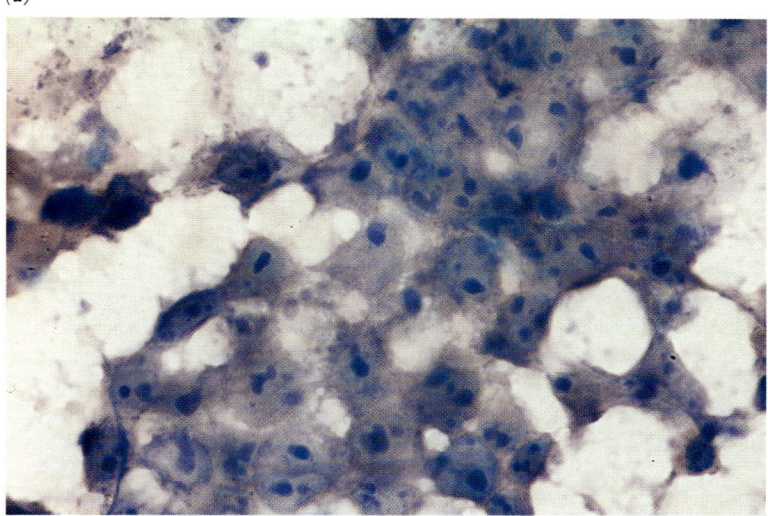

10. Lymph nodes

The procedure for fine needle aspiration of a palpable lymph node and the preparation of smears is identical with that of the breast (Ch. 2). Interventional radiology is employed to obtain diagnostic material from deep seated lymph nodes and the methodology is as for aspiration of intrathoracic and sub-diaphragmatic lesions.

Lymph node enlargement may be due to benign reactive hyperplasia, neoplastic proliferation of one or more cell lines of a lymph node (malignant lymphoma) or metastatic cancer.

The appearance of benign reactive hyperplasia varies with the type of immune response to foreign material. It may consist of paracortical hyperplasia of T-lymphocytes when the immune response is cell mediated, follicular hyperplasia of B lymphocytes in a humoral immune response or sinus catarrh due to proliferation of the sinus-lining phagocytic cells. The diagnosis is based on morphological assessment of the proliferative element and, in doubtful cases, immunocytochemical localisation of polytypic lymphoid cells; it requires intact node architecture in either a section or an imprint smear of the cut surface of a resected node. A needle aspiration of a reactive node contains the various cell types in random distribution. The multiplicity of cells seen is at best suggestive of benign hyperplasia, but the diagnosis is unlikely to be definitive.

The presence of multinucleated epithelioid cells in an aspirate may be indicative of a granulomatous lesion, but the diagnosis is again of limited value without supplementary histology or microbiology as it does not discriminate between the different types of granulomas.

Diagnosis of malignant lymphomas has become progressively more precise with the introduction and application of monoclonal antibodies, and at the same time, increasingly complex. There is, to date, no international agreement on a single classification and different terms are used in different centres to designate the same pathological entity. In current practice a diagnosis on which treatment and prognosis may be based requires information regarding the pattern of growth and immunological sub-typing of the neoplastic cell line.

Cytodiagnosis of a lymphoma is often feasible in a fine needle aspiration of a node, but may be more tentative than a similar diagnosis on a serous or pulmonary specimen for the following reasons. Distinction between a mixed centrocytic-centroblastic lymphoma and benign reactive hyperplasia may not be clear cut. An abundance of large mononuclear lymphoid cells may reflect a focus of transformed reactive lymphocytes rather than a high grade non-Hodgkin's lymphoma. In cases in which the neoplastic character of the cells is obvious on cell morphology, the all-important distinction between a Hodgkin's and a non-Hodgkin's lymphoma may not be possible in the absence of Reed-Sternberg cells. Furthermore, the pattern of growth whether diffuse or nodular cannot be determined by this technique. Histological and/or immunocytochemical confirmation of a provisional cytological diagnosis of a lymphoma in a lymph node is consequently advisable. Once the diagnosis is established cytology is helpful in monitoring the course of the disease.

The major contribution of FNA cytology of lymph nodes is in the diagnosis of metastatic cancer.

LYMPH NODES 181

MALIGNANT LYMPHOMA

Fig. 10.1 Malignant lymphoma: centrocytic-centroblastic

MGG ×720: abdominal lymph node

This micrograph illustrates discrete neoplastic lymphoid cells from a para-aortic abdominal lymph node of a histologically confirmed case of a low grade B-cell lymphoma. The predominant cell is small. Note that unlike mature lymphocytes which are non-nucleolated and more or less the same size, the neoplastic cells of centrocytic origin contain one to four nucleoli and exhibit a gradation in size which at one end approaches the few large cells in the field. These are centroblasts with more reticular chromatin and several nucleoli located near the nuclear membrane. The marked preponderance of centrocytes over centroblasts accords with a low grade lymphoma.

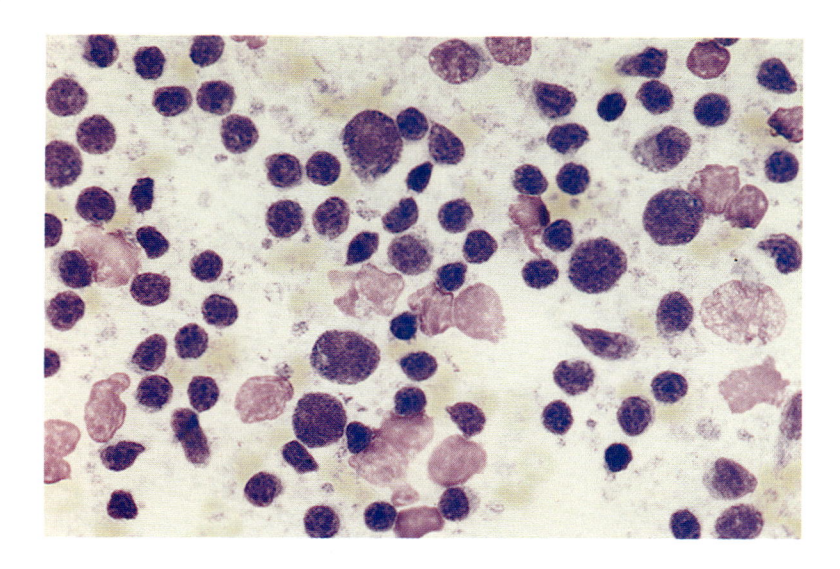

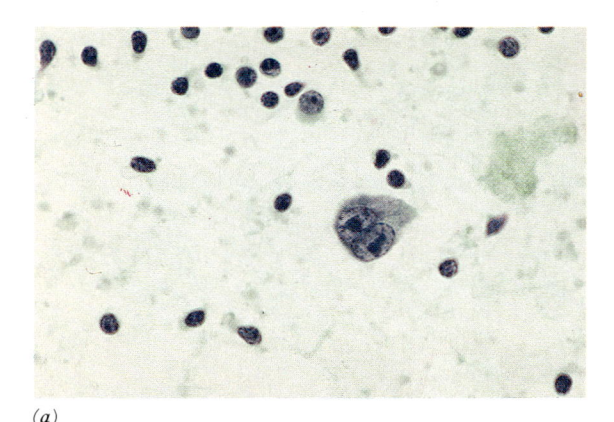

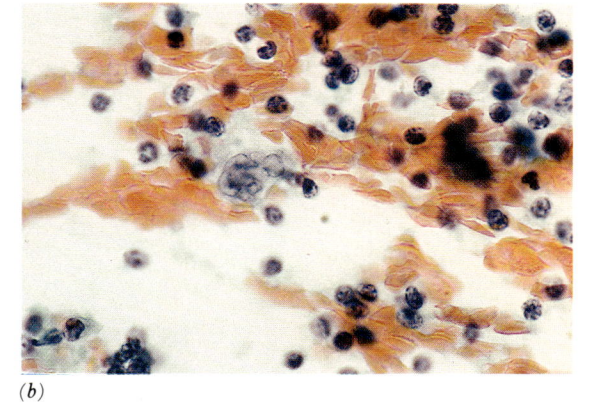

(a) (b)

Fig. 10.2 Hodgkin's lymphoma

Papanicolaou ×525 (a) cervical node (b) axillary node: another case

The two cases of Hodgkin's lymphoma illustrated in these micrographs demonstrate both the usefulness and limitations of cytology in this field. Micrograph (a) shows a large neoplastic cell accompanied by small reactive lymphocytes. The tumour cell has a flimsy histiocytic type of cytoplasm and two mirror image nuclei, each of which contains a macronucleolus, linked by fine strands of chromatin to the nuclear membrane. The appearance is that of a classical Reed-Sternberg cell and in conjunction with benign lymphocytes is diagnostic of a Hodgkin's lymphoma. The patient, a 14-year-old boy from the Middle East presented with cervical lymphadenopathy which was clinically suggestive of tuberculous lymphadenopathy.

The second case (b) is of a post-menopausal woman with a mass which appeared clinically to be a carcinoma of the axillary tail of the breast. There were three features of note in the aspirate: absence of mammary tissue, abundance of small, mature lymphocytes and the presence of scattered discrete neoplastic non-epithelial cells. These had scanty cytoplasm and a single large nucleus which was either polylobated or had a deep cleft. As discussed in Chapters 3 and 4, this type of cell may occur in both Hodgkin's and non-Hodgkin's lymphoma. The benign character of the associated lymphocytes favours in this case a diagnosis of the former; the presumptive cytological diagnosis of lymphocyte-predominant Hodgkin's disease was established by resection biopsy histology.

182 DIAGNOSTIC CYTOPATHOLOGY

METASTATIC TUMOURS

(a)

(b)

(c)

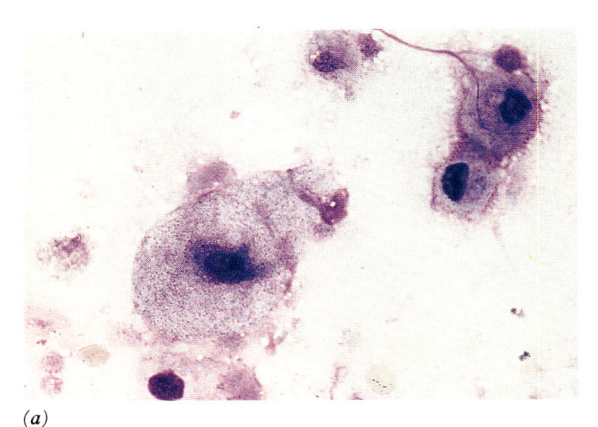

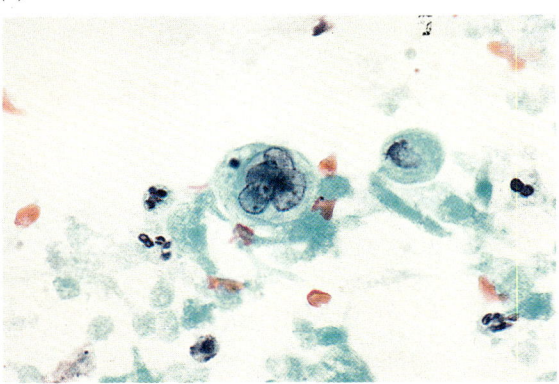

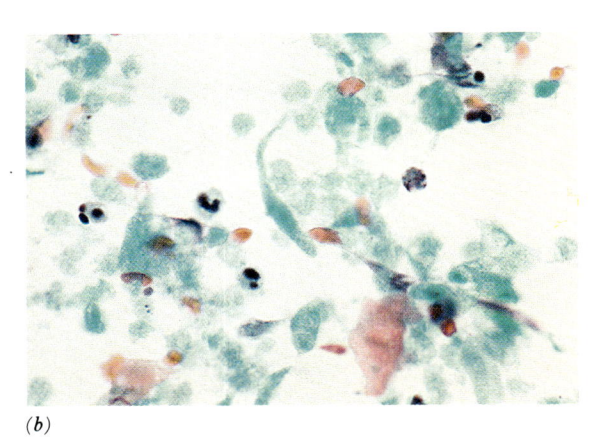

Fig. 10.3 Metastatic squamous cell carcinoma

(a) MGG ×525: cervical lymph node; carcinoma of tongue
(b) Papanicolaou ×525: cervical lymph node; carcinoma of larynx (c) same smear as (b); another field

In suspected metastatic disease of lymph nodes, surgical resection may be avoided by the use of FNA cytology. Since lymph nodes do not contain epithelial cells, a diagnosis of metastatic carcinoma is generally easy and reliable. Whilst in most cases, the cell type is identifiable, it is not possible to determine the source of the primary. The cells in (a) from a carcinoma of tongue have the pallid cytoplasm of keratinized cells stained by the Romanowsky method, and dark condensed nuclei. The necrotic tumour tissue in (b) and (c) is a common feature of a well differentiated squamous cell carcinoma, but may occur with other cell types. Evidence of squamous origin is seen in the fibre-shaped cells in (b) and the large round cell with firm cyanophilic cytoplasm and a bizarre nucleus in (c).

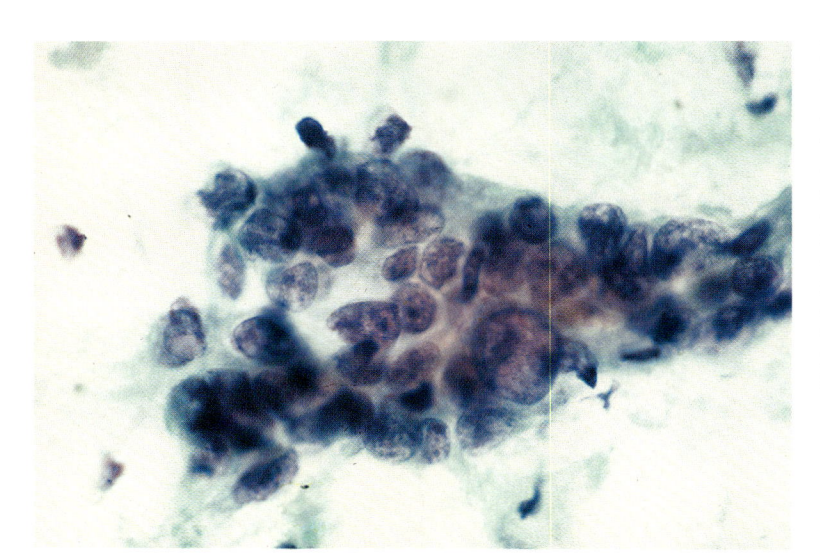

Fig. 10.4 Metastatic transitional cell carcinoma

Papanicolaou ×720: cervical lymph node

This micrograph illustrates a large cluster of cohesive cells which show obvious stigmata of malignancy. The cells are poorly differentiated and the cytological diagnosis is of metastatic carcinoma, cell type uncertain. The patient had a history of bladder carcinoma and as there was no evidence, clinical or radiological of another primary, the node metastasis was assumed to be of transitional cell origin.

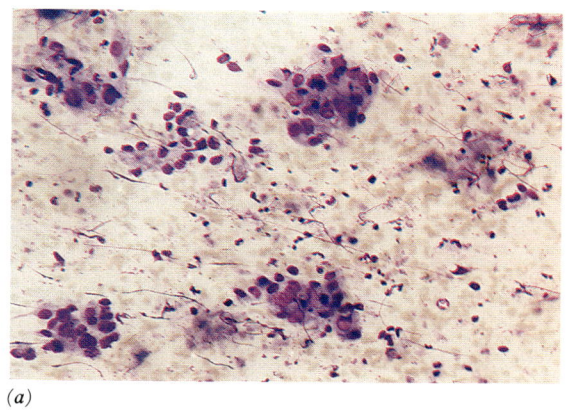

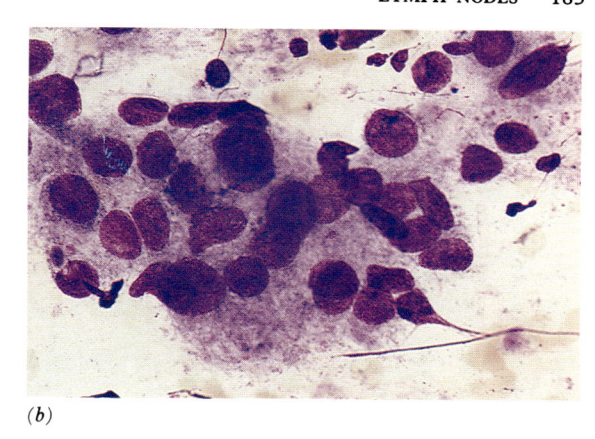

Fig. 10.5 Metastatic adenocarcinoma
MGG (a) ×133: intrathoracic lymph node (b) ×525: same smear; another field

A lymph node may be virtually replaced by secondary deposits with few lymphoid cells remaining (a). Amorphous debris and a variable number of neutrophils may be present. The tumour cells in this example form large clusters with some peripheral orientation of nuclei (a). The cytoplasm is variable in amount and relatively abundant (b). The appearance, suggestive of adenocarcinoma, is consistent with but not proof of spread from an endometrial carcinoma from which the patient suffered.

Fig. 10.6 Metastatic carcinoma of lung
MGG ×183: cervical lymph node

Enlargement of one or more lymph nodes may be the presenting symptom of malignant disease. In the case illustrated, an aspirate of a cervical node shows numerous large, poorly differentiated carcinoma cells. A lung mass, subsequently demonstrated on a chest X-ray, is considered to be the likely primary.

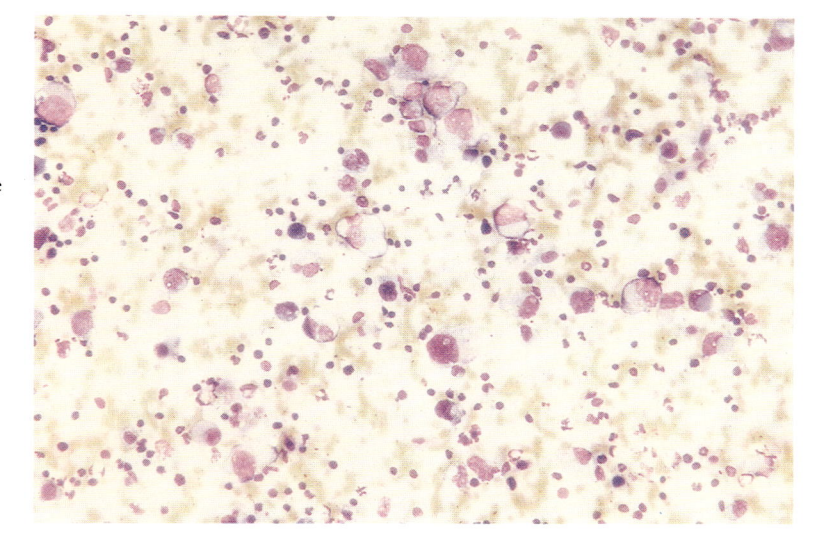

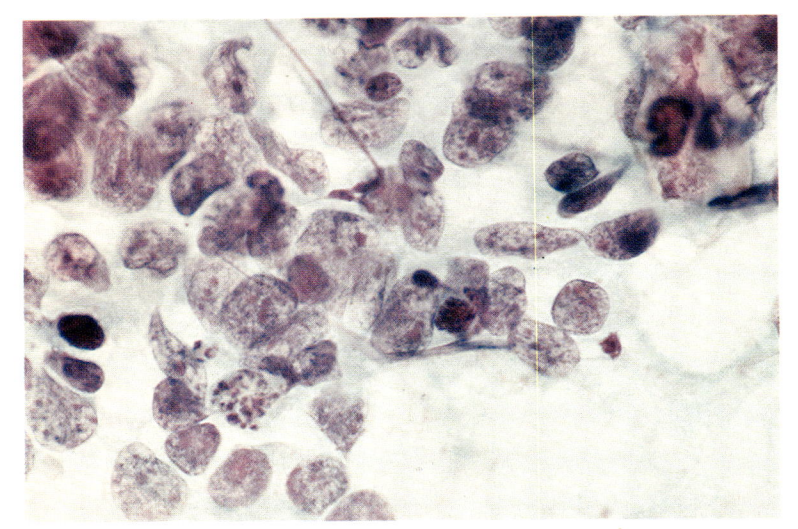

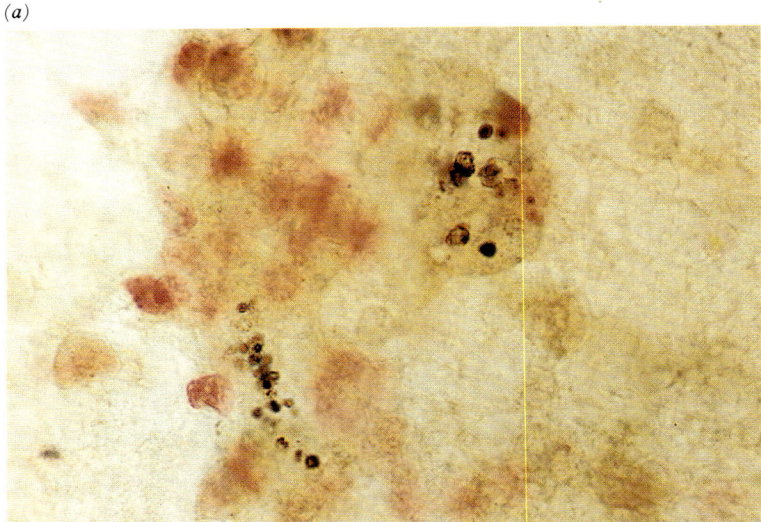

Fig. 10.7 Metastatic melanotic melanoma

(a) Papanicolaou ×720: axillary lymph node (b) Masson Fontana ×720: same specimen; another smear

Melanoma, a highly malignant tumour of melanocytes spreads rapidly to regional lymph nodes. The melanotic form does not as a rule present a diagnostic problem, but the amelanotic variety which is devoid of pigment is not usually identifiable as a melanoma, although its malignant nature is never in doubt. The tumour nuclei in (a) exhibit marked variation in shape and size and contain several eosinophilic nucleoli. The cell morphology, whilst diagnostic of malignancy, is non-specific as to type. The nature of the tumour is established by demonstration of intracytoplasmic melanin in the tumour cells (b).

11. Bone

Large bore needle biopsy of the sternum or the iliac crest is a well-established procedure in haematology. The usual indication for obtaining diagnostic material from bone or marrow for cytopathology is suspected malignancy. A neoplastic lesion in bone may be osteolytic due to destruction of bone trabeculae and stimulation of osteoclasts in the surrounding bone. Some of the commoner cancers which produced lytic lesions are multiple myelomatosis, non-Hodgkin's lymphomas and metastatic deposits from kidney, thyroid and lower bowel. Stimulation of osteoblasts resulting in new bone formation by Hodgkin's lymphoma or metastases from a carcinoma of the prostate result in osteosclerotic lesions with increased radiodensity. Carcinoma of the breast is associated with both osteolytic and osteosclerotic lesions. The latter type of lesion requires the use of thick needles if adequate material is to be obtained.

NORMAL CELLS

(a)

(b)

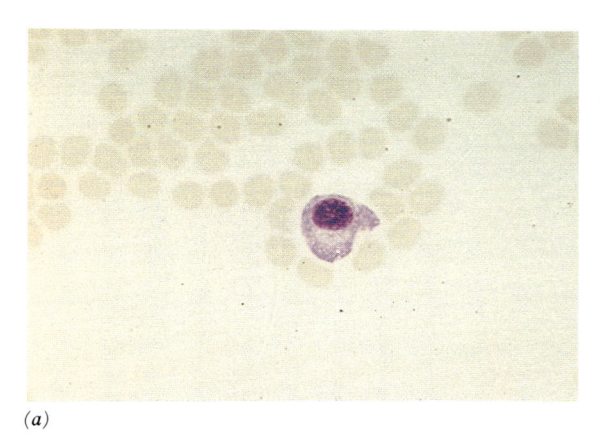

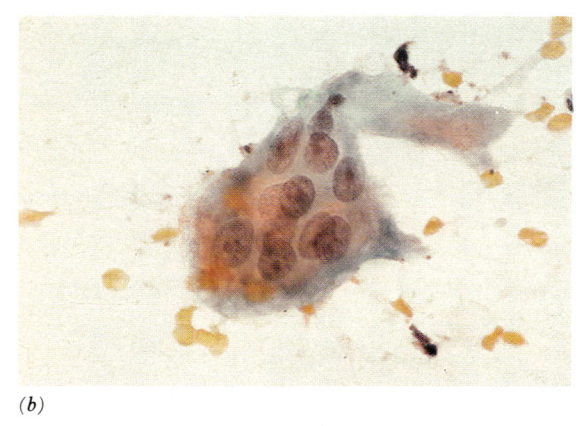

Fig. 11.1 Osteoblast: osteoclast

(a) MGG ×525: lumbar vertebrum; osteoblast (b) Papanicolaou ×525: lumbar vertebrum; osteoclast

Two types of bone cells concerned with maintaining the integrity of the skeletal system by continuous dynamic remodelling of bone may be met with in a needle aspiration of bone. Each has a different function which is reflected in its morphology.

The osteoblast, derived from a precursor cell probably of the stromal cell system, synthesizes and secretes osteoid, the non-mineralized extracellular matrix of bone. It is a mononuclear cell of moderate size and has a basophilic cytoplasm which stains less intensely in its central portion due to the presence of a large paranuclear Golgi apparatus. This gives the osteoblast a superficial resemblance to another actively secretory cell, the plasma cell, The latter is smaller in size and has a clock face nucleus.

The osteoclast is responsible for the resorption of osteoid, and its precursor, like the precursors of other phagocytic cells, is probably of haematopoietic origin. The osteoclast is a large cell, and may contain one or many nuclei, in which form it resembles a giant multinucleated histiocyte. Its cell outline is often indistinct or irregular and with the Papanicolaou stain, its cytoplasm is generally amphophilic. The nuclei are oval or round, and each contains an eosinophilic nucleolus.

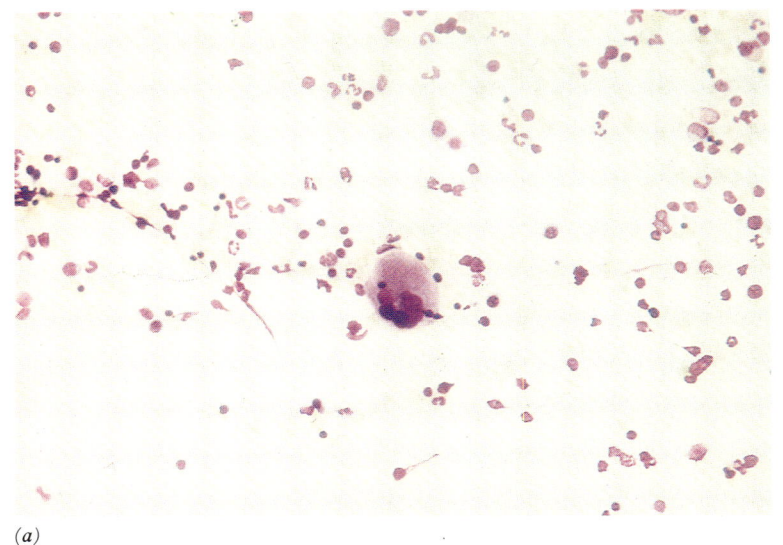

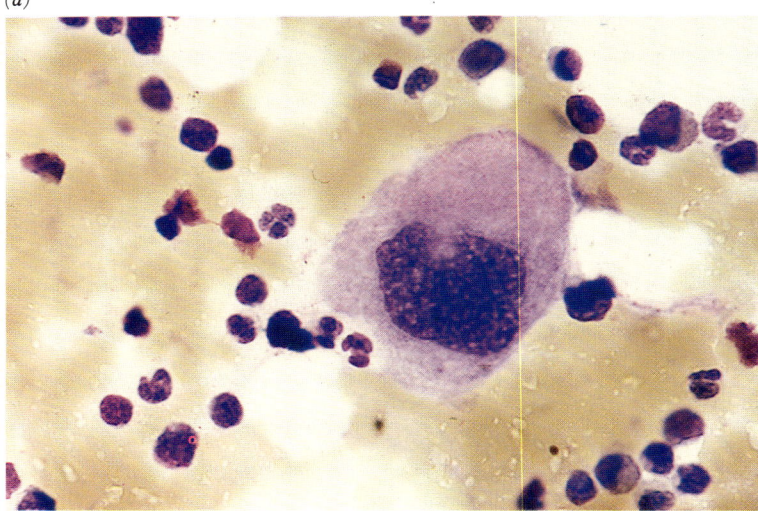

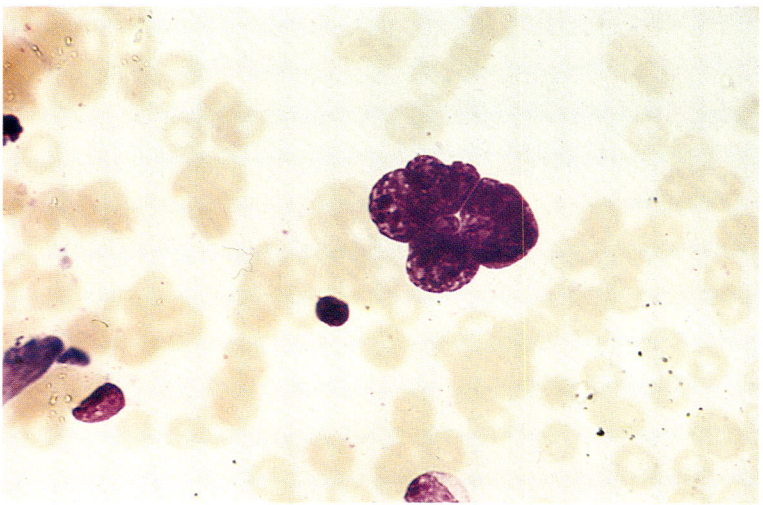

Fig. 11.2 Haematopoietic cells

*MGG: lumbar vertebrum (a) ×183
(b) ×720: same smear; another field
(c) ×720: another specimen*

Haematopoietic tissue present in the intertrabecular spaces of bone consists of both red and white blood cells in various stages of maturation, and of the platelet-forming megakaryocytes (a). Whilst it is not necessary for the cytopathologist to be able to identify each red and white cell precursor, familiarity with the overall appearance of haematopoietic tissue is required if a misdiagnosis of a small celled malignancy is to be avoided. The megakaryocyte with its coarsely reticulated, giant polyploid nucleus (b) needs to be distinguished from a bizarre carcinoma or sarcoma cell. The nucleus of the megakaryocyte is occasionally seen stripped of its cytoplasm (c), and in this form mimics a group of oat cells. Distinguishing features are the indentation and lobulation of the megakaryocyte nucleus rather than moulding of adjacent separate nuclei, its coarsely reticulated chromatin and the absence of any cytoplasm round it.

PRIMARY TUMOURS

Fig. 11.3 Plasmacytoma
MGG ×720: sacrum

Plasmacytoma, a neoplasm of plasma cells in the marrow, is a localized form of multiple myelomatosis. Unlike the latter, a plasmacytoma is not generally associated with anaemia and hypercalcaemia and gammopathies are either absent or occur in a milder form. The tumour may be single or multiple and produces lytic lesions in bone. Focal collections of neoplastic plasma cells are seen in aspirates of these lesions. The cells may be similar in morphology to normal plasma cells, or they may be larger and less mature as in the example illustrated.

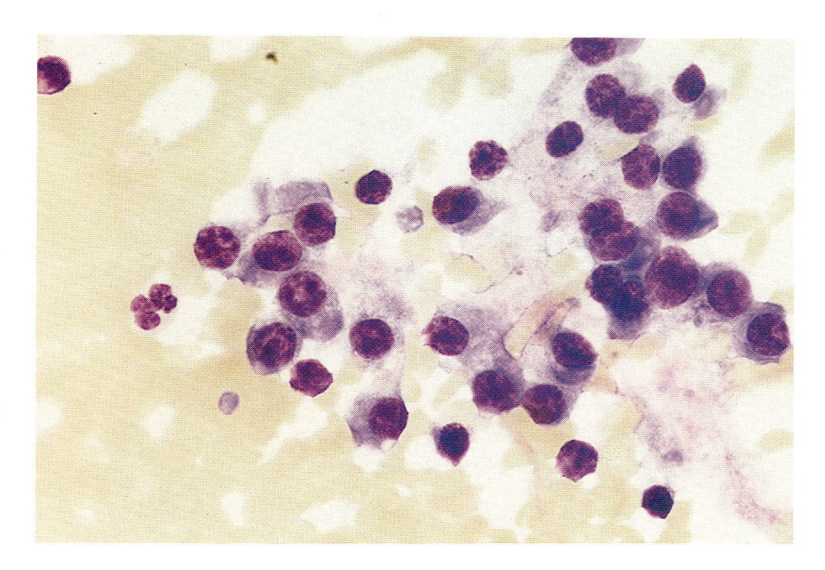

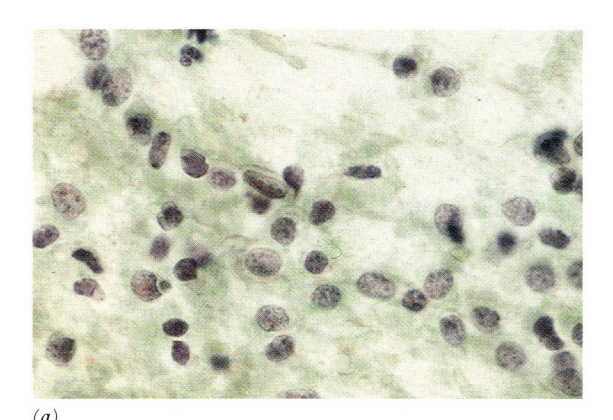

(a)

(b)

Fig. 11.4 Ewing's tumour
(a) Papanicolaou ×525: sacrum (b) MGG ×525: femur; same case (c) PAS ×525: same specimen as (b); another smear

Ewing's tumour is a highly aggressive, small celled sarcoma which originates in the medullary cavity, usually of the midshaft of long bones, and metastasizes rapidly and extensively. The cell of origin is unknown. The tumour affects mainly children and adolescents. Specimens from two separate sites in a 16-year-old male are illustrated, stained by the Papanicolaou method (a) and MGG (b) to allow comparison of the differences in appearance produced by different methodologies. The neoplastic cells are uniform in size and their size may be assessed by comparing them with the single neutrophil present in (a) and in (b). The cytoplasm is sparse and ill-defined. The round or oval nuclei have finely stippled chromatin and one or more small nucleoli in (a); in (b) the chromatin is arranged in fine bands and nucleoli are not clearly seen. The cells of Ewing's tumour may be distinguished from other small celled cancers, particularly non-Hodgkin's lymphoma, by the presence of moderate to abundant intracytoplasmic granules of glycogen (c).

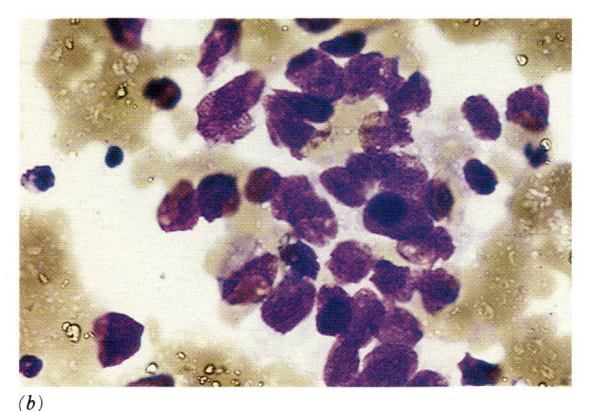

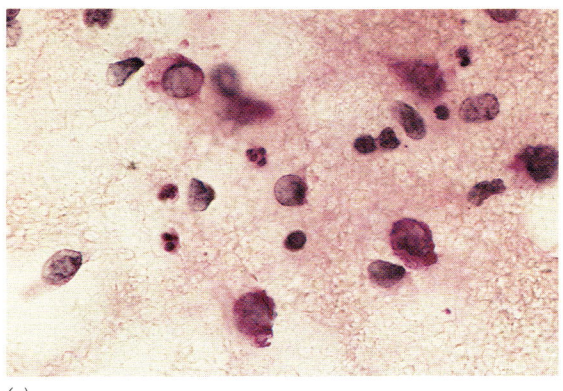

(c)

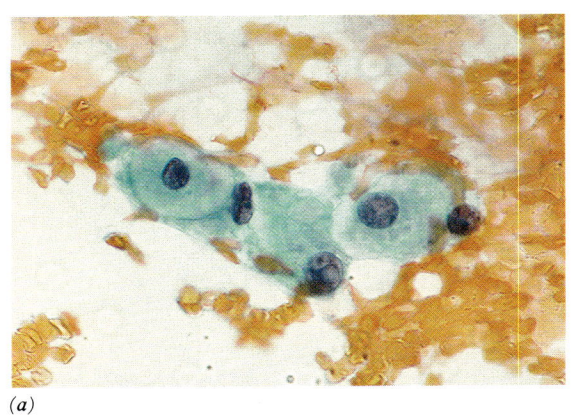

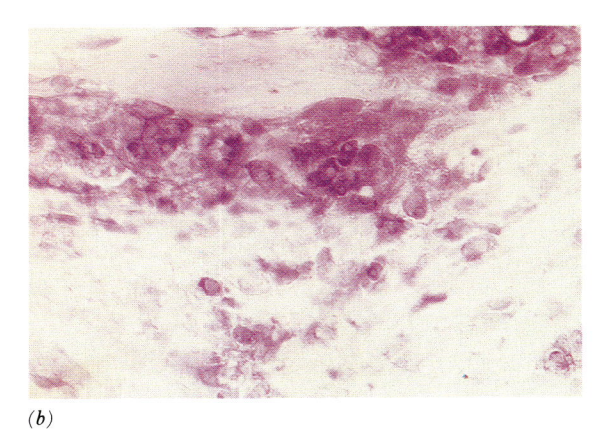

Fig. 11.5 Chordoma

(a) Papanicolaou ×525: lumbosacrum (b) PAS ×133: same specimen; another smear

A chordoma is a locally invasive, jelly-like tumour which develops from the notochord, essentially an embryonic structure which persists in the adult in the central pulp of the intervertebral discs. Microscopically, the tumour has a characteristic appearance, being composed of large, clear, epithelium-like cells. The nuclei, usually one per cell, occasionally multiple, are small and bland and contain one or two pin-point nucleoli (a). The abundant cytoplasm contains many intracytoplasmic granules of glycogen and the cells are embedded in a mucoid substance which also is PAS-positive (b). A chordoma may develop from any part of the vertebral canal, the lumbo-sacrum and the base of the cranium being the commonest sites.

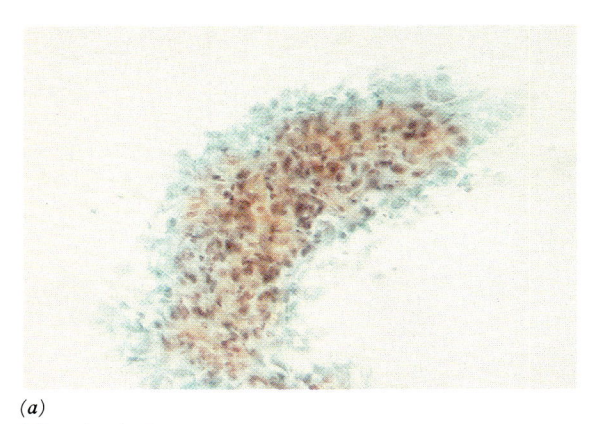

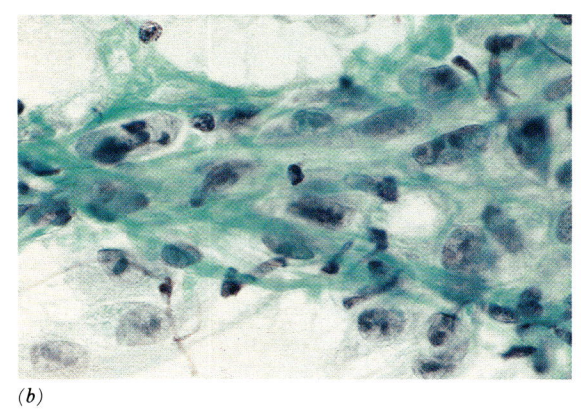

Fig. 11.6 Osteosarcoma

Papanicolaou: neck of femur (a) ×133 (b) ×525: same smear; another field

This rare but important primary cancer of bone is derived from osteoblasts or possibly osteoprogenitor cells. It affects mainly young subjects, the usual sites being the lower end of the femur or the upper end of the tibia. In the older patient, it is usually a complication of a predisposing disorder such as Paget's disease of the bone or fibrous dysplasia. The case illustrated is of a 56-year-old male with long standing polyostotic fibrous dysplasia and a recent pathological fracture of the neck of the femur. Large fragments of softish tissue were obtained in a needle aspirate of the fracture site (a). At higher magnification (b) the tissue is seen to consist of pleomorphic cells with ill-defined cell borders, and high nuclear cytoplasmic ratios. The plump nuclei are markedly variable in shape and size and contain one or several prominent macronucleoli. The preponderance of fusiform or sausage-shaped malignant nuclei and the absence of epithelial type cell borders is consistent with a diagnosis of sarcoma. The type of sarcoma, whether for example, an osteosarcoma or a fibrosarcoma, is identified by its characteristic extracellular matrix. Osteoid was identified in a tissue section of part of the aspirate.

BONE 189

Fig. 11.7 Undifferentiated sarcoma

Papanicolaou ×720: lumbar vertebrum

In the absence of a typical matrix or of other morphological or functional features such as the cross striations of a rhabdomyosarcoma, the nature of a sarcoma may not be identifiable. The location of the tumour may also be unhelpful as a bone tumour may form a mass in adjacent soft tissues.

An example of an undifferentiated sarcoma, the origin of which remained uncertain, is illustrated in this micrograph. The cellular presentation in an aspirate of a fractured lumbar vertebrum consisting of highly pleomorphic nuclei, many of which are spindle-shaped, and absence of cell-limiting membrane is characteristic of sarcoma. Post-mortem histology of a soft tissue mass continuous with the tumour in the vertebrum confirmed undifferentiated sarcoma but whether a soft tissue sarcoma had eroded bone or an osteosarcoma had extended outwards could not be ascertained.

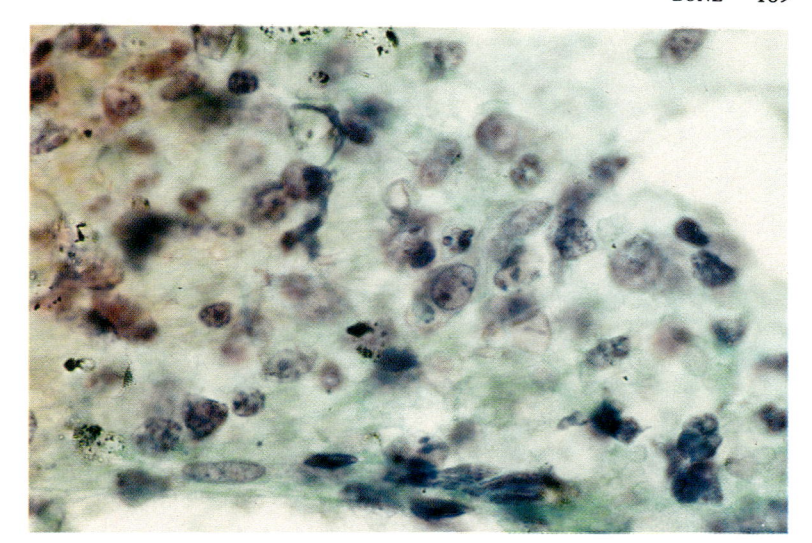

METASTATIC TUMOURS

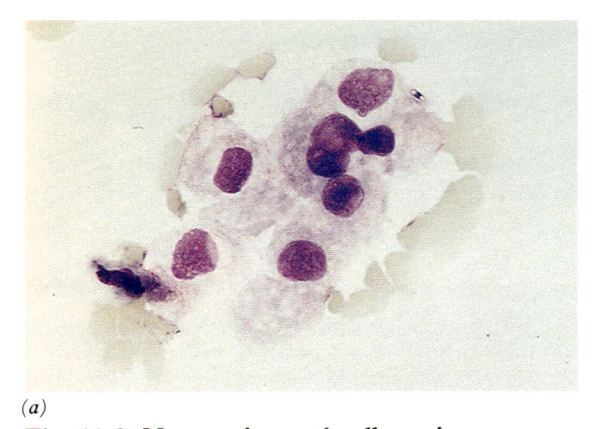

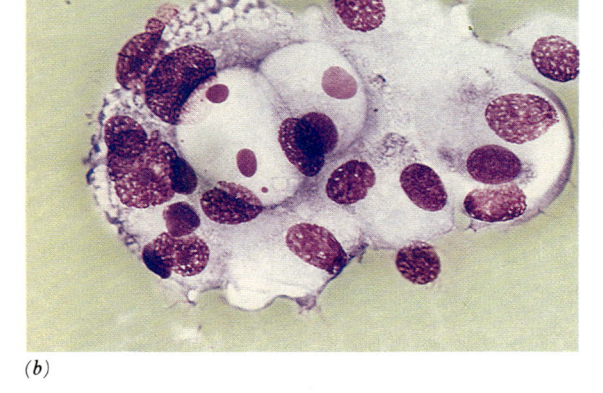

(a)   (b)

Fig. 11.8 Metastatic renal cell carcinoma

Papanicolaou ×525: (a) lumbar vertebrum (b) renal aspirate; same case

Bone is a common site of blood-borne metastases and metastatic disease which is much more common than primary cancer is the most frequent indication for FNA cytology. The diagnosis of secondary carcinoma based on recognition of neoplastic epithelial cells is relatively simple. Comparison with the cells of the primary lesion is helpful. The large, circumscribed epithelial cells with abundant clear cytoplasm, relatively small nuclei and prominent nucleoli in (a) are comparable with the cells from a primary carcinoma of kidney (b).

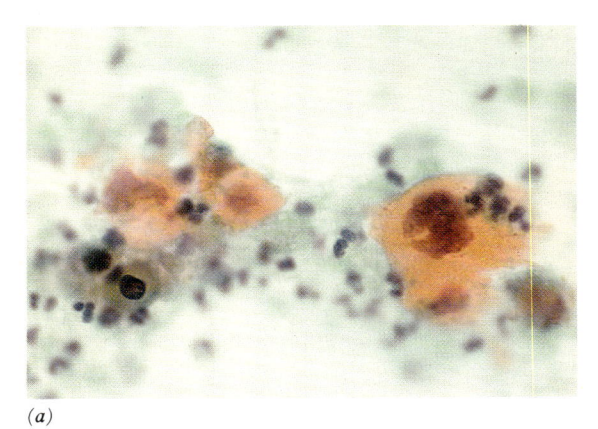

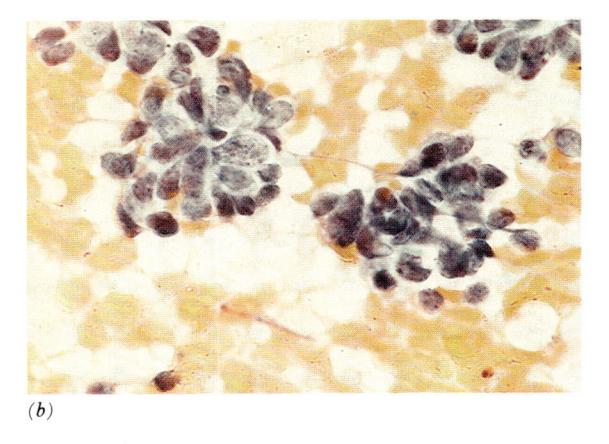

Fig. 11.9 Metastatic bronchogenic carcinoma

Papanicolaou ×525: lumbar vertebra (a) squamous cell carcinoma (b) small cell carcinoma

Bronchogenic carcinoma is one of the commonest sources of metastatic deposits in the skeleton. Micrograph (a) illustrates well differentiated, large, variable, orangeophilic malignant squamous cells obtained from a vertebrum of a male with lung carcinoma.

The cells in (b) are small and virtually filled with nuclei which mould one another and have a 'salt and pepper' chromatin. The appearance is so typical of a small cell carcinoma that a bronchogenic origin may be easily deduced from the secondary tumour.

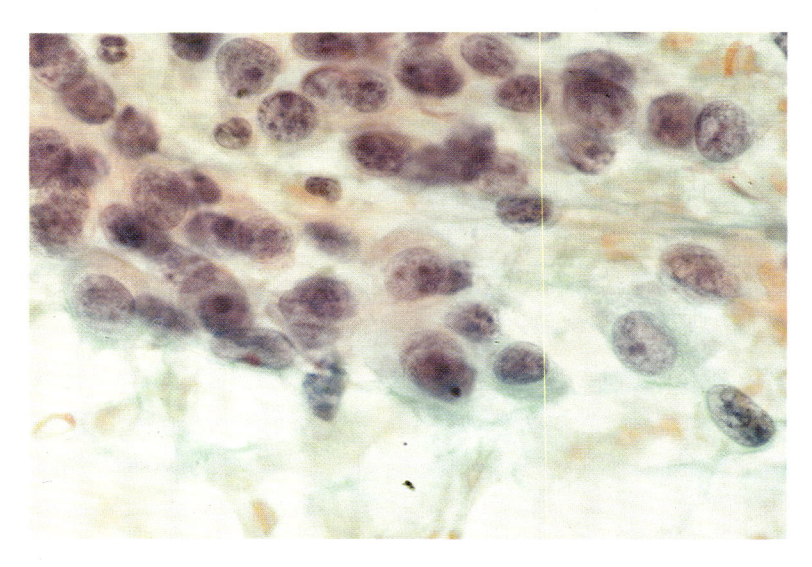

Fig. 11.10 Metastatic carcinoma of unknown origin

Papanicolaou ×720: rib

There remains a proportion of cases in which the patient presents with evidence of widespread metastatic disease, but the primary remains unidentified. The case illustrated in this micrograph is of a middle-aged male with numerous osteolytic lesions, and a provisional diagnosis of multiple myelomatosis. The neoplastic cells in an aspiration of a rib lesion are cohesive, have vesicular nuclei, and their morphology is consistent with adenocarcinoma. Since the treatment of carcinomatosis involving the skeletal system is palliative (the cell type having been identified) a further search for the site of the primary is not indicated.

12. Skin and sub-cutaneous lesions

The role of cytology in the field of dermatological pathology is fairly limited. Fungal lesions may be identified by incubating a scraping of the affected skin or hairs detached from the lesion in 10% KOH until the epidermal elements are dissolved and hyphae become microscopically visible. Viral lesions are identified by their cytopathic effects in cells obtained from the base of a vesicle (Tzanck test). Round or oval parabasal cells with prominent eosinophilic nucleoli, seen in fluid aspirated from a bullous lesion are suggestive of pemphigus, a disorder characterized by dissolution of the intercellular bridges, or acantholysis, in the lower epithelium. These cells, often referred to as Tzanck cells, may also be seen in bullous pemphigoid. Immunofluorescent demonstration of IgG antibodies to intercellular antigen at the precise site of acantholysis is necessary to distinguish pemphigus, a serious condition, from the less significant pemphigoid. Keratoacanthoma is usually identifiable in a cytological preparation, but caution is indicated to avoid a false positive diagnosis of squamous cell carcinoma. The many other benign lesions of the skin, whether topical or manifestations of systemic disorders, are outside the scope of cytopathology.

As regards the primary cancers of the skin, cytology is of particular value in the diagnosis of basal cell carcinoma. Melanotic melanoma is distinguished from benign pigmented lesions by its frankly malignant cellular features (see Figs. 5.8 and 10.7). Sensitivity for squamous cell carcinoma is lower as the cell yield from these tumours is often inadequate.

Diagnostic material may be obtained by direct scrape or by fine needle aspiration. The former is preferred for ulcerated lesions and the latter is used to sample sub-cutaneous nodules and soft tissue masses. Permanent preparation may be made by either the Papanicolaou or Romanowsky methods.

Fig. 12.1 Sebaceous epithelial cells

MMG ×720: percutaneous needle aspiration

Cells from the skin or its appendages may enter a needle during its passage through the skin. Squamous cells are easily recognized and unlikely to cause confusion. This micrograph illustrates epithelial cells from a sebaceous gland. These cells secrete oily sebum and their abundant cytoplasm is distended with lipid. This is removed by ethanol in a wet-fixed preparation leaving a clear cytoplasm. In the air-dried, methanol-fixed smear illustrated, a few clear cells with small nuclei are seen; others contain amorphous eosinophilic material which obscures the nuclei.

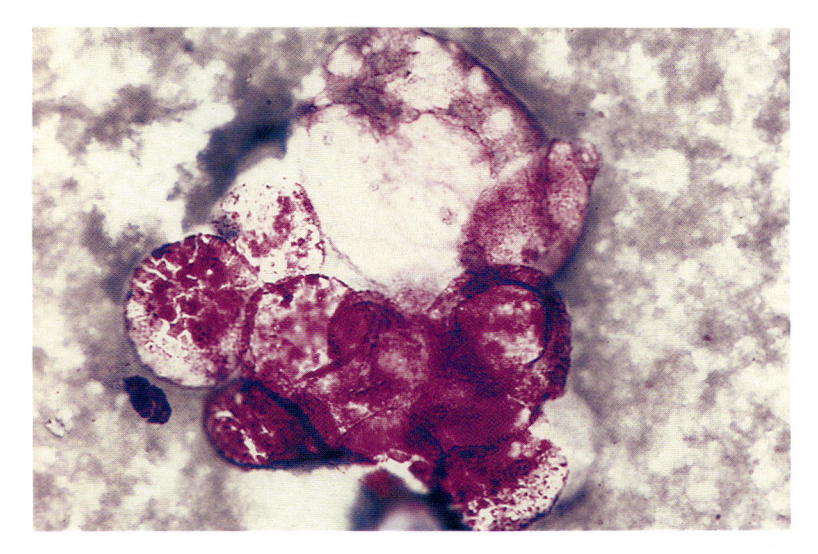

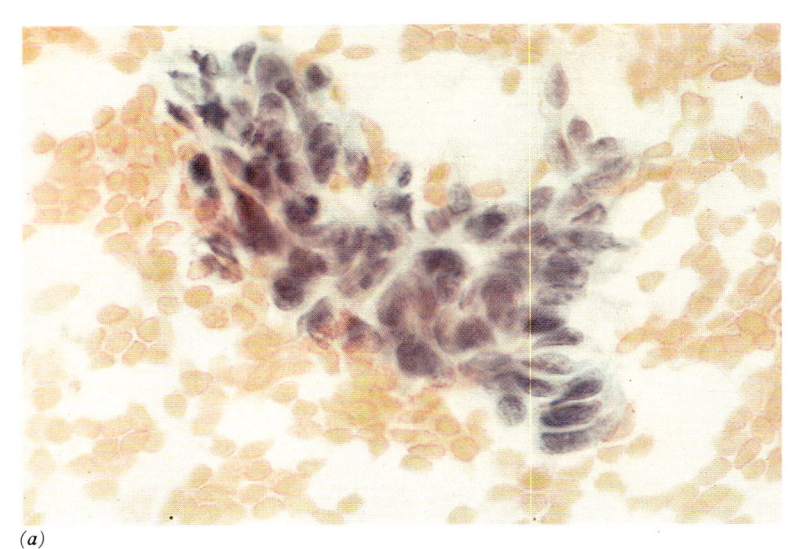

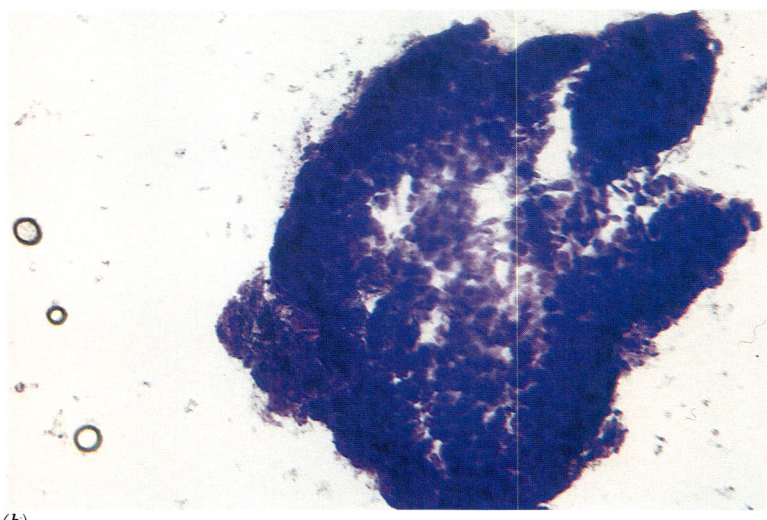

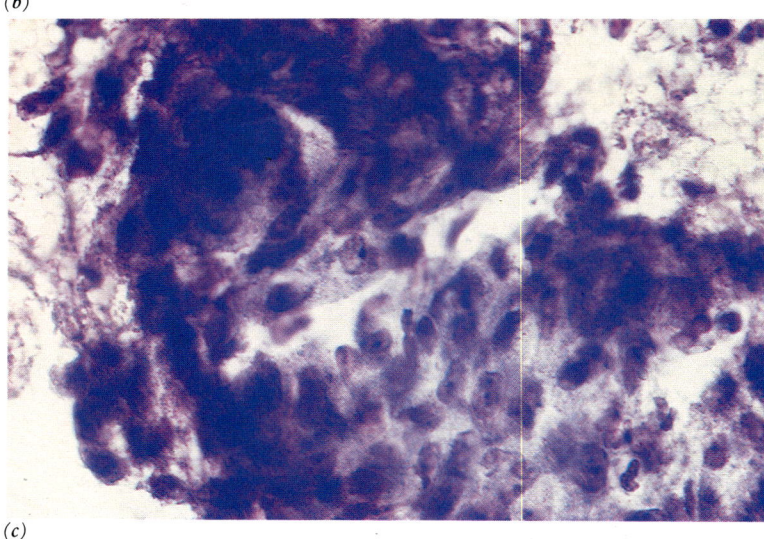

Fig. 12.2 Basal cell carcinoma (BCC)

(a) *Papanicolaou ×720: skin scrape*
(b) *aqueous methylene blue ×183: skin scrape; another case* (c) *×458: same field as (b)*

The commonest primary cancer of the skin is a basal cell carcinoma, which, as its name implies, develops from the basal cells of the epidermis and its appendages. It occurs on areas exposed to sunlight or ultraviolet light, particularly the face in fair skinned subjects. The tumour is of low grade malignancy and infiltrates the sub-epithelial tissues but almost never metastasizes. It forms a nodular lesion which frequently ulcerates, hence it is popularly referred to as a rodent ulcer.

Diagnostic material may be obtained from a basal cell carcinoma either by needle aspiration of the nodule or by direct scrape of the base of the ulcer after the crust has been gently levered off with the back of a scalpel blade or a fine spatula. A permanent preparation may be stained by the Papanicolaou method (a) or MGG. An alternative rapid out-patient procedure is to suspend the cells in a drop or two of 1.0% aqueous methylene blue (b), (c), flatten them under a cover slip and examine the wet preparation with the microscope.

The characteristic cellular presentation consists of sheets of cohesive basal cells, the fragments of tissue appearing as microbiopsies (b). The cells have little or no apparent cytoplasm and consist largely of round or, more often, ovoid nuclei with finely granular chromatin (a). A somewhat greater amount of cytoplasm is evident in some cases and the cells may approximate in size to small parabasal cells and the tumour cells may show a basisquamoid morphology (c). Nucleoli are variable in number and size. Generally inconspicuous or absent in the smaller cells (a), they are usually evident in the cells with a greater volume of cytoplasm (c).

The neoplastic cells of BCC do not exhibit the usual criteria of malignancy and the diagnosis is based on the characteristic appearance of sheets of cohesive basal cells.

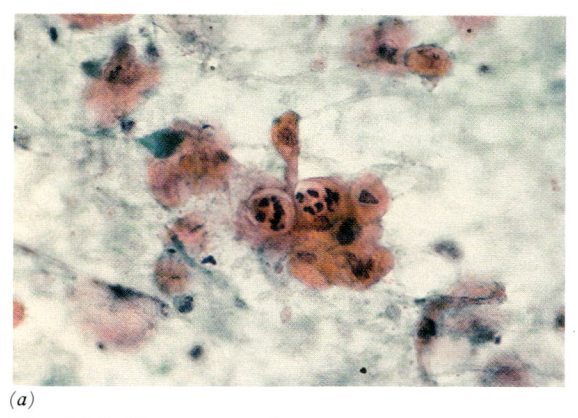

SKIN AND SUB-CUTANEOUS LESIONS 193

(a) 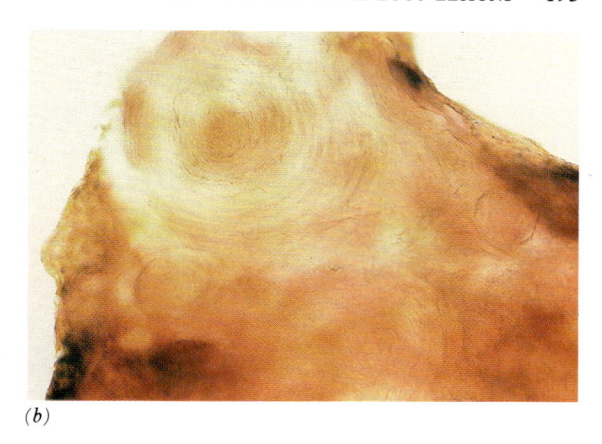   (b)

Fig. 12.3 Keratoacanthoma
Papanicolaou ×525: skin scrape (a) dyskeratotic cells (b) keratin

Keratoacanthoma, a disease of unknown aetiology, produces a nodular lesion with a central crater. The cells from the base of the crater are generally atypical in appearance (a). Although similar in size to the prickle cells, the intensely eosinophilic or orangeophilic cytoplasm indicates premature keratinization. Other features commonly associated with dyskeratosis, such as abnormality of shape and pyknotic degeneration of the nucleus are also seen. The dyskeratotic atypical cells should not be overdiagnosed as squamous carcinoma cells. The presence of masses of keratin (b) which may be arranged in a concentric manner similar to that seen in squamous papilloma (see Fig. 1.20 e), facilitates recognition of keratoacanthoma.

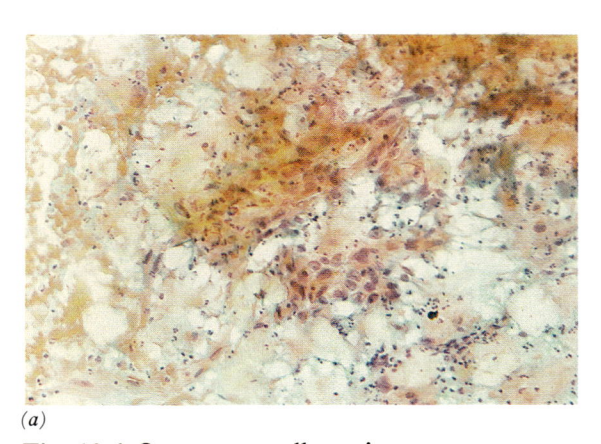

(a) 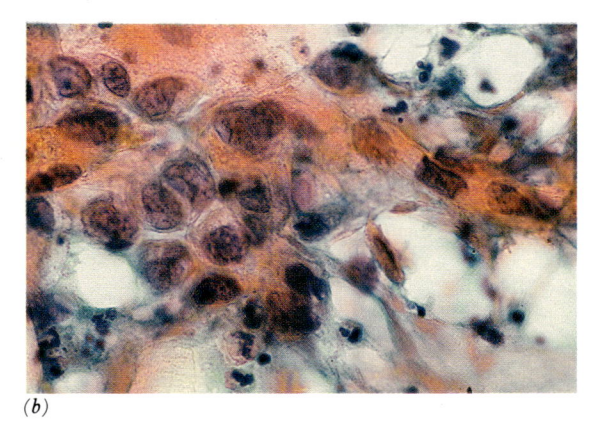   (b)

Fig. 12.4 Squamous cell carcinoma
Papanicolaou (a) ×133: skin scrape (b) ×525: same smear

Squamous cell carcinoma of the skin is much less common than basal cell carcinoma, but carries a graver prognosis as it spreads to the regional lymph nodes via the lymphatics. These tumours are generally well differentiated with abundant keratin formation. Because of this, they are difficult to scrape and the cell yield is often sparse and may be insufficient for a definitive diagnosis. Minor atypias of nucleus and abnormality of cell shape and keratinization, which occur in benign skin lesions such as keratoacanthoma (Fig. 12.3a) are discounted in arriving at a diagnosis which is based on the presence of a sufficient number of cells (a) with unequivocal malignant characteristics (b) and morphological features of squamous origin (b).

194 DIAGNOSTIC CYTOPATHOLOGY

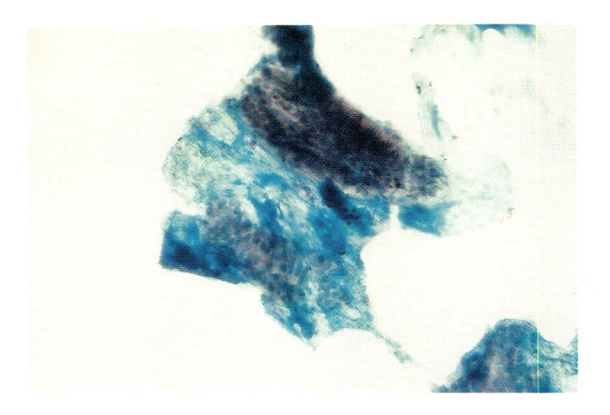

Fig. 12.5 Metastatic adenocarcinoma
Alcian blue ×133: FNA; Sub-cutaneous nodule on chest wall

Metastatic deposits in the skin and sub-cutaneous tissues are not uncommon, the most frequent sources being lymphomas and carcinomas of lung, breast, thyroid, ovary, stomach and kidney. Occasionally, a sub-cutaneous nodule of a metastatic deposit may be the first presenting symptom of an underlying carcinoma as in the case illustrated in this micrograph of a mucus-secreting adenocarcinoma of lung with a secondary deposit on the chest wall.

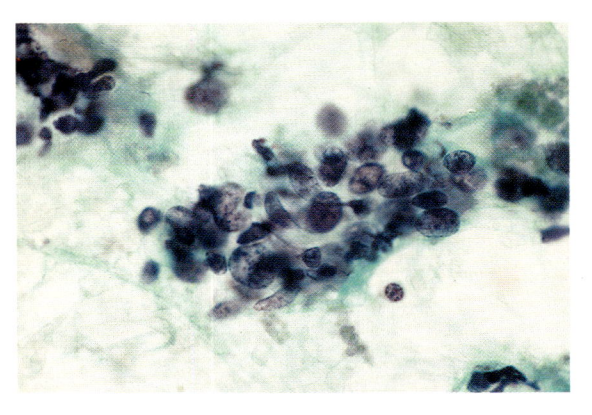

Fig. 12.6 Malignant fibrous histiocytoma
Papanicolaou ×525: FNA; sub-cutaneous nodule on thigh

Malignant fibrous histiocytoma is an aggressive neoplasm of soft tissue which occurs on the extremities, particularly the thigh and leg. The tumour forms an ill-defined, multinodular sub-cutaneous mass easily sampled with a fine needle. The neoplastic cells are pleomorphic and may include giant forms with grossly aberrant nuclei and histiocytic cells with abundant foamy or granular cytoplasm. This micrograph illustrates round and spindle-shaped cells. The latter provide a clue to the sarcomatous nature of the lesion, but a definitive diagnosis of a malignant fibrous histiocytoma is not feasible on cytology, and is established by tissue pathology.

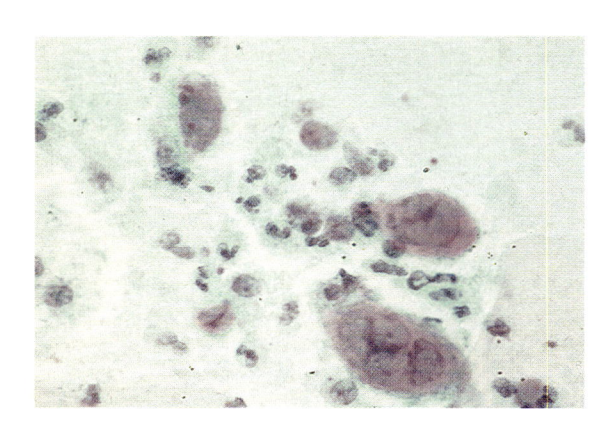

Fig. 12.7 Herpes zoster
Papanicolaou ×525: skin scrap

The cellular presentation of herpes zoster is identical with that of herpes simplex (see Figs. 1.19 and 3.29) and consists of mono- or multinucleated cells with moulded ground glass nuclei and margination of the nuclear chromatin. The vesicular lesions of Herpes zoster have a segmental distribution and appear on the skin along the course of the spinal or cranial nerve infected by the virus.

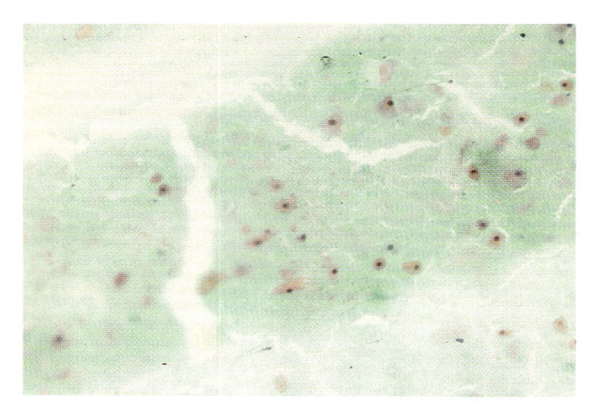

Fig. 12.8 Branchial cyst
Papanicolaou ×133

An anomaly of the branchial or visceral clefts which develop from the side of the embryonic pharynx may present in later life as a palpable or visible swelling at the angle of the mandible. Probably derived from the pharyngeal endoderm, the lining cells of a branchial cyst are usually large polyhedral squamous cells with pyknotic nuclei. Abundant sub-epithelial lymphoid tissue is present in the cyst wall and lymphocytes may be seen in the cyst fluid. A columnar cell lining may occur but is less common.

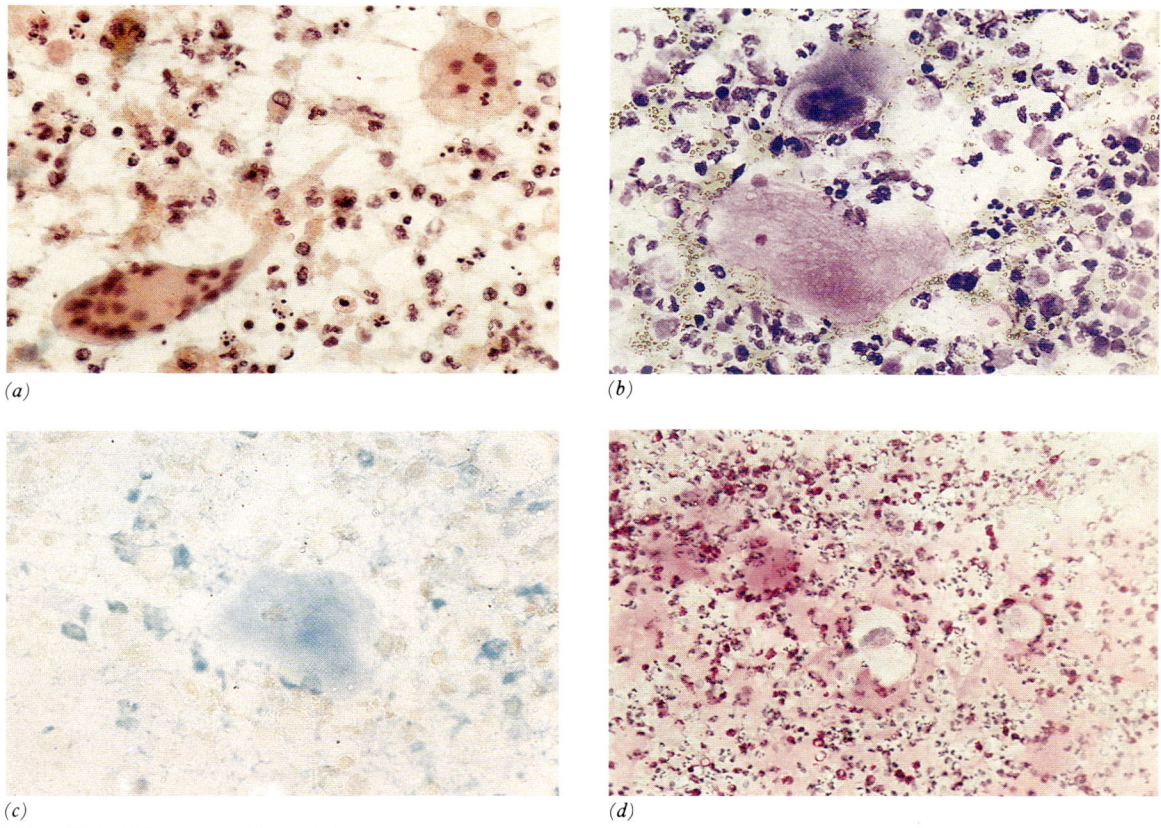

Fig. 12.9 Rheumatoid nodule

(a) Papanicolaou ×333: FNA; subcutaneous nodule on calf (b) MGG ×333: same specimen; another smear (c) Alcian blue ×133: same specimen; another smear (d) PAS ×133: same specimen; another smear

These micrographs illustrate the several components of a typical fully developed rheumatoid nodule (see also Fig. 4.18). The cells to note are the characteristic fish shaped (a) and the round multinucleated giant epithelioid cells (a), (b), (d), the shift to the right and the pyknotic degeneration of the abundant neutrophils (a) and the moderate number of lymphocytes (b). The necrobiotic fibrinoid core of the nodule is represented in the MGG smear by violet-coloured amorphous debris with a foamy honeycomb appearance (b). Being derived from collagen, it stains positively with alcian blue (c) and PAS (d).

13. Thyroid

There are few areas of pathology in which cytomorphological evaluation has to be gauged in the context of clinical, functional and biochemical data to the same extent as in diseases of the thyroid.

The most likely indication for aspiration cytology is a solitary nodule which is 'cold' on scintiscan. A neoplastic lesion with frankly malignant cells from a papillary or an anaplastic carcinoma is unlikely to pose diagnostic difficulties. A high grade non-Hodgkin's lymphoma may require supplementary immunocytochemical studies to distinguish it from a small cell anaplastic carcinoma, but its neoplastic nature is seldom in doubt. A tumour with a well developed follicular pattern, on the other hand, may be indistinguishable from a focus of benign hyperplasia, and discrimination between a follicular adenoma and a follicular carcinoma requires histological evidence of invasion.

Cytology is generally useful in providing confirmatory evidence of Hashimoto's lymphocytic thyroiditis. A benign cystic lesion may be simultaneously diagnosed and cured by needle aspiration. Since however, cystic changes occur more often in carcinomatous lesions a careful follow-up is indicated in these cases, and a recurrence calls for repeat cytology and a cutting needle or excision biopsy with frozen section examination of tissue.

The procedure for aspiration of the thyroid and preparation of smears for microscopic examination is identical to that for breast or palpable lymph nodes.

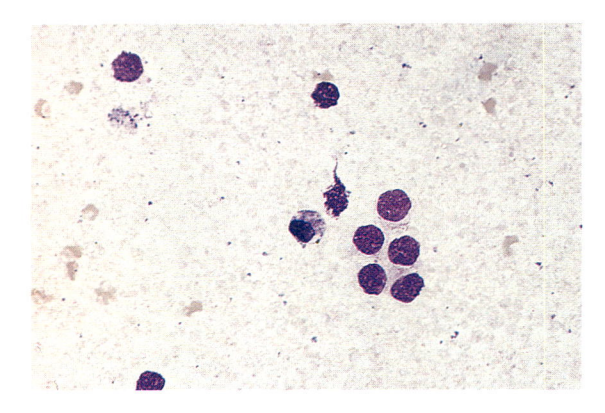

Fig. 13.1 Thyroid follicle cells
MGG ×133

The epithelial lining of the acini or follicles of the thyroid consists of a single row of cuboidal cells. In an aspiration smear, these cells usually appear in flat sheets, often in a monolayer. They have sparse cytoplasm, round or spherical nuclei which approximate in size to large lymphocytes, and the nuclear cytoplasmic ratio is high. The nuclear chromatin is compact and nucleoli are not usually discernible. The acinar cells may be disrupted by the suction applied during aspiration and it is usual to see some stripped nuclei.

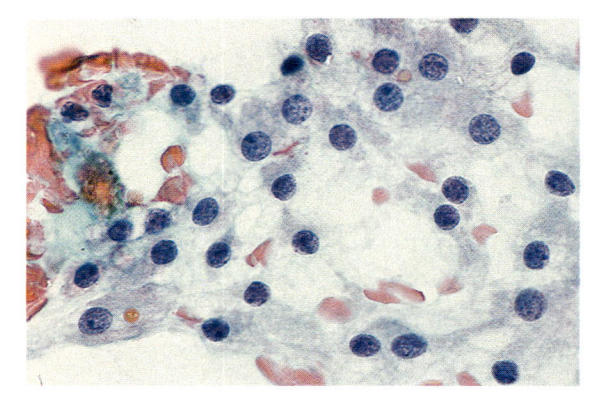

Fig. 13.2 Askanazy cells
Papanicolaou ×525

The acinar cells may undergo alteration into substantially larger cells, referred to as Askanazy, Hürthle or oncocytic cells. The increase in size is due to a greater volume of cytoplasm which is often finely granular and/or contains multiple small vacuoles. The cells are strongly eosinophilic with H & E and amphophilic with the Papanicolaou stain. The round nuclei are similar in size to the nuclei of acinar cells, but have a more open chromatin and contain one prominent or two or three small nucleoli. Variations occur in the number of nuclei and the size of cells. Askanazy cells are generally plentiful in Hashimoto's thyroiditis, in which they are accompanied by numerous lymphocytes. Occasionally, they may form a localized adenoma.

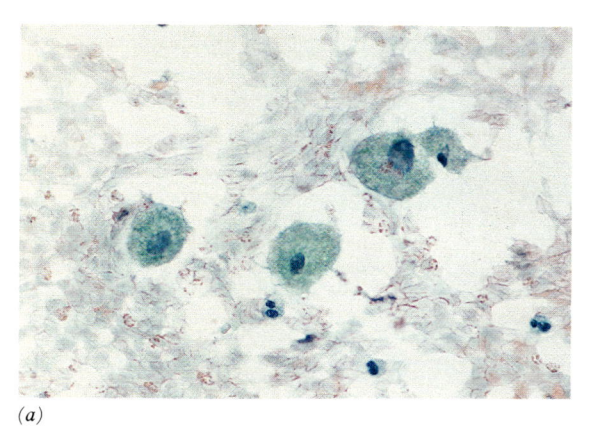

THYROID 197

(a)

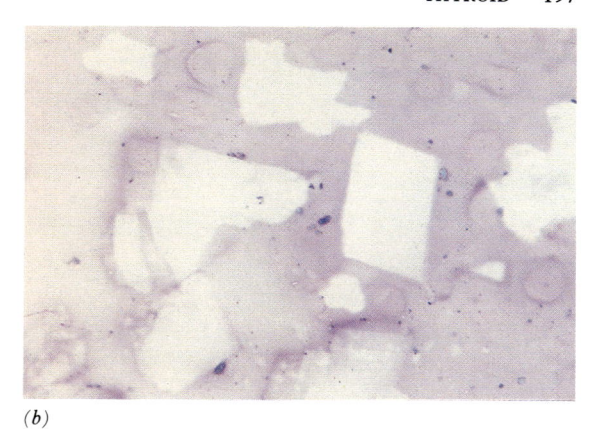

(b)

Fig. 13.3 Cyst

Papanicolaou ×525 (a) foam cells (b) cholesterol crystals

Foam cells are degenerate, swollen, benign acinar cells. The cytoplasm contains fine or large hydropic vacuoles and the nuclei are crenated or pyknotic (a). Intracytoplasmic particles, suggestive of phagocytic activity, may be present. The appearance of foam cells is similar to epithelium-derived foam cells seen in breast and renal cysts.

The plate-like crystals of cholesterol seen against a sheet of violet-staining material similar to colloid (b) develop in long standing cysts. Epithelial or foam cells are usually not seen in these specimens.

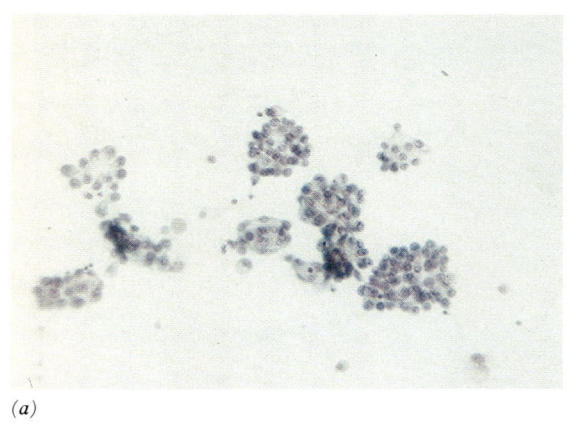

(a)

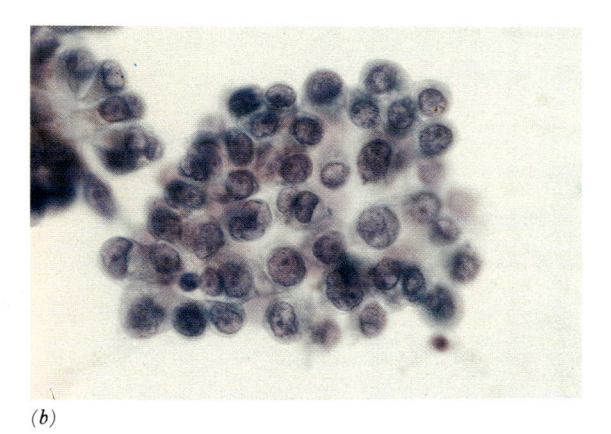

(b)

Fig. 13.4 Hyperplastic follicle cells

Papanicolaou (a) ×133 (b) ×525: same smear

Hyperplastic follicle cells are taller than normal follicle lining cells. They have more cytoplasm, larger nuclei and usually contain one or more nucleoli. A moderate degree of anisonucleosis is generally evident. The cells are usually seen in large clusters (a), with some depth of focus (b), and their arrangement suggests a papillary outgrowth of the lining epithelium. Cells of this type may be recovered from a hyperplastic thyroid or a benign adenoma and distinction between the two lesions is not feasible on the cellular characteristics.

198 DIAGNOSTIC CYTOPATHOLOGY

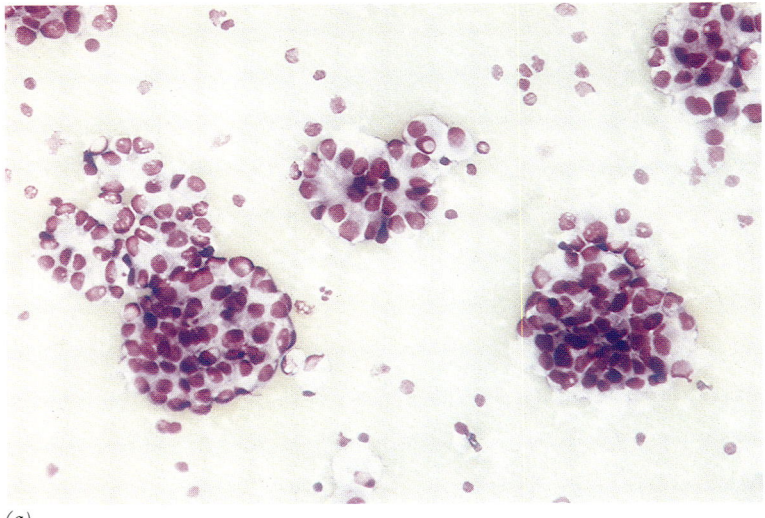

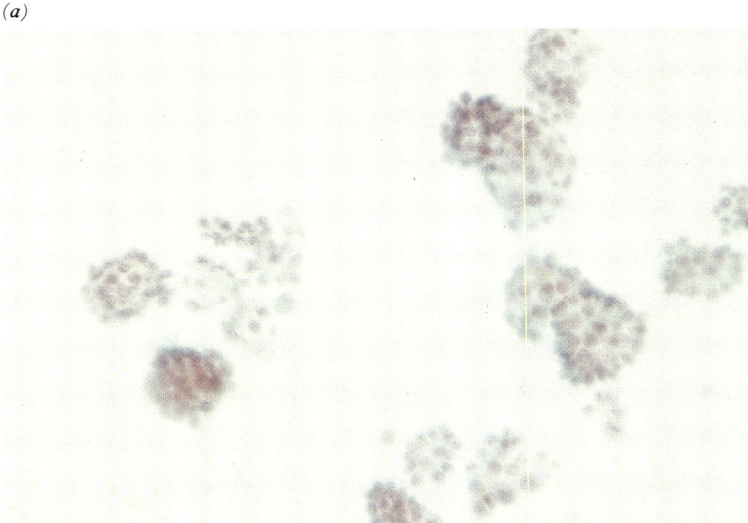

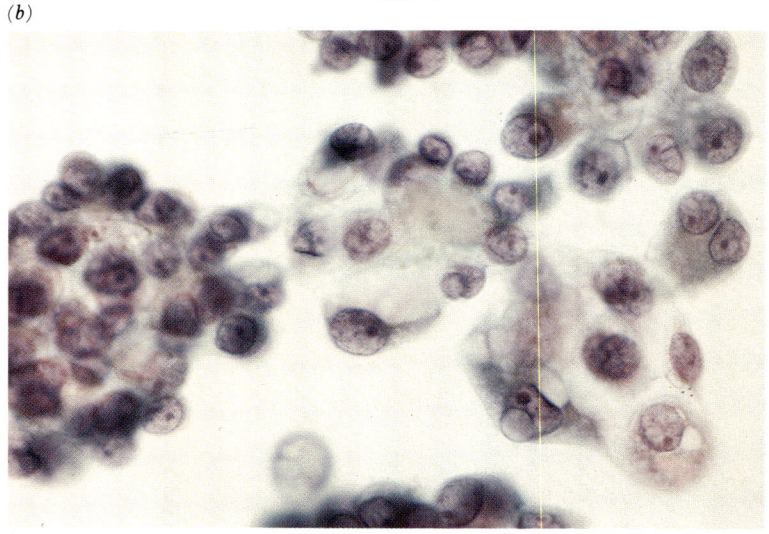

Fig. 13.5 Follicular carcinoma

(a) *MGG* ×183 (b) *Papanicolaou* ×183: same specimen (c) *Papanicolaou* ×720: same smear as (b)

A well recognized area of difficulty in thyroid pathology is distinction between a benign follicular adenoma and a carcinoma with a well developed follicular pattern and well differentiated cells. In histopathology, the problem is resolved when penetration of the capsule or invasion of a lymph or blood vessel by tumour cells is demonstrated.

These micrographs illustrate cells from a histologically-proven folliculr carcinoma of thyroid and demonstrate the diagnostic difficulty met with in cytological material from a lesion of this type. The alignment of the cells on the periphery of a clear central space in the top centre cluster in (a) indicates a follicular arrangement. The majority of cells form three-dimensional clusters (a), (b). Compare these with the cells in Figure 13.4 (a) and note the similarity in size, shape and arrangement. At high magnification (c) the neoplastic cells are seen to be marginally larger than the benign hyperplastic cells in Figure 13.4 (b), and to have more cytoplasm which is vacuolated in some cells. The nuclear cytoplasmic ratio, however, is lower in the neoplastic cells aspirated from the tumour and the nuclei are more regular in size and shape.

(a)

(b)

(c)

THYROID 199

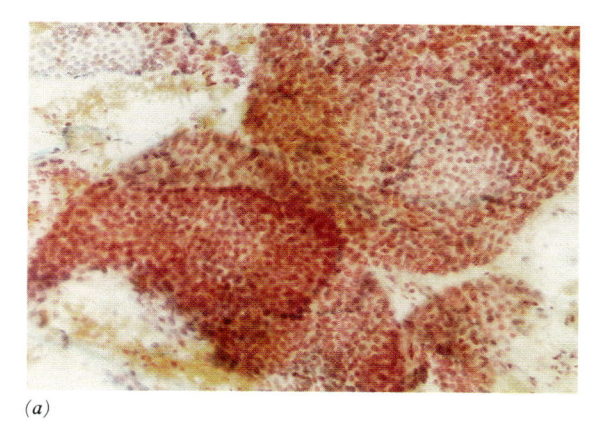

(a)
(b)

Fig. 13.6 Papillary carcinoma

Papanicolaou (a) ×133: follicle cells (b) ×133: foam cells and follicle cells (c) ×525: follicle cells (d) ×525: carcinoma cells (e) ×525: carcinoma cells

Papillary adenocarcinoma of the thyroid develops, like follicular carcinoma, from the follicle lining epithelium and forms frond-like projections with a central fibrous core covered with neoplastic cells. Some areas of the tumour may retain a follicular pattern. Cystic change is common. Papillary adenocarcinoma is the commonest type of carcinoma seen in the thyroid and has a bimodal frequency, occurring before 40 years of age and in later life.

A histologically-proven papillary carcinoma, part cystic, part solid, is illustrated in these micrographs. Numerous small regular follicle cells organised into large spheroidal clusters are seen in (a) and a similar smaller fragment of tissue is seen in (b). Higher magnification of a sheet of follicle cells in another field show round, regular, bland nuclei containing pin point nucleoli, and surrounded by moderate amounts of cytoplasm. The epithelial cells in the three fields do not display features of malignancy and it is likely that they represent areas of benign hyperplasia.

The foam cells in (b) suggest an area of cystic change. Note the particulate matter within the cytoplasm of some of the foam cells.

The cells in (d) and (e) form tight aggregates and have more deeply staining basophilic cytoplasm. The nuclei are crowded together, hyperchromatic and exhibit a considerable variation in size and some irregularity of shape and outline. The morphological atypia is gross enough for a firm diagnosis of malignancy. Papillary adenocarcinoma of the thyroid frequently contain many psammoma bodies, not seen in these micrographs.

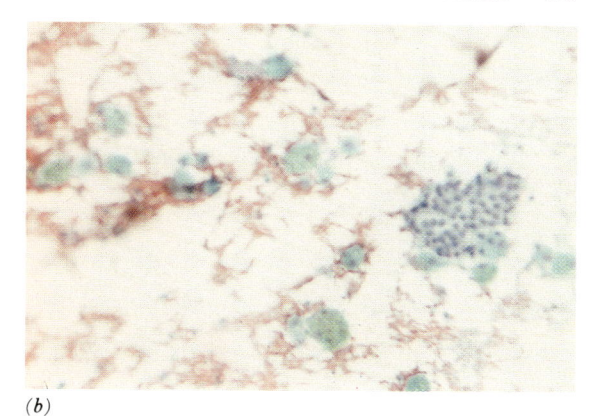

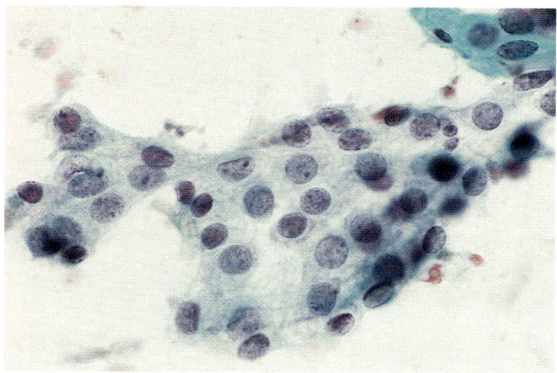

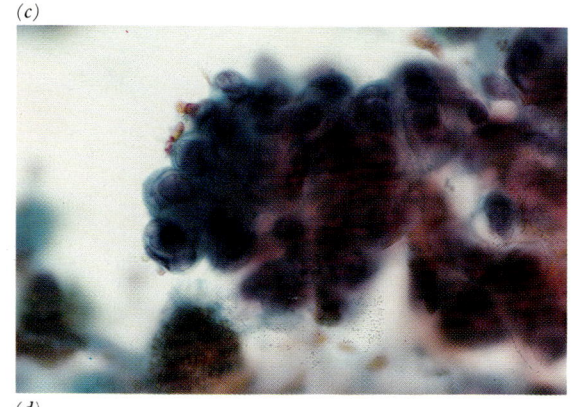

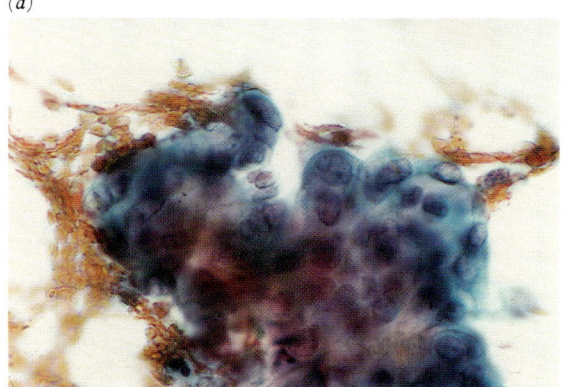

(c)

(d)

(e)

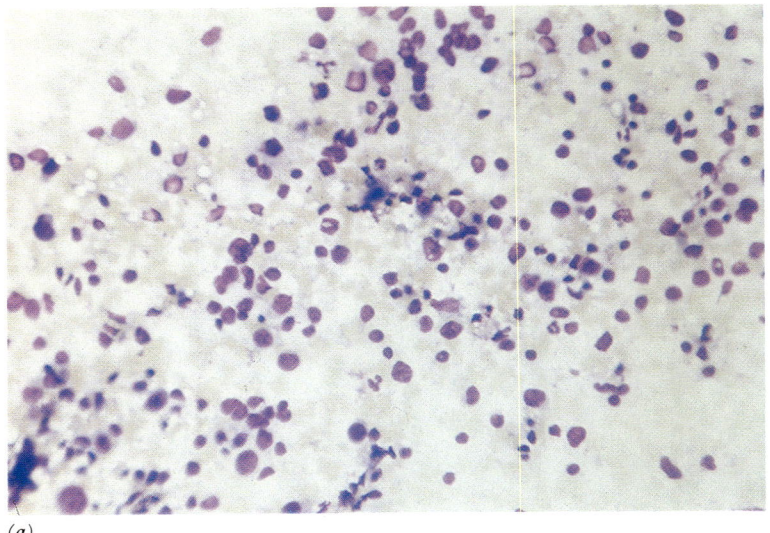

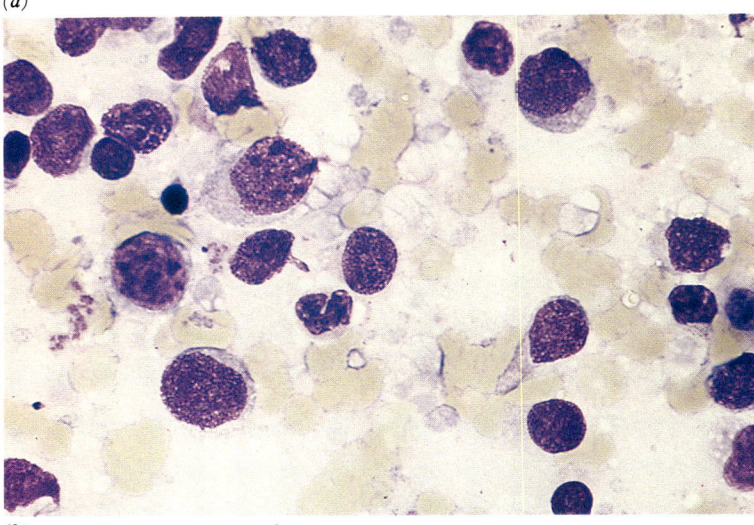

Fig. 13.7 Non-Hodgkin's lymphoma

MGG (a) ×183 (b) ×720: same smear

Non-Hodgkin's lymphoma of the thyroid may occur as a primary lesion or it may form part of a more diffuse disease. A low grade lymphoma composed of differentiated small lymphocytes or prolymphocytes may appear similar to lymphoid cells seen in Hashimoto's disease. A high grade lymphoma, as in the example illustrated, needs to be distinguished from an anaplastic carcinoma. Lymphoma cells are recovered in large numbers and are discrete (a). At a higher magnification, the cells have very little cytoplasm and the disproportionately large nuclei contain from one to five nucleoli. Note that the nucleoli lie close to the nuclear membrane, a characteristic repeatedly noted in centroblastic cells. The tumour cells in the case illustrated were shown to be B-lymphocytes.

14. Cellular changes due to treatment

A variety of therapeutic agents, the most important of which are the anti-cancer agents, alter the morphology of cells. There is often a loss of the distinctive cytoplasmic features that help in the identification of the cell type. Benign cells may be so altered by ionizing radiation that distinction from malignant cells becomes exacting. Neoplastic cells may show features of complete necrosis, partial degeneration which raises the question of possible or probable viability or may remain virtually unaffected. The success or failure of treatment may be assessed to some degree by the number and the morphological features of tumour cells in a post-treatment specimen. Some of the commoner treatment induced changes in cell morphology and smear pattern are considered in this chapter.

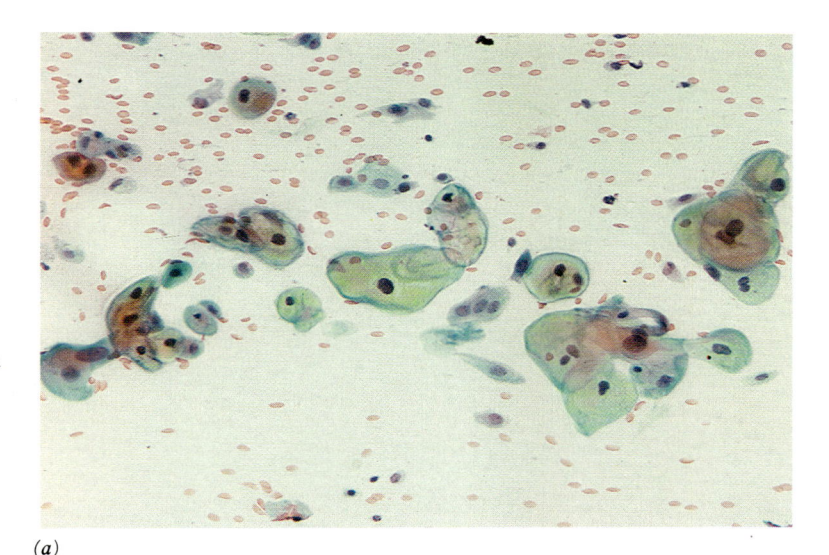

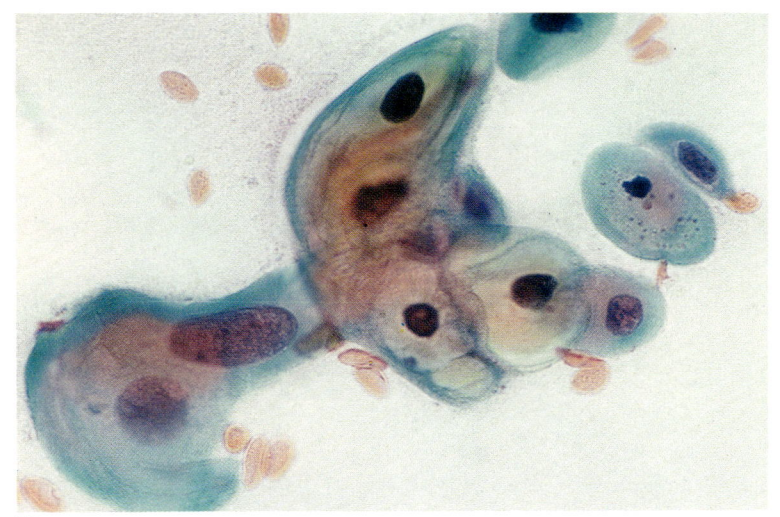

Fig. 14.1 Radiation effects: polychromasia

Papanicolaou (a) ×183: vaginal smear
(b) ×720: same smear

A Papanicolaou smear of a woman with a good response to recent radiotherapy has a dramatic appearance. This is due to marked changes in the tinctorial properties, shape and size of the benign cells.

Benign cells in a vaginal smear taken 6 weeks after completion of a course of caesium for invasive squamous carcinoma of the cervix are illustrated in this and the next three figures.

The immediate impact is of the polychromasia of the cytoplasma and the vividness of the colours (a). The peripheral portion of the cells is essentially basophilic and the central part acidophilic (a), (b). The basophilia ranges from bright blue to yellowish green and a corresponding range of shades from salmon pink to apricot is displayed by the acidophilic part of the cells. The nuclei are small and the majority are condensed and hyperchromic (b).

(a)

(b)

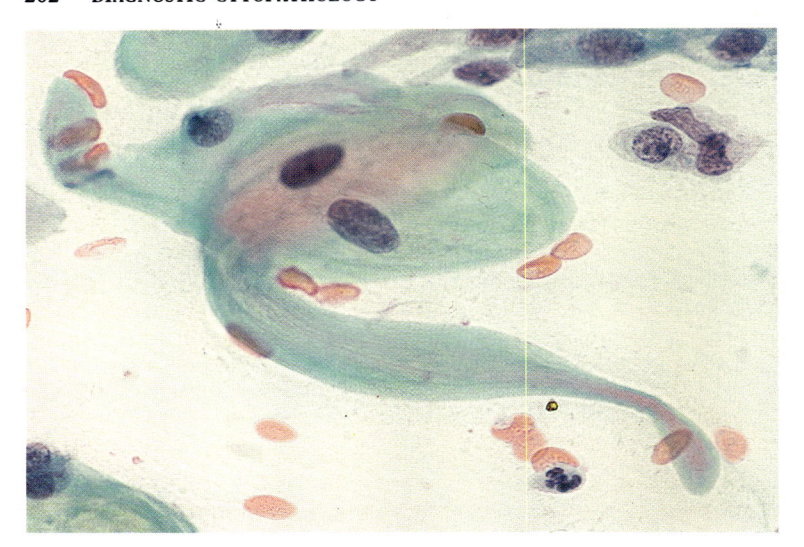

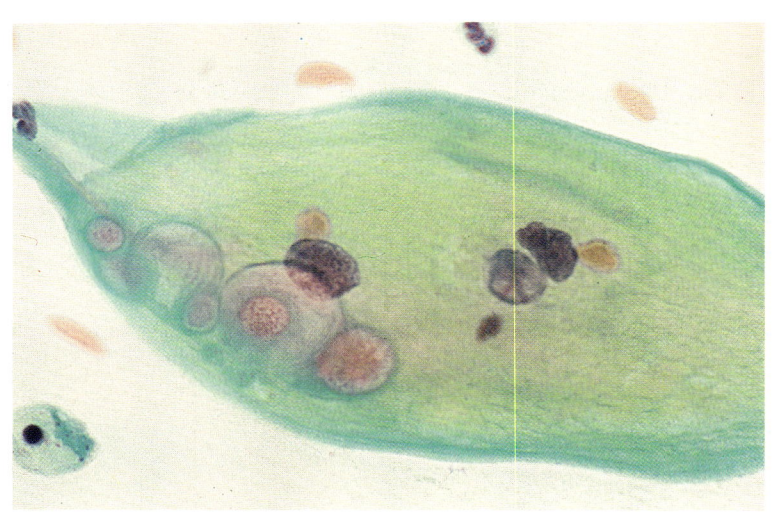

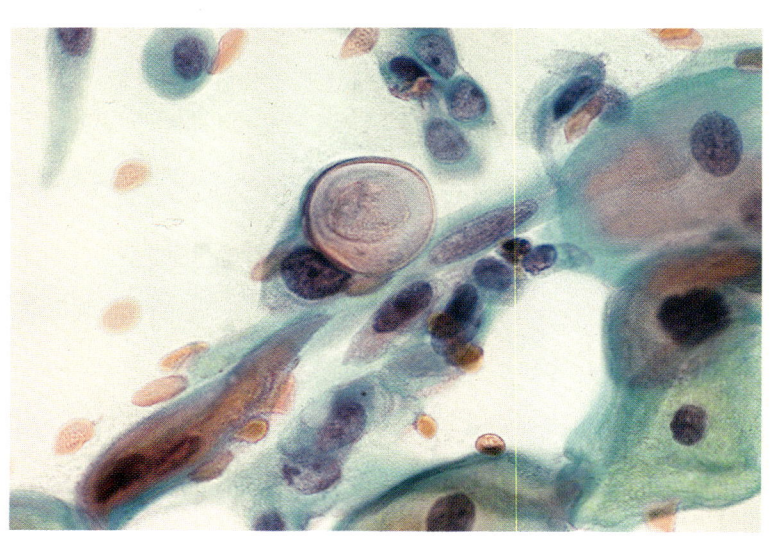

Fig. 14.2 Radiation effects: abnormal shapes

Papanicolaou ×720: same smear as in Figure 14.1

The two cells in this field have tail like extensions of the cytoplasm which terminate in club shaped expansions; the cells are similar in appearance to caudate cells frequently met with in well differentiated squamous cell carcinoma. A suggestion of a Herxheimer spiral is seen in the lower cytoplasmic process. Compare these cells with normal squamous cells (Figs. 1.1–1.3) and note their larger size and the substantial increase in the volume of their cytoplasm. The nuclei of irradiated benign cells remain normal in size or enlarge to a lesser extent than the cytoplasm, the nuclear to cytoplasmic ratio is reduced.

Fig. 14.3 Radiation effects: macrocytosis

Papanicolaou ×720: same smear as in Figure 14.1

The increase in the volume of the cytoplasm may be so gross that the cell cannot be assigned to any of the layers of normal stratified squamous epithelium. The giant cell in this micrograph has the ovoid shape of a navicular cell but it extends beyond one high power field and is several times the size of any normal squamous cell. It also shows two other features commonly met with in irradiated cells, multinucleation and intracytoplasmic vacuoles. The vacuoles may form a fine honey-comb (right) or they may be circumscribed with central zones of condensation or inclusions. (lower left).

Fig. 14.4 Radiation effects: vacuolisation

Papanicolaou ×720: same smear as in Figure 14.1

A sharply outlined vacuole, especially one with central condensation, may mimic a large intracellular mucin globule. It is seen here in a parabasal squamous cell which has acquired a resemblance to a glandular cell.

CELLULAR CHANGES DUE TO TREATMENT

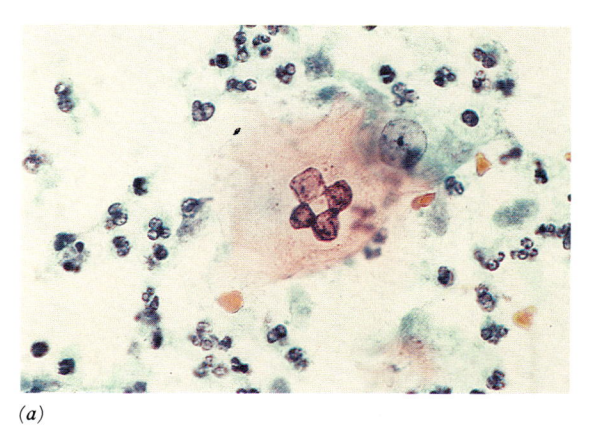

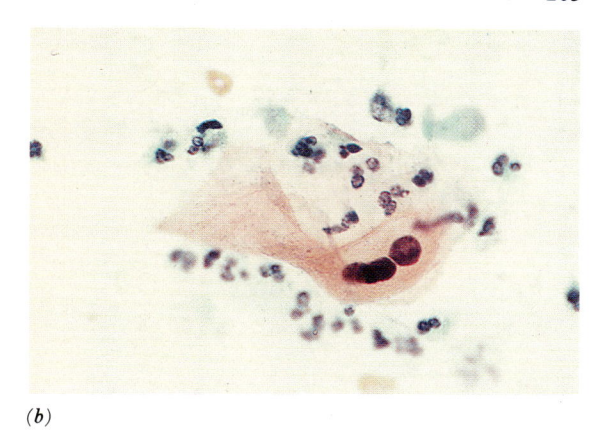

(a) (b)

Fig. 14.5 Radiation effects: long term

Papanicolaou ×525: vaginal smear (a) pseudoesoinophilia; multinucleation (b) vacuolization of cytoplasm

As a general rule, the changes induced in benign cells by ionizing radiation gradually fade and disappear within 3–6 months after treatment. In a small proportion of cases, they last longer and in a few individuals, persist for life: marked irradiation effects have been seen by the author in follow-up smears for 10 years or more.

This micrograph illustrates changes seen 12 months after caesium therapy. Polychromasia and macrocytosis are no longer present, but multinucleation (a) and binucleation and some abnormality of shape remain. The size and shape of the cells, the pseudoeosinophilia, loss of definition of cell outline and vacuolisation of the cytoplasm (b) is consistent with non-specific inflammatory change in a mature squamous epithelium: in an older or castrated woman with an atrophic epithelium, it is more often associated with previous radiotherapy.

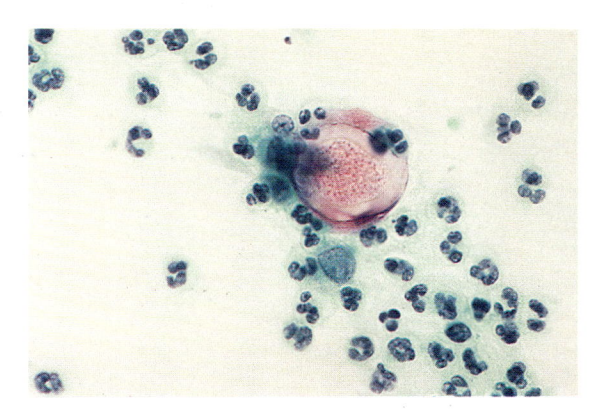

Fig. 14.6 Radiation effects: long term

Papanicolaou ×525: vaginal smear

The vacuolated parabasaal cell with the appearance of a mucin-secreting columnar cell, shown in this micrograph, was seen in a vaginal smear 2½ years after caesium treatment for a cervical squamous carcinoma.

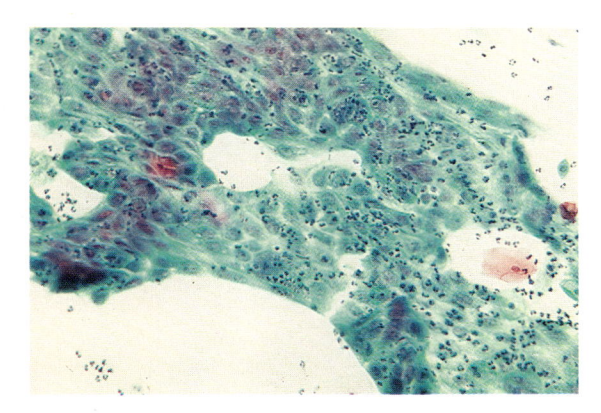

Fig. 14.7 Radiation effects: increased exfoliation

Papanicolaou ×133: vaginal smear

The cellularity of a post-radiotherapy smear varies. There is generally an increase of exfoliation during and for some months after the course of treatment. Thereafter the cell yield diminishes and in the majority of cases, the smear reverts to an atrophic pattern and may indeed become quite sparse. In exceptional cases, massive exfoliation may persist for longer periods. This micrograph shows a representative field in a follow-up smear 12 months after treatment. A microbiopsy of hypertrophic immature metaplastic squamous cells is seen together with an occasional mature squamous cell.

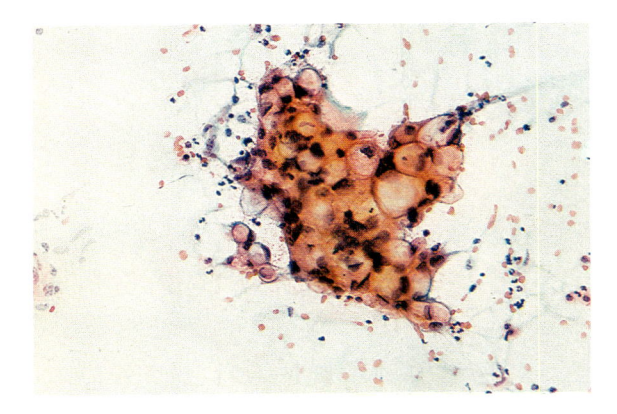

Fig. 14.8 Radiation effects: apparent alteration of cell type

Papanicolaou ×133: vaginal smear

A combination of continued irradiation change and excessive exfoliation may produce a problematical appearance. The vacuolated parabasal cells in a sheet illustrated in this micrograph are suggestive of signet-ring cell carcinoma. They were seen in a vaginal smear over a year after total hysterectomy and radiotherapy for a squamous cell carcinoma. This case illustrates the importance to the cytopathologist of relevant clinical data which should include details of the therapeutic protocols and information about the cell type of the original tumour.

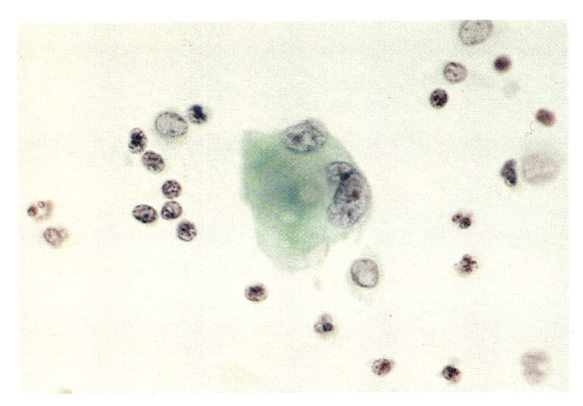

Fig. 14.9 Radiation effects in metastatic malignant cell

Papanicolaou ×525: ascitic fluid

Treatment induced changes of morphology are also seen in malignant cells which are the target of cancer therapy. Persistence or recurrence of disease is indicated by the presence of intact cells the nuclei of the which retain malignant characteristics. The cell illustrated in this micrograph was one of several present in the ascitic fluid of a woman previously treated for cervical squamous carcinoma by radiotherapy. The finely stippled, irregularly distributed chromatin, characteristic of malignancy is indicative of metastatic squamous carcinoma despite the peripheral alignment of the nuclei more commonly seen in cells which originate in glandular tissue.

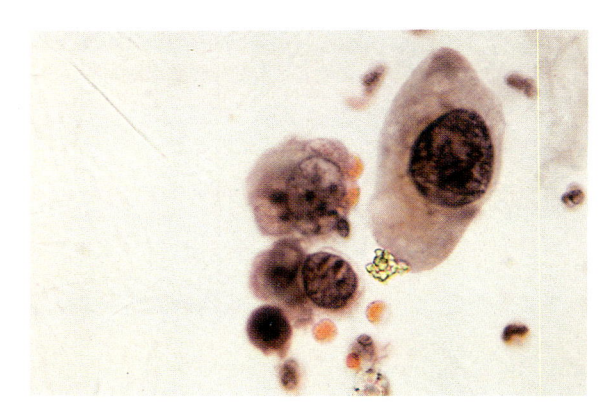

Fig. 14.10 Radiation-resistant carcinoma cells

Papanicolaou ×525: urine

This micrograph illustrates cells which continued to exfoliate after a course of radiotherapy for a carcinoma of bladder. The coarse granularity of the nuclear chromatin, the high nuclear-cytoplasmic ratio and the anisocytosis are indicative of persistent tumour. The large size of the cell to the right probably reflects minimal radiation change but the majority of the tumour cells appear to be unaffected.

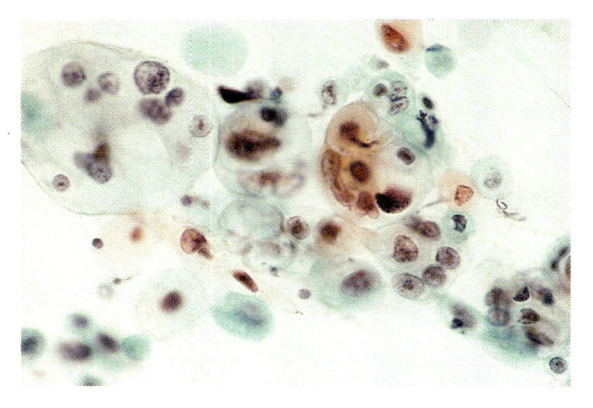

Fig. 14.11 Degenerative changes in irradiated carcinoma cells

Papanicolaou ×525: sputum

The probable viability of severely altered cancer cells seen soon after completion of treatment is difficult to assess. The abnormal cells seen here are derived from a squamous carcinoma of lung treated by deep X-irradiation (DXR). Degenerative changes are seen in the cytoplasm which is swollen in some cells and in the nuclei several of which are fragmented. Note the three prominent nucleoli near the centre of the field. Large nucleoli may occur in both benign and malignant irradiated cells and are not helpful in the assessment of malignancy in a post-treatment specimen. Continued exfoliation of cells of the type illustrated would be suggestive of persistent tumour.

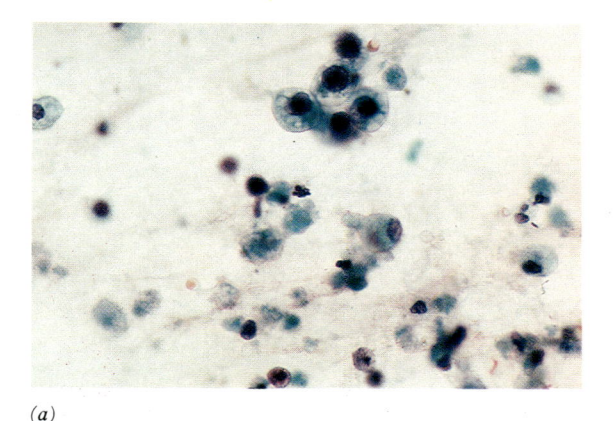

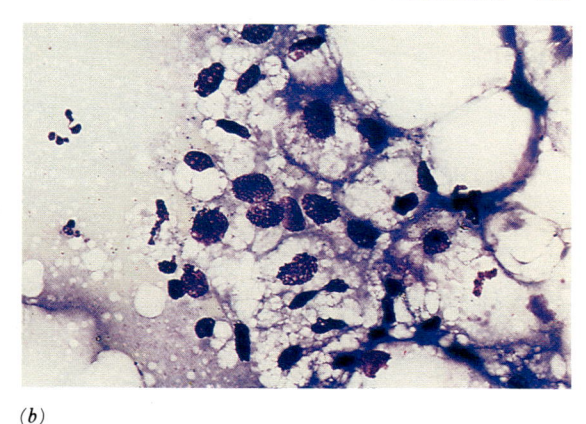

Fig. 14.12 Necrosis of irradiated carcinoma cells

(a) *Papanicolaou* ×525: FNA; breast (b) MGG ×525: same specimen; another smear

The patient whose cells are illustrated in this micrograph had been treated for carcinoma of the breast by DXR. There are no viable well preserved tumour cells in this post-treatment specimen which shows necrotic change. In (a), this consists of pyknotic degeneration in the few recognizable cells and cytoplasmic remnants of disintegrated cells. The cells in (b) are foamy and histiocytic in appearance and the nuclei condensed or crenated.

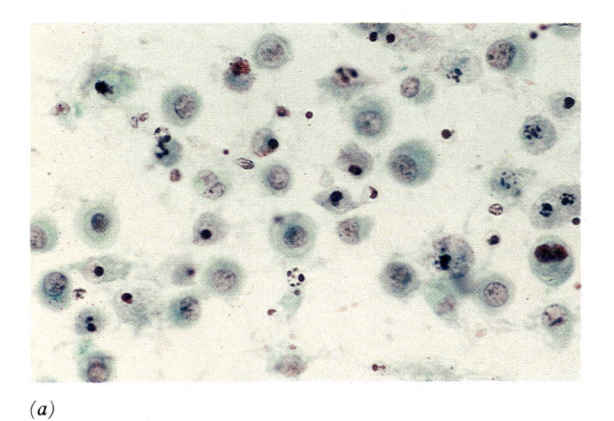

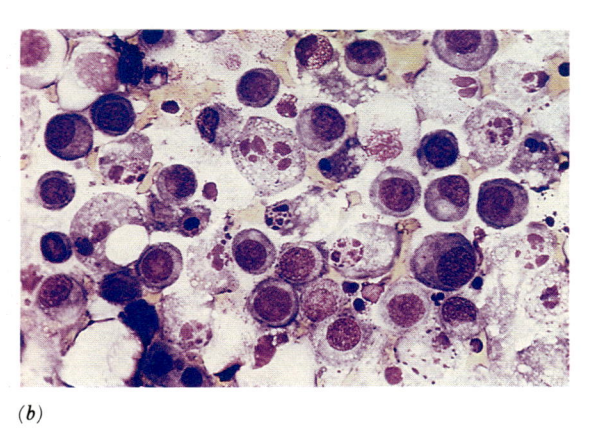

Fig. 14.13 Incomplete response to adriamycin

(a) *Papanicolaou* ×525: pleural fluid (b) MGG ×525: same specimen; another smear

Both well preserved and necrotic tumour cells are seen in the pleural fluid of a woman treated for disseminated carcinoma of breast with adriamycin. The viable tumour cells have basophilic cytoplasm and stippled nuclei (a). A high nuclear cytoplasmic ratio is evident in the air dried smear (b). The necrotic tumour cells show either karyopyknosis or karyorrhexis. In addition, there are several tiny fragments of cytoplasm with pin-point chromatin inclusions such as are seen in apoptosis (see Fig. 1.13).

206   DIAGNOSTIC CYTOPATHOLOGY

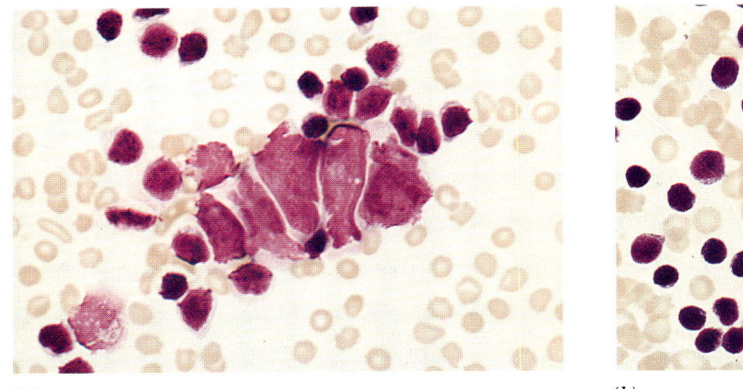

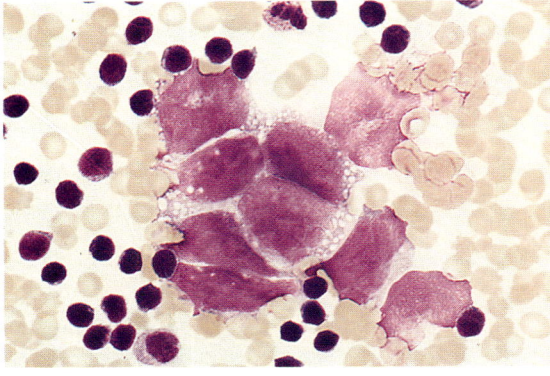

(a)   (b)

Fig. 14.14 Chemotherapy-induced change in small cell carcinoma

MGG ×525: pleural fluid (a) pre-treatment specimen (b) post-treatment specimen

One effect of combined chemotherapy administered for small cell carcinoma of the lung illustrated above in Figure 3.60 is the emergence of a refractory large cell carcinoma. Another effect which is occasionally met with is a substantial increase in the size of cells with the characteristic morphology of oat cells. Compare the appearance of the tumour cells (a) before and (b) after treatment and note the increase in the volume of the cytoplasm of the post-treatment cells. The three morphological features of oat cells stained by the MGG method, namely violet coloration and a smudged appearance of the nuclei and fine internuclear clefts are seen in both specimens.

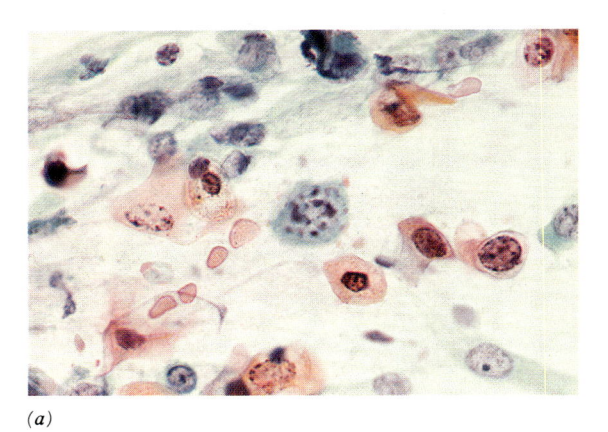

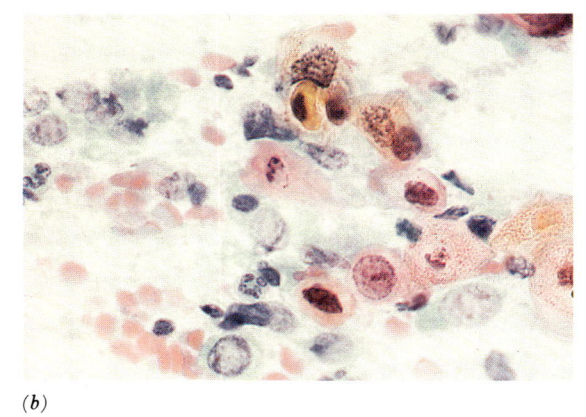

(a)   (b)

Fig. 14.15 Squamous metaplasia after laser therapy

Papanicolaou ×525: bronchial brush (a) abnormal shapes (b) dyskeratosis

Two representative fields from a bronchial brush smear obtained after laser treatment for a bronchogenic squamous cell carcinoma are illustrated in these micrographs. The size and shape of the cells seen is similar to that of atypical but benign metaplastic squamous cells with degenerate nuclei (compare with Figs. 3.36–3.40).

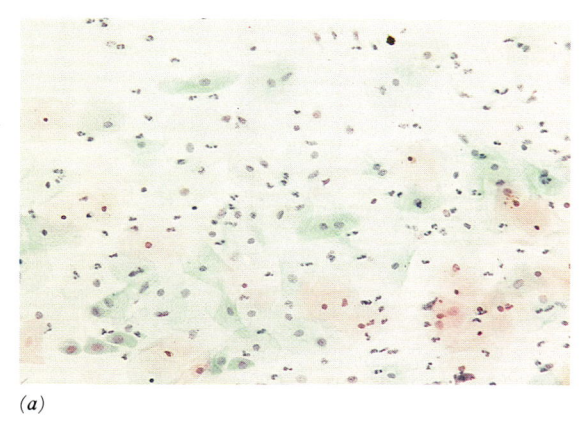

(a)

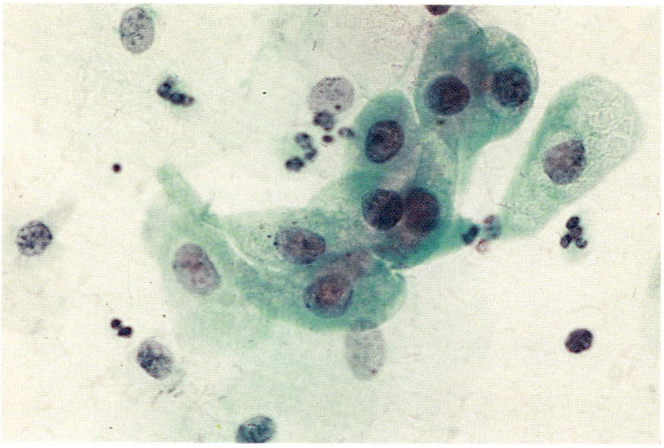

(b)

Fig. 14.16 Effect of hormones

(a) Papanicolaou ×133: cervical smear; mature squamous cells (b) ×525: same smear; squamous metaplasia

The smear illustrated in these micrographs demonstates the effect of female sex hormones on the atrophic epithelium of a 55-year-old post-menopausal woman receiving hormone replacement therapy. Maturation of the epithelium is indicated by the abundance of oestrogenized eosinophilic superficial cells and their precursors, the cyanophilic intermediate squamous cells (a). Further evidence of hormone-induced change is provided by metaplastic squamous cells (b) not normally seen in a post-menopausal smear.

Index

References are to page numbers, main references are in bold type

Abscess, breast, 44
  psoas, 163
Acantholysis, 191
Acid fast bacilli, *see* Mycobacterium tuberculosis
Acinic cell, **51**
Acquired immune deficiency syndrome (AIDS), 80, 81
ACTH, 91
Actinomyces israeli, 16
Actinomycetes spp., **16**, 75
Actinomycetoma, 16
Adenocarcinoma, 2, **106**, **144**, **160**, **190**
  of breast, 107, 124, 126, 129, 140, 144
  in CSF, **144**
  of colon, 37, 106, 107, 128, 154, 163
  diagnostic features of, **33**
  of endometrium, 32, **33–34**, 108, 183
  of endocervix, 29, 33, **35–36**
    in situ, 29
  of Fallopian tube, 32
  of lung, 86, 88, **99–102**, **123–124**, 140, 194
  of pancreas, 108, 124, 127, 162
  papillary, 37, **126**, **127**
  of prostate, **177**, **178**
  of stomach, 127, 128, 149, 153
Adenoma, of thyroid, 196, 197, 198
  villous, of colon, 155
  see also Fibroadenosis of breast
Adenosis, of cervix, 32
  of vagina, 32
ADH (antidiuretic hormone), 91
Adrenal gland, 163, 175
Adriamycin, 205
AIDS, *see* Acquired immune deficiency syndrome
Alpha-fetoprotein, 2
  and hepatocellular carcinoma, 2, 158
  and teratoma, malignant undifferentiated, 179
Alveolar cell carcinoma, *see* Broncho-alveolar carcinoma
Antenatal smear, 11
Antibodies, monoclonal, 112, 123, 180
  demonstration, immunocytochemical, of **138–140**
Anticoagulants, for effusions, serous, 113
Anucleate squamous cells, benign, 7, 18, **67**
  malignant, 26, **86–87**, 106
Apocrine metaplasia, *see* Metaplasia, apocrine; Fibroadenoma; Gynaecomastia
Apoptosis, **14**, 205
APUD system cells, 68, 91
Asbestos, 74, 136

Asbestos body, *see* Ferruginous body
Ascites, 113
Askanazy cells, **196**
Aspergilloma, 77
Aspergillosis, bronchopulmonary, 77
  and calcium oxalate crystals, 77
Aspergillus fumigatus, **77**
Aspergillus spp., **78**
Asthma, bronchial, 73, 84, 119
  and Creola bodies, 84
Astrocytoma, 142
Atrophic squamous epithelium, **7**
Atrophic vaginitis, *see* Vaginitis, atrophic

Barr body, 17, 80
Bartholinitis, 19
Basal squamous cells, 4, **7**
Basement membrane, 8, 20, 43, 53
Basophil, 118
Bence Jones protein, 112
  see also Myeloma, multiple
Benign cystic mastopathy, *see* Fibroadenosis of breast
Benign mammary dysplasia, *see* Fibroadenosis of breast
Bile, 156, 159
Bile pigment, **157**, **159**
Bilharziasis, *see* Schistosomiasis
Bird's eye cell, **58**, **128**, **137**
Bladder, adenocarcinoma, 178
  carcinoma, squamous cell, primary, **169**
    secondary, **170**
  transitional cell, metastatic, **133**, **182**
    primary, **167**, **168**, **204**
    in situ, 168
  cytopathia, viral, **171**
  metaplasia, squamous, 169, 172
  reconstructed, **170**
  see also Transitional epithelium
Blastomyces, 75
Bone, aspiration, indications for, 185
  cells of, **185**
  haematopoietic tissue in, **186**
  tumours, metastatic, **189–190**
    primary, **187–189**
Branchial cyst, **194**
Breast, adenocarcinoma, metastatic, **107**, **124**, **126**, **129**, **140**, **144**, 185
  carcinoma, 44, 45, **54–63**, 181, 205
    apocrine, **60**
    ductal, 54, **56–58**, **61**
    inflammatory, 44
    intracystic, **55**

    intraduct, 45, 54, **55**
    intralobular, 54, 61
    lobular, 54, 58, **61**
    of male, **63**
    medullary, 43, **57**
    with metaplasia, **63**
    necrosis in, **56**, **205**
    tubular, **54–55**
  cells, acinic, **51**
    ductal, 43, **44**, 45, 46
    myoepithelial, 43, 53
  cyst, 39, **46–48**, 55
    apocrine metaplasia of, 46, **48**, **49**
    malignant, 55
    papillary, **47**
    simple, **47**
  duct ectasia, 45, **46**, 173
  fat necrosis, **44**
  fibroadenoma, 49, **52–53**, 54, 55
  fibroadenosis, 45, **49**
  fibrofatty tissue, **43**
  fibrosarcoma, 54
  granuloma, **44**
  gynaecomastia, **50**, 55
  hyperplasia, lobular, 54
    papillary, 45
  lactating, 44, **51**
  metastases to, 64
  nipple, 43
    Paget's disease, **62**
  papilloma, 45
  phyllodes tumour, 54
  sentinel nuclei in, **53**, **56**
  specimens, types of, 43
Broncho-alveolar carcinoma, 86, 99, **103–104**, 108
Broncho-alveolar cells, 67, **69**, 70
Bronchus, carcinoid, 91, **96–98**
  carcinoma, 74, **86–96**, 112, **190**, 194
  metaplasia, squamous, **82–83**
  specimens, types of, **65–66**
  see also Lung; Respiratory epithelium
Brush border, 114, 115, 153
  see also Microvilli
Bull's eye cell, 58

Caecocystoplasty, *see* Bladder, reconstructed
Caecum, carcinoma, **154**
Caesium, *see* Radiation, ionizing
Calcium, 36, 54, 73, 120
Calcospherite, **54**, **58**, **73**
  see also Psammoma body
Cancer diathesis, 25, **26**, 29, 30, **36**
Candida albicans, **16**, 76, 78
Candida parapsilosis, **76**
Candida spp., 76, **81**, **147**, 178

INDEX

Candidiasis, broncho-pulmonary, 76
  oesophago-gastric, **147**
  oral, 76
  vulvo-vaginal, **16**, 76
Capillaries, in breast aspirate, 43
  in CSF, ventricular, **141**
Carcino-embryonic antigen (CEA), 2, 137
  demonstration, immunocytochemical, of, **138–140**
Carcinoid, bronchial, 91, **96–98**
  intestinal, 96
Carcinoma, basal cell, 191, **192**, 193
  bronchogenic, 74, **86–96**, 112, 190, 194
  clear cell, 32, 108, 173
  endometrioid, 32
  gastro-intestinal, 99
  hepatocellular, **158**
  oat cell, 91, **95**, 96
  renal cell, **108**, 169, **173–174**, 178, **189**
  signet-ring, 117, **151**, 204
  small cell, 70, 86, **91–96**, 111, **130–131**, **190**, **206**
  in situ, 20, 168
  transitional cell, **133**, **167–169**, 182, **204**
  see also named organs and tissues
CAT, *see* Computerized axial tomography
Caudate cell, benign, irradiated, **202**
  malignant, **26**, 30, 83, **86–87**, 90, 169
  metaplastic, atypical, 83
Cell block, 114
Central nervous system, 141–145
  meningitis, carcinomatous, **144**
    cryptococcal, **145**
  tumours, metastatic, **143–145**
    primary, 142–143
Cerebriform cell, **134**
Cerebro-spinal fluid, preparation of, 141
  specimens, types of, 141
Cervical intraepithelial neoplasia (CIN) 20, 30, 31
  CIN 1, 20, **21**
  CIN 2, 20, **22**
  CIN 3, **23–24**, 25, **28**, **29**, 30, 31
  and Condyloma acuminatum, flat, 22
  differential diagnosis, 29
  grading of, **20**
Cervicitis, **11–12**
  follicular, **14**
  trichomonal, **15**
  see also Endocervicitis
Cervix uteri, 3
  carcinoma, clear cell, 32
    in situ, 20
    squamous cell, 31
      metastatic, **163**, **170**, **204**
      microinvasive, **30**
      primary, 2, **25–27**, **29**, 30
  ectropion, 8
  epithelial lining, 2, 3, **4–5**, **6–7**
  erosion, 8
  pars vaginalis, 3

squamo-columnar junction, 3, 6, 8, 11, 20
squamous metaplasia, *see* Metaplasia, squamous
  stroma, 8
  transformation zone, 8
Charcot-Leyden crystals, 73
Chemotherapy, effect, of, 201
  on breast carcinoma, **205**
  on small cell carcinoma, **96**, **206**
Chlamydia trachomatis, 19
Cholangiocarcinoma, **159**
Cholangiocyte, **156**, 159
Cholangiography, percutaneous, transhepatic, 159
Cholesterol crystals, 120, **162**, **197**
Chordoma, **188**
Choroid plexus, 141
Ciliocytophthoria, 82
CIN *see* Cervical intraepithelial neoplasia
Cirrhosis, **158**
Clara cell, 68, 86, 99
Clue cells, **16**
Coal miner's lung, 74
Coccidiodes, 75
Coelom, 113
Colitis, ulcerative, 155
Colloid, **197**
Colon, adenocarcinoma, metastatic, 37, 106, **107**, **128**, **163**, 185
  primary, 154
  mucosa, in Franzen needle aspiration, **177**
  polyp, 155
    dysplasia of, 155
Colostrum, 51
Colposcopy, 20, 29
Computerized axial tomography (CAT), 134, 156, 160, 163
Condyloma acuminatum, 18
  flat, (plane wart), **18**, 22
Conjunctivitis, inclusion, 19
Contraceptive, oral, 8, 16
Corpora amylacea, 72, 73, **176**
Corpus albicans, 3, 5
Corpus luteum, 3
Corpus uteri, 3
Creola body, 84
Cryptococcoma, 79
Cryptococcus neoformans, in CSF, **145**
  in lung, 79
Curschmann spiral, 72
Cyst, branchial, *see* Branchial cyst
  breast, *see* Breast, cyst
  ovary, *see* Ovary, cyst
  renal, *see* Kidney, cyst
  thyroid, *see* Thyroid, cyst
Cystadenocarcinoma of ovary, **126**
  mucinous, **40**, 125
  serous, **41**, **129**, **130**
    mucous metaplasia in, 41, **129**
    pseudo-ciliated cells of, **130**
Cystadenoma of ovary, mucinous, **41**
  serous, 42
Cystic mammary dysplasia, *see* Fibroadenosis of breast

Cystosarcoma phyllodes, *see* Breast, phyllodes tumour
Cytocentrifuge, use of, 141
Cytolysis, 5
Cytolytic pattern, **5**
Cytomegalovirus (CMV), **80**, 81
Cytopathia, viral, of bladder, **171**
  of bronchial mucosa, **79–80**
  of cervical epithelium, **17–18**
  of skin, **194**

Diethylstilboesterol (DES) 32
DNA synthesis, 1
Doderlein's bacilli, **5**
Duct ectasia, **45**, **46**, 173
  see also Fibroadenosis of breast
Dyskaryosis, definition of, 20
  intermediate squamous cell, 20, **21**
  navicular cell, **22**
  in Paget's disease of nipple, **62**
  parabasal squamous cell, 20, **22**, **23**, 31
  poorly differentiated squamous cell, **30**
  undifferentiated cell, **24**
Dyskeratosis, 13, **18**, **22**, 30, **62**, **83**, **86**, **106**, **193**
Dysplasia, cervical, 18, 20
  fibrous, of bone, 188
  of mucosa, gastric, intestinalized, **151**
  of polyp, colonic, 155

Echinococcus granulosus, **81**, **164**
Ectocervix, 2, 3, 4
  epithelial lining of, 2, **4–5**, **6**, **7**
Ectropion, 8
Effusion, serous, 113
  benign, **114–122**, 178
  malignant, **123–140**, 161
    carcinoma, metastatic, **123–133**, **140**, **206**
    leukaemic infiltrate, **134**, **136**
    lymphoma, **135**
    mesothelioma, **136–139**
    myeloma, **135**
    sarcoma, **134**
  preparation of, 113–114
  types of, 113
Empyema, streptococcal, **122**
  tuberculous, **122**
Endocervicitis, 12, 19
Endocervix, 3
  adenocarcinoma, **29**, 32, **33**, **35–36**
    in situ, 29, 32
  canal, 3
  pH of, 8
  epithelium, columnar, 3, 6, **9**
    degenerating, **12**
    hyperplastic, **12**
Endometriosis, 39
Endometrium, 3, 5
  adenocarcinoma, metastatic, **108**, **183**
    primary, 32, **33–34**

INDEX

cells, glandular, **6, 9**
  stromal, **6**
cyclical changes, 3
direct sampling, 32
hyperplasia, 33
Endoscopic retrograde cholangio-pancreatography (ERCP), 146
Endoscopy, fibreoptic, of digestive tract, **146**
  respiratory tract, **65–66**
  urinary tract, **165**, 166
Entamoeba gingivalis, **16**
Eosinophilia, pulmonary, primary, 73
Eosinophils, **73**, 118, **119**
Ependyma, 142
Ependymoma, **142**
Epidydimitis, 19
Epithelial pearl, benign, 18, **67**
  malignant, 26, 30, **31**, 86, **106**
Epithelioid cell, *see* Macrophage, epithelioid
Epitheliosis, *see* Fibroadenosis of breast
Erosion, cervical, 8
Euchromatin, 1
Ewing's tumour, **187**
Exodus, and menstrual smear, 6
Exudate, characteristics of, 113, 123
  see also Effusion, serous

Fallopian tube 3, 32, 113
  adenocarcinoma 32
  epithelial lining, 3
Ferruginous body, **74**
Feyrter cell, 68, 91
Fibroadenoma, **52–53**
  apocrine metaplasia in, 52
Fibroadenosis of breast, **45–49**, 52, 54, 55
Fibrocystic disease of breast, *see* Fibroadenosis of breast
Fibrosarcoma, 54, 188
Fibrosis, *see* Fibroadenosis of breast
Filter, membrane, 141, 165
Fine needle aspiration (FNA), of bone, 185
  of breast, 43
  of lung, 66
  of lymph node, 180
  of ovary, 40
  of prostate gland, 177
  of skin, 190
  of sub-cutaneous tissues, 190
  sub-diaphragmatic, 156
  of testis, 179
  of thyroid, 196
  transbronchial, 66
  of urinary system, 165
Fluid, serous, *see* Effusion, serous
FNA, *see* Fine needle aspiration
Foam cells, 39, **45, 46**, 49, 173, **197, 199**
Follicle cells,
  of ovary, *see* Granulosa cells
  of thyroid, 196, 197, 199
Follicle centre cell, 135

Follicle stimulating hormone (FSH), 3
Follicular carcinoma of thyroid, **198**
Follicular cervicitis, *see* Cervicitis, follicular
Foreign body giant cell, **44, 46**
Franzen needle aspiration, **177**

Galactorrhoea, 45
Gall bladder, adenocarcinoma, metastatic, **126**
Gardnerella vaginalis, **16**
Gastritis, *see* Stomach
Germ cell tumour, 106, **179**
Germinoma of pineal gland, 143
Giardia lamblia, **146**
Glioma, **142**
Gliosis, 142
Glycogen, 5, 136, 157
  in chordoma, **188**
  in Ewing's tumour, **187**
  in renal cell carcinoma, **174**
Goodpasture's syndrome, 71
Graffian follicle, 3, 6, 38, 42
Granuloma, **44**, 70, 73, 180
Granulosa cells, 3, **38**, 39
Granulosa lutein cells, 3, **38**, 39
Gynaecomastia, **50**, 55
  apocrine metaplasia, in, **50**

Haematopoietic tissue, **186**
  extra medullary, **119**
Haemosiderin, extracellular, **71**
  in ferruginous body, **74**
  in siderophages, **71**
Haemosiderosis, pulmonary, idiopathic, 71
Hashimoto's disease, *see* Thyroiditis, Hashimoto's
Heart failure cells, *see* Macrophage, iron-laden
Heparin, 118
Hepatocellular carcinoma, 2, **158**
Hepatocyte, 156, **157**
Hepatoma, *see* Hepatocellular carcinoma
Herpes genitalis, *see* Herpesvirus simplex
Herpesvirus simplex, cytopathia of, **17, 79, 176**, 194
  in cervix uteri, **17**
  on penis, **176**
  in respiratory tract, **79**
  type 1, 17
  type 2 (herpes genitalis), 17, 176
  and carcinoma, cervical, 17
Herpes zoster, **194**
Herxheimer spiral, **90, 202**
Heterochromatin, 1
Histamine, 118
Histiocyte, in urine, **171**
  see also, Macrophage
Histiocytoma, fibrous, malignant, **194**
Histoplasma, 75

Hodgkin's disease, **109–110**, 180, **181**
  and Hodgkin's cell, **109**, **181**
  nodular sclerosing, 110
  and lacunar cell, **110**
  and Reed-Sternberg cell, **109–110**, 180, **181**
Hormone replacement theraphy (HRT), 32
  effect on squamous epithelium, atrophic, **207**
Human chorionic gonadotrophin (HCG), 179
Human papilloma virus (HPV), **18, 22**
  and condyloma acuminatum, **18**
  flat (plane wart), **18, 22**
  DNA sequence of, and carcinoma, cervical, 18
  and koilocytosis, **18, 22**
Hürthle cell, 196
Hyaluronic acid, 123, 136, 137
Hyaluronidase, 123, 136, 137
Hydatid cyst, in lung, **81**
  subdiaphragmatic, **164**
  see also Echinococcus granulosus
Hydrocoele, 176, **178**
5-Hydroxytryptamine, *see* Serotonin
Hyperkeratosis, 7, **18, 67**, 193
Hypernephroma, *see* Renal cell carcinoma

Immunoblast, 135
Immunocytochemistry, 16, 123, 143, **138–140**, 161, 179, 180, 191, 196
Inflammation, effect on cells, epithelial, 11
Intermediate squamous cells, **4, 5, 6**, 9, 20, **207**
  inner, 5, 20
  outer, **4, 6, 9**, **207**
  see also, Cervix uteri, epithelial lining
Intestinal metaplasia, *see* Metaplasia, intestinal
Intrauterine contraceptive device (IUCD), 6
  and Actinomyces israeli, 16
Intrinsic factor, 151

Karyolysis, 11, 13, 15, **147**
Karyopyknosis, 11, **13**, 82, **147**, 205
Karyorrhexis, 11, **13**, 14, **82**, **147**, 205
Keratin, 2, 6, 26, **86**, **193**
Keratoacanthoma, 191, **193**
Keratohyaline granules, 67
Kidney, cyst, 39, **173**
  embryonal tumour (nephroblastoma), 134, 161, **175**
  renal cell carcinoma, metastatic, **108**, 185, **189**, 194
  primary, 169, **173–174**, 178, **189**
  transitional cell carcinoma, **168–169**
Koilocyte, **18, 22**
Kultschitsky cell, 68, 91

212   INDEX

Kupffer cell, **157**

Lactic acid, in vagina, 5
Lacunar cell, **110**
Large cell undifferentiated carcinoma of lung, 86, **96**, 99, 100, 102, **104–105**, **132**, **183**
Laser treatment, effect of, **206**
Larynx, carcinoma, metastatic, **106**, **182**
  primary, **106**
LE cell, *see* Lupus erythematosis
Legionnaire's disease, 76
Leiyomyoma, of stomach, **154**
Leiyomyosarcoma, 154
Leptomeninges, **141**
Leucoerythroblastic anaemia, 119
Leukaemia, T-cell, **134**
  myeloid, **136**
Lipofuscin, 173
Lipid, 39
  in macrophages, **71**
  in renal cell carcinoma, **174**
Lipophage, *see* Macrophage, fat-laden
Liver, adenocarcinoma, metastatic, in, **160**
  cholangiocarcinoma, intrahepatic, **159**
  cholangiocytes, **156**
  cirrhosis, **158**
  hepatocellular carcinoma, **158**
  hepatocytes, 156, **157**
  Kupffer cells, **157**
  lymphoma, metastatic, **161**
Lung, adenocarcinoma, metastatic, of, **123–124**, **140**, **194**
  primary, 86, 88, **99–102**
  carcinoma, broncho-alveolar, 86, 99, 102, **103–104**, 108
    large cell, metastatic, of, **132**, **183**
      primary, 86, 96, 99, 100, 102, **104–105**
    small cell, metastatic, of, **130–131**, **190**, **206**
      primary, 70, 86, **91–96**, 111
    squamous cell, metastatic, of, **132–133**, **144**, **163**, **175**, **190**
      primary, **86–90**, **96**, 102
  cyst, hydatid, 81
  infections, bacterial, 75
    fungal, **76–79**
    opportunistic, **75–81**
    parasitic, **80–81**
    viral, **79–80**
  lymphoproliferative disorders, **108–112**
  metaplasia, squamous, **82–83**
  metastases, in, **106–112**
  specimens, types of, **65–66**
Lupus erythematosis (LE), 122
  cell, **122**
Luteal phase, smear pattern in, 5
Luteinising hormone (LH), 3, 38
Lymph node, metastases, in, 180, **182–184**

hyperplasia, benign reactive, 180
lymphoma, malignant, **181**
Lymphoblasts, **14**, 118, **134**
Lymphocytes, in breast aspirate, **43**, 44, **57**
  in cervicitis, follicular, **14**
  in effusions, serous, 118, **123**
  in Hodgkin's disease, **109**
  in respiratory tract specimens, **69**, **99**, **109**
Lymphogranuloma inguinale, 19
Lymphoma, non-Hodgkin's, malignant, 43, 54, 64, 128, **134**, **143**, 175, 180, **185**, **187**
  B-cell, **153**, **161**, **181**, **200**
  centroblastic, **111**, **135**
  centrocytic-centroblastic, **135**, 180
  T-cell, 136
  see also named types
Lymphoplasmacytoid cell, **118**

Macronucleolus, 2, **63**, **109**, 123, **143**, **179**, **181**, **188**, **204**
  see also, Nucleolus, large
Macrophage, 6, 44, 46, 67, **118**, **124**, **147**
  alveolar, pulmonary, 67, 69, **70–71**, 74
  anthracotic, **70**, 74
  cohesive, **70**
  epithelioid, **70**, **120–121**, 180
  fat-laden (lipopophage), **71**
  giant, multinucleate, **44**, **70**, **121**, **185**, **195**
  iron-laden (siderophage), 39, 42, **71**, **173**
Malignancy, cytodiagnosis of, **1–2**
  cytoplasmic features, 2
  nuclear features, 1–2
Mast cells, **118**, **123**
Megakaryocyte, **186**
  stripped nucleus of, **119**, **186**
Meig's syndrome, 125
Melanin, Masson-Fontana stain for, **145**, **184**
Melanoma, amelanotic, **64**
  melanotic, **145**, **184**, **191**
Membrane, serous, 113
  parietal, 113
  visceral, 113
Meningitis, carcinomatous, **144**
  cryptococcal, 79, **145**
Menstrual cycle, 3, 4, 6, 8
Menstrual smear, **6**, **34**
Mesonephroid carcinoma of ovary, **108**, **125**
Mesothelial cell, **114–117**, **128**, **131**
  active/reactive, **115–116**
  degenerate, **117**
  hyperplastic, **178**
  malignant, *see* Mesothelioma, malignant
  in metaphase, **116**
  multinucleate, **115**
Mesothelioma, benign, 136
  malignant, **136–139**

asbestos, and, 74, 136
differential diagnosis, **136–137**
hyaluronic acid in, 136, 137
hyaluronidase, for diagnosis of, 136, 137
immunocytochemistry, for diagnosis of, 137, **138–139**
Metaplasia, apocrine, **48–49**, **50**, 52, 60
  intestinal, of stomach, **150–151**
  mucous, of serous tumours, 41
  myeloid, **119**
  squamous, of bladder, 169, 172
  of cervix, 8, **9**, 12, 20, 26, 29, **203**, **207**
  of respiratory epithelium, **82–83**, **206**
Microinvasive carcinoma, cervical, 30
Microvilli, 2
  in malignant cells, 2, 102, **130**, **153**
  in mesothelial cells, 114, **115**
  in metaplasia, apocrine, **48**
  intestinal, **150**
  in polyp, colonic, **155**
  see also Brush border
Midcycle smear, **4**
Midsecretory smear, 5
Millipore filter *see* Filter, membrane
Mitoses, abnormal, 2
  in benign cells, 2, 9, **14**, 38, 53, 116, **150**
  in tumours, malignant, 2, **94**, **112**, **125**, **135**, **139**, **143**, **148**, **153**
Monocyte, 70, 118
Mucin, demonstration, biochemical, **40**, **58**, **59**, **100**, **127**, **129**, **160**, **163**
Mucus, 71
  cervical, 11
Mycobacterium tuberculosis, **75**
Mycosis fungoides, 134
Myeloblast, 134, 136
Myelocyte, **119**
Myelofibrosis, 119
Myeloid metaplasia, *see* Metaplasia, myeloid
Myeloma, multiple, **112**, **135**, **185**, **187**, 190
Myoepithelial cell, 43, 53
  see also Sentinel nuclei
Myosarcoma, 161

Navicular cell, **5**, **7**
  see also Intermediate squamous cell
Nephroblastoma, 134, **161**, **175**
Neuroblastoma, 134, **161**, **175**
Neutrophils, 11, **15**, 44, 46, **118**
Nipple, Paget's disease of, **62**
Nocardia, 75
Normoblast, **119**, **136**
Notochord, 188
  see also Chordoma
Nucleolus, large, **25**, **85**, **88**, **105**, **125**, **151**, **153**, **173**, **177**
Nucleus, cerebriform, **134**

INDEX

convoluted, **143**
malignant, characteristics of, 1–2

Oat cell carcinoma, 64, 94, **96**
  combined, **95**
  see also Small cell carcinoma
Oesophagus, adenocarcinoma, 149
  infections, opportunistic, **147**
  squamous cell carcinoma, **148**
Oestrogen, 3, 4, 7, 8, 13
  see also Ovarian cycle
Osteoblast, **185**, 188
Osteoclast, **185**
Osteoid, 185, 188
Osteosarcoma, **188**
Ovarian cycle, **3**
Ovary, carcinoma, 32, **36–37**, 58, 194
  mesonephroid, metastatic, **108**, 125
  cyst, chocolate, **39**
    corpus luteum, **39**, 42
    follicular, **38**
    germinal inclusion, **39**, 42, 173
    luteinized, post-ovulatory, **38**
  cystadenocarcinoma, mucinous,
    metastatic, **125**
    primary, **40**
    serous, metastatic, **37**, **126**, **129**, **130**
    primary, **41**
  cystadenoma, mucinous, **41**
    serous, **42**
Oviduct, *see* Fallopian tube

Paget's disease, of bone, 188
  of nipple, **62**
Pancreas, carcinoma, metastatic, **108**, **124**, **127**
  primary, **162**
  cells, acinar, 156, **162**
  pseudocyst, **162**
Pancreatitis, 147
Paneth cell, 150
Papilloma, squamous, 18, 22, 193
  see also Human papilloma virus
Parabasal squamous cell, 4, **7**, **9**, **11**, **13**, 20, 23
  see also Cervix uteri, epithelial lining
Parakeratosis, **18**, **24**
Parapromyelocyte, **136**
Pearl, squamous, *see* Epithelial pearl
Pemphigoid, 191
Pemphigus, 191
Pericardium, 113
Peritoneum, 39, 113
Pernicious anaemia, **151**
Pinealoma, **143**
Plasma cell, **44**, 118, 120, 153, 187
  neoplastic, **112**, **135**, **187**
Plasmacytoid cell, 118, 135
Plasmacytoma, 112, **187**
  see also Myeloma, multiple
Pleura, 113
Pneumoconiosis, **74**
Pneumocystis carinii, **80–81**
Pneumocyte, 68, 70, 86, 99

Pneumonia, infant, 19
  lipoid, 71
Pollen, **172**
Polyoma virus, 171
Polyp, colonic, **155**
Polyposis coli, 155
Post-coital smear, **10**, 14
Post-menopausal smear, **7**
Pouch of Douglas, 82, 114
Pregnancy, 3, 5, 16
Prekeratin, 86
Premenstrual smear, **5**
Progesterone, 3, 5, 6
  see also Ovarian cycle
Prolymphocyte, **14**, 118
Promyelocyte, **136**
Prostate gland, 176
  adenocarcinoma, **177**, **178**, 185
  cells, epithelial, **177**
  corpora amylacea in, 176
  hyperplasia, benign nodular, 176
Protein, nuclear, 1
Psammoma body, **36**, **37**, **42**, 199
  see also Calcospherite
Psoas, abscess 163
  muscle, metastases in, **163**
Pulmonary alveolar microlithiasis, 73

Radiation, ionizing, 200
  effect on cell morphology, 200–205
Rectum, mucosa, **177**
Reed-Sternberg cell, *see* Hodgkin's disease
Reiter's syndrome, 19
Renal cell carcinoma, **108**, 169, **173–174**, **178**, **189**
Renal pelvis, carcinoma, **168–169**
Reserve cell, 8, 9, 12
  hyperplasia, 9, 12, **28**, **29**, 82
Respiratory epithelium, **68–69**
  hyperplasia, **84–85**
  metaplasia, squamous, **82–83**
    atypical, **83**
Rhabdomyosarcoma, 134, 175, 189
Rheumatoid disease, 113, 120
  effusion, serous, in, **120–121**
  nodule, 120, **195**
Rodent ulcer, 192

Saliva, **67**
Salpingitis, 19
Sampling techniques, *see* Techniques, sampling
Sarcoidosis, 69
Sarcoma, 106, 187
  undifferentiated, **134**, **189**
Schistosomiasis, 165, 169, 172
  haematobium, **172**
  japonica, 172
  mansoni, 172
Sclerosing adenosis, *see* Fibroadenosis of breast
Sebaceous gland, cells, **191**
Seminoma, 57, 179
Sentinel nuclei, **53**, 56

Serous effusion, *see* Effusion, serous
Serous membrane, *see* Membrane, serous
Sexually transmitted diseases (STD), **15–16**, **17–19**
Sezary's syndrome, **134**
Siderophage, *see* Macrophage, iron-laden
Signet ring carcinoma, 117, **151**, 204
Skin, carcinoma, basal cell, 191, **192**, 193
  squamous cell, 191, **193**
  fungal lesions, diagnosis of, 191
  herpes zoster, **194**
  keratoacanthoma, 191, **193**
  pemphigus, diagnosis of, 191
Small cell carcinoma of lung, 70, 86, **91–96**, 111, **130–131**, 190, 206
  classification of, **91**
Spermatocoele, 176
Spermatozoa, 6, **10**, 176, 178
Spider cell, 9
Sputum, collection of, **65**
Squamo-columnar junction, *see* Cervix uteri
Squamous cell carcinoma, of bladder, **169**
  of bronchus, **86–90**, **96**, 102, **132–133**, **144**, **163**, **175**, 190, 206
  of cervix uteri, 2, **25–27**, **29**, **30**, **163**, **170**, 204
    microinvasive, **30**
  of larynx, **106**, **182**
  of oesophagus, 148
  of skin, 191, **193**
  of tongue, **182**
  of vagina, **31**, **170**
Squamous epithelium, cervico-vaginal, **4–5**
  oral, **67**
  of respiratory tract, upper, **67**
Squamous metaplasia, *see* Metaplasia, squamous
Stomach, adenocarcinoma, metastatic, **127**, **128**, 194
  primary, **149**, **153**
  carcinoma, signet ring, **151**
  gastritis, 150, 151
  infections, opportunistic, **147**
  leiomyoma, **154**
  leiomyosarcoma, 154
  lymphoma, primary, **153**
  mucosa, atrophic, 150, 151
    intestinalized, **150–151**
    normal, **149**
    regenerating, **150**
  and pernicious anaemia, 151
  ulcer, slough on, **147**
Streptococcus, haemolyticus, **122**
  pneumoniae, 110
Superficial squamous cell, 4, 5, **7**, 22, **207**
  see also Cervix uteri, epithelial lining

Tadpole cell, *see* Caudate cell

Techniques, sampling, breast, **43**
  CSF, **141**
  digestive tract, **146**
  ovary, **40**
  respiratory tract, **65–66**
  skin, 191
  sub-cutaneous tissues, 191
  sub-diaphragmatic lesions, **156**
  urinary system, **165**
Teratoma, 143
  malignant, undifferentiated, **179**
Testis, tumours of, 176, **179**
Theca externa, 3
Theca interna, 3
Thyroid, adenoma, follicular, 196, 197, 198
  carcinoma, follicular, 185, 194, 196, **198**, 199
    papillary, **199**
  cells, 196,
    hyperplastic, **197, 199**
  lymphoma, **200**
Thyroiditis, Hashimoto's, 196, 200
Tongue, squamous carcinoma, metastatic, **182**
Trachoma, 19
Transformation zone, *see* Cervix uteri
Transitional cell, **165–166**
  carcinoma, metastatic, **133, 182**
    primary, **167–169, 204**
    in situ, 168

Transitional epithelium, 165, 166
Transudate, characteristics of, 113, 123
  see also Effusion, serous
Trichomonas vaginalis, 15
Trichomoniasis, 15, 165
Tuberculosis, 118, 163, 181
  AFB in 75
  empyema, **122**
Tzanck cell, 191
Tzanck test, 191

Ultrasonography, 156, 160, 175
Umbrella cell, **165, 166**
Undifferentiated cells, 20, **29**
  diagnostic problems, **29**
Urethra, transitional cell carcinoma, 135
Urethral syndrome, 19
Urethritis, non-gonococcal, 19
Urine, collection and preparation, 165
Urothelium, *see* Transitional epithelium
Uterus, 3, 32

Vagina, 3, 8
  adenosis, 32
  carcinoma, clear cell 32

  intraepithelial (VAIN), 31, 170
    squamous cell, metastatic, **170**
    primary, **31**
  epithelial lining, 3, 4–5
  pH, 5
  posterior fornix, 32
Vaginal intraepithelial carcinoma, *see* Vagina
Vaginitis, atrophic, **13,** 14
  fungal, **16,** 76
  trichomonal, 15
Vanillymandelic acid (VMA), 134
Vulva, 3
  carcinoma, 31
Vulvovaginitis, 16

Wart, cervical, **18, 22**
  virus, *see* Human papilloma virus
Wegner's granuloma, 73, 113
Wilm's tumour, *see* Nephroblastoma

Zymogen granules, 162